THE OCCUPATIONAL THERAPY EXAMINATION REVIEW GUIDE, Edition 2

Caryn R. Johnson, MS, OTR/L, FAOTA
Academic Fieldwork Coordinator
Department of Occupational Therapy
Thomas Jefferson University
Philadelphia, Pennsylvania

Arlene Lorch, MS, OTR/L, CHES
Clinical Instructor
Department of Occupational Therapy
Thomas Jefferson University Philadelphia, Pennsylvania

Tina DeAngelis, MS, OTR/L
Department of Occupational Therapy
Thomas Jefferson University
Philadelphia, Pennsylvania
and
Occupational Therapist
Crozer Chester Medical Center
Upland, Pennsylvania

Debra N. Anderson, OTR
Administrative Director of Occupational Therapy
Frye Regional Medical Center
Hickory, North Carolina
and
Adjunct Instructor
Department of Occupational Therapy
Lenoir-Rhyne College
Hickory, North Carolina

Mary Kathryn Cowan, MA, OTR, FAOTA
Professor of Occupational Therapy
University of Texas-Pan American
Edinburg, Texas

Jolene Marie Jacobson, OTR
Occupational Therapist
Health South
Northern Kentucky Rehabilitation Hospital
Edgewood, Kentucky

Jean Steffan Smith, MS, OTR
Associate Professor
Department of Occupational Therapy
Eastern Kentucky University
Richmond, Kentucky

 F. A. DAVIS COMPANY • Philadelphia

F. A. Davis Company
1915 Arch Street
Philadelphia, PA 19103
www.fadavis.com

Printed in the United States of America

0-8036-0776-8

Last digit indicates print number: 10 9 8 7 6 5 4 3 2 1

Acquisitions Editor: Margaret Biblis
Developmental Editor: Colleen Ward
Cover Designer: Louis J. Forgione

As new scientific information becomes available through basic and clinical research, recommended treatments and drug therapies undergo changes. The author(s) and publisher have done everything possible to make this book accurate, up to date, and in accord with accepted standards at the time of publication. The author(s), editors, and publisher are not responsible for errors or omissions or for consequences from application of the book, and make no warranty, expressed or implied, in regard to the contents of the book. Any practice described in this book should be applied by the reader in accordance with professional standards of care used in regard to the unique circumstances that may apply in each situation. The reader is advised always to check product information (package inserts) for changes and new information regarding dose and contraindications before administering any drug. Caution is especially urged when using new or infrequently ordered drugs.

PREFACE

The purpose of this review guide is to give candidates for the National Board for Certification in Occupational Therapy (NBCOT) certification examination a general review of the profession and study tools to use while preparing to take the exam. It will also serve as an excellent review for occupational therapists reentering the field or changing areas of practice.

This book's format encourages users to synthesize and *apply* knowledge and become comfortable with the format of the NBCOT exam. The questions in the certification exam are designed to require students to call upon their knowledge of occupational therapy practice and to apply that knowledge to realistic practice situations. The questions in this book are designed to evoke these same thought processes. The reader will find that basic knowledge combined with reasoning will lead to the best answer; the questions in this book do not test basic knowledge alone. While the majority of questions in the *Occupational Therapy Exam Review Guide* have been written in a style that simulates the NBCOT exam, some have been written to maximize review of important content areas.

The textbooks referenced for most answers are those most commonly required for purchase by students in occupational therapy programs across the United States. In some cases, the authors cite less well-known references because they provide the best rationales. Students can access these books through their school's occupational therapy libraries or libraries of other occupational therapy programs. In addition, many of the books cited are available from the Wilma West Library at AOTA headquarters.

Please keep in mind that this workbook will *not:*

- be a comprehensive guide to practicing as an occupational therapist,
- replicate the examination or any of the questions on the examination, or
- offer the student a guarantee of passing the examination.

This workbook *will:*

- provide a general review of occupational therapy practice,
- help readers identify the strengths and weaknesses in their knowledge of occupational therapy,
- acquaint the reader with the format of questions used on the examination,
- help the reader organize and set priorities for study time, and
- provide the reader with a reference list from which further study may be pursued.

THE AUTHORS

Caryn R. Johnson, MS, OTR/L, FAOTA, serves as Academic Fieldwork Coordinator for the Occupational Therapy Program at Thomas Jefferson University in Philadelphia, Pennsylvania, where she has taught since 1983. Caryn received her Bachelor's degree in Occupational Therapy from Tufts University in 1978 and an advanced Masters Degree in Occupational Therapy from Thomas Jefferson University in 1991. In addition, she is president of Occupational Therapy Associates, a private practice specializing in aquatic rehabilitation. Caryn's special interests include developing fieldwork opportunities in non-traditional community settings and in the development of professional behaviors in OT and OTA students. In her free time, Caryn works with a wide variety of craft media.

Arlene Lorch, MS, OTR/L, CHES received a Bachelor of Science degree in Occupational Therapy from the University of Pennsylvania and a Master of Science in Health Education from Beaver College. She has been a practicing occupational therapist in acute care, rehabilitation, and long-term care settings for 25 years. Since 1996, Arlene has been a clinical instructor involved in teaching occupational therapy courses and labs in evaluation, intervention, occupation, group dynamics and environmental adaptation at the Thomas Jefferson University College of Health Professions. A Certified Health Education Specialist, Arlene is interested in combining knowledge of occupational performance and environmental assessment with health education approaches to assist in the development of accessibility and injury prevention programs. Other special interests include occupational performance and quality of life issues in the elderly population, falls prevention, and the role of the environment in supporting occupation and development of wellness programs.

Tina DeAngelis, MS, OTR/L, has worked part time in the Department of Occupational Therapy at Thomas Jefferson University teaching selected courses and managing federally funded grant projects. In addition, she is a practicing occupational therapist at Crozer Chester Medical Center in Upland, Pennsylvania, where she has been employed full and part time since 1991. She has experience in burn care, orthopedic, and neurological conditions. Tina received her Associate's degree in Occupational Therapy from Harcum College in 1987, her Bachelor's degree in Occupational Therapy from College Misericordia in 1992, and her advanced Master's degree in Occupational Therapy from Thomas Jefferson University in 1997. She is currently enrolled in a doctoral program in Higher Education Leadership at Widener University in Chester, Pennsylvania. Tina is also the public relations co-chair of the Pennsylvania Occupational Therapy Association's District V and the mother of two school-age girls.

ACKNOWLEDGMENTS

The input and enthusiasm of many individuals has made this book possible. We especially want to thank Margaret Biblis and Lynn Borders Caldwell for their guidance and support. We also want to thank Janice Burke for her support and tolerance over the course of the work. Our deepest thanks to friends and family, for tolerating us, present and absent, while we lost ourselves to this project for the last year.

CONTRIBUTORS

Each of the following individuals has called upon her years of experience and wealth of knowledge to develop well-researched and well-written questions. Their contribution to the *Occupational Therapy Exam Review Guide* has been invaluable.

Florence Hannes, MS, OTR/L
Chair, Occupational Therapy Assistant Program
Orange County Community College
Middletown, New York

Catherine Verrier Piersol, MS, OTR/L
Academic Fieldwork Coordinator
Department of Occupational Therapy
Philadelphia University
Philadelphia, Pennsylvania

Brittany Duling, OTR/L
Pediatric Occupational Therapist
Thomas Jefferson University Hospital
Philadelphia, Pennsylvania

E. Adel Herge, MS OTR/L
Instructor
Department of Occupational Therapy
Thomas Jefferson University
Philadelphia, Pennsylvania

Kerstin Potter, MA, OTR/L
Associate Professor and Program Director
Occupational Therapy Assistant Program
Harcum College
Bryn Mawr, Pennsylvania

REVIEWERS

Finally, we would like to recognize the efforts of those educators and practitioners from across the country who painstakingly reviewed, critiqued, and validated every question to ensure accuracy and appropriateness.

Kristie P. Koenig, MS, OTR/L
Assistant Professor, Fieldwork Coordinator
Temple University
Department of Occupational Therapy
Philadelphia, PA

Judith Vestal, PhD, OTR
Associate Professor
School of Allied Health Professions
Louisiana State University
Health Sciences Center
Shreveport, LA

Debra A. Tupe, MPH, MS, OTR/L
Director Occupational Therapy, Incarnation Childrens Center
Clinical Instructor in Occupational Therapy
Columbia University
New York, NY

Stacey Bunch-Harrison, OTR/L
Thomas Jefferson University Hospital
Department of Rehabilitation Medicine
Philadelphia, PA

Julia Waggoner, OTR/L
Occupational Therapy Clinical Coordinator
Magee Rehabilitation Hospital
Department of Occupational Therapy
Philadelphia, PA

Jane Case-Smith, EdD, OTR/L, BCP, FAOTA
Associate Professor
Ohio State University
School of Allied Medical Professions
Department of Occupational Therapy
Columbus, OH

Carol L. Heisner, OTR/L
Operations Manager Rehabilitation Services
Delaware County Memorial Hospital
Drexel Hill, PA

Robert W. Gibson, MS, OTR/L
Instructor
University of Florida
College of Health Professions
Department of Occupational Therapy
Gainesville, FL

Joanne Opperman, MS, OTR/L
Occupational Therapist Hospital of the University
of Pennsylvania
Department of Occupational and Physical Therapy
Philadelphia, PA

Gretchen Reeks, MA, OTR
Assistant Professor
School of Allied Health Professions
Louisiana State University
Health Sciences Center
Shreveport, LA

CONTENTS

PREPARING FOR THE EXAMINATION

WHAT IS THE NBCOT EXAMINATION?

Successful completion of the certification examination is required for anyone who wants to practice as an occupational therapist. Passing the NBCOT examination is the culmination of academic and fieldwork study. The examination tests your depth of knowledge and ability to apply that knowledge to practice. The questions require you to apply knowledge of occupational therapy or synthesize bits of knowledge to select the correct answer. The purpose of the examination is to identify those candidates who demonstrate entry-level competence for practicing as an occupational therapist. Once candidates have successfully completed the examination, they are certified as occupational therapists. The examination is offered at designated times throughout the year. Examinations are given for both certified occupational therapy assistant (COTA) and registered occupational therapist (OTR) candidates.

Beginning September 2001, the exam will only be delivered by computer. The computerized exams will be offered over a period of 18 days four times a year (January, April, July, and October). Both the NBCOT exams and practice exams will be offered at hundreds of centers around the country. Only those registered for the NBCOT exam are eligible to take practice exams. More information on the computerized exams and practice exams is available at www.nbcot.org.

WHO CAN TAKE THE CERTIFICATION EXAMINATION?

The NBCOT oversees the certification examination and eligibility of candidates. Candidates must be graduates of an accredited occupational therapy education program and have successfully completed the required fieldwork. Candidates are required to submit either an official transcript or the NBCOT Academic Credential Verification form from their occupational therapy programs. Many states require students to sit for the first exam offered once they have become eligible; however, this is no longer an NBCOT requirement.

In cases where graduation is not scheduled until after the examination date, students must be cleared for graduation (both academically and financially) by the institution's registrar. If complete official transcripts cannot be submitted, the student must have the "NBCOT Academic Credential Verification Form" completed by the registrar and submitted to the NBCOT. Deadlines are strictly enforced. An official transcript must be submitted *no later* than 90 days after the date of the examination. Failure to do so may result in loss of certification.

Individuals who are not recent graduates (within one year) of an accredited U.S. program and international candidates seeking to take the examination must contact NBCOT for additional information.

ABOUT THE NBCOT CANDIDATE HANDBOOK

The NBCOT Candidate Handbook contains the application for the exam. Detailed and critical information is included in the NBCOT Candidate Handbook, which the candidate should read from cover to cover before completing the application form. The handbook is available online at www.nbcot.org. Students may also request a hard copy of the Candidate Handbook by writing to NBCOT at: NBCOT Candidate Handbook, PO Box 70, Waldorf, MD 20604-0070. You must include a self-addressed, pressure-sensitive label with your request. Candidates may contact NBCOT by phone at (301) 990-7979.

The handbook includes an application for the examination, eligibility requirements, deadlines, and information about test administration and scoring. Read this handbook thoroughly and save it until after you have received your test scores.

HOW TO APPLY FOR THE EXAMINATION

Applications to take the exam are actually submitted to the Professional Examination Service (PES), not NBCOT, and may be submitted online or by mail. Applying online significantly reduces the possibility of submitting an incomplete application and is strongly encouraged. Candidates should contact PES at (877) 314-0786 for questions concerning the online application. The fee for taking the examination (at the time of this writing) is approximately $325. There is an additional charge to have reports of scores sent to state regulatory agencies and for each notice of Confirmation of Eligibility requested. These items are frequently required in order to obtain a license to practice.

The Candidate Handbook and application forms are usually available online 3-4 months prior to the exam. The application deadline is usually about two months before the exam date. There is no longer a late registration deadline and deadlines are strictly enforced. Candidates can check the status of their applications online. Those mailing applications to PES may include a self-addressed postcard, which PES will return to the candidate as confirmation that the application was received. The postcard confirms receipt of the student's application, but does not provide information regarding the status, such as whether the application is complete. Candidates may wish to send the application by certified mail to receive a "returned receipt" from the Post Office. Candidates requiring special accommodations need to submit a request by the designated deadline.

WHAT IS THE FORMAT OF THE EXAMINATION?

The certification examination is composed of 200 multiple-choice questions that use the four-option format. No combination or "K" questions are used. Questions are designed as brief practice scenarios, and require you to decide what you should *do* based on your application of occupational therapy *knowledge*. You have 4 hours to complete the examination. Each item has the same weight in scoring, and every question on the examination has only one correct answer. There is not a penalty for guessing, so you should *never* leave a question unanswered. In fact, the computerized format allows you to "flag" questions you have difficulty answering and may want to return to later.

WHAT DOES THE EXAMINATION COVER?

The exam covers the following seven categories. Additional information is available at www.nbcot.org.

1. Evaluation

This portion comprises approximately 22% of the exam, or about 44 questions. These questions apply to tasks related to your ability to evaluate the individual, analyze the data, and identify problem areas. You must be familiar with multiple methods for collecting data, such as: observation, chart review, screening, interviewing, and standardized and non-standardized assessments (although few will actually be identified by name). You will also need to understand how to interpret results, prioritize strengths and weaknesses, and document results. This category corresponds to NBCOT's "Domain A."

When studying for this category, be sure to review a variety of methods for evaluating sensation, motor performance, cognition (especially Allen's Cognitive Levels), psychosocial performance, and development (both standardized and non-standardized). Familiarize yourself with the proper techniques for administering evaluations in general. Be certain to review normal and abnormal human development and pathological conditions. You should also review your basic sciences (anatomy, kinesiology, psychology, and neuroscience), and finally, effects and side-effects of medications.

2. Treatment Planning

This portion comprises approximately 14% of the exam, or about 28 questions. These questions will test your ability to plan interventions based on evaluation results and theory. It will address tasks such as collaborating with the individual, caregivers, and team members and selecting the *most appropriate* frame of reference and setting goals. It will test your ability to adapt or modify tasks or the environment and to select and/or design occupation-based interventions that establish or restore function or prevent negative outcomes. You will also need to know how to select the *most appropriate* intervention, perform activity analysis, and select appropriate environments and contexts for treatment. Finally, this portion will test your ability to document treatment/intervention plans and write goals. This category corresponds to NBCOT's "Domain B."

Questions in this category will require you to design treatment for individuals of all ages with a wide range of abilities and disabilities, so familiarity with human development, pathology and the basic sciences is again important. Good clinical reasoning skills and knowledge of the basic tenets of occupational therapy will be critical for success in this section. You will need to be able to select and document the *best* theory-based treatment plan and project the outcomes. Knowledge of a wide range of therapeutic media, purposeful activities, and relevant precautions and contraindications will be essential.

3. Treatment Implementation

This portion comprises approximately 37% of the exam, or about 74 questions—more than any other category. These questions apply to tasks related to providing occupation-based interventions for individuals and/or their caregivers once the treatment plan has been developed. You will need to show you know when, where, and how to provide treatment, while applying good therapeutic use of self and effective communication skills. You will need to recognize when and how to grade and adapt activities and environments, and be able to select, construct, and provide the *most appropriate* devices, including adaptive equipment, splints, and technology. These questions will also test you on your ability to instruct individuals and others on subjects such as joint protection, time management, and care of assistive devices. There will also be questions related to documenting intervention. This category corresponds to NBCOT's "Domain C."

Review for this category will also require familiarity with the basic sciences, pathology, and human development. You will need to be familiar with a wide range of therapeutic media, adaptive equipment, splints and splinting methods, physical agent modalities, and some technology. You will also need to understand group theories, how groups develop and function, and how to lead groups. The emphasis in this portion is on how you can *most effectively* implement occupation-based treatment, your therapeutic use of self, how to respond to various behaviors, and your ability to assess the individual's response to the intervention and react as needed.

4. Effectiveness of Treatment and Discharge Planning

This category comprises approximately 11% of the exam, or about 22 questions. These questions apply to tasks associated with monitoring and modifying the treatment plan and with discharge planning. Questions in this category will address the task of evaluating and reevaluating continuously to determine if goals and treatment methods are appropriate and realistic, and revising the treatment plan when necessary. This category also deals with discharge planning and its associated tasks such as identifying the need for and selecting the *most appropriate* follow-up services and recommending equipment for home use and developing and instructing the individual and others in home programs. This area will also cover discharge documentation and timely and appropriate termination of services. This category corresponds to NBCOT's "Domain D."

Study for this portion is similar to the three categories previously identified. In addition, you should be familiar with service delivery models available to individuals after discharge, such as home health, outpatient services, and other community resources.

5. Occupational Therapy for Populations

This category comprises approximately 4% of the exam, or about 8 questions. These questions apply to provision of occupational therapy to groups of people rather than individuals (often underserved, at-risk, or well populations) through preventive, supportive, or remediative services in select settings. Examples of such settings include adult day programs, schools, homeless shelters, and work environments. Questions in this category address tasks such as assessing the needs of the organization or population, recommending and implementing interventions, measuring outcomes, and consulting. This category corresponds to NBCOT's "Domain E."

Study for this portion is similar to the first three categories previously identified. In addition, you should be familiar with community service delivery models, consultation skills, and the characteristics and needs of underserved, at-risk, and well populations.

6. Service Management

This category comprises approximately 9% of the exam, or about 18 questions. Questions in this section apply to tasks relating to management and service delivery, such as: developing, coordinating and promoting occupational therapy services, program evaluation, and supervision of staff and students. This category corresponds to NBCOT's "Domain F."

Study for this portion will involve basic principles of management, leadership, supervision, budgeting, and marketing. Review of AOTA documents such as the Standards of Practice and Occupational Therapy Roles, and documents related to supervision of occupational therapy and non-occupational therapy personnel is recommended. You also need to know methods for evaluating services, such as quality assurance and utilization review. Finally, it is important to understand how provision of occupational therapy services varies from one setting or service delivery model to another.

7. Professional Practice

This category comprises approximately 3% of the exam, or about 6 questions. Questions in this section apply to tasks relating to practicing competently, legally, ethically, and professionally. You may be asked about promoting occupational therapy to the public, applying and engaging in research, presenting and publishing, and fieldwork education. This category corresponds to NBCOT's "Domain G."

Study for this category will require familiarity with AOTA documents such as the Occupational Therapy Code of Ethics and Standards of Practice. You should also review concepts related to licensure, methods for maintaining competency, laws that affect the practice of occupational therapy, and role delineation between OTRs and COTAs. Because the exam is designed for a national audience, no state-specific information is included.

THE DAY OF THE EXAMINATION

At the time of this writing, little information is available about the computer-delivered exam. However, the following checklist should help you on the day of the exam:

[ ] Double-check the date and time.

[ ] Know where you are going, how to get there, and where you will be able to park.

[ ] Bring your admission ticket.

[ ] Bring two forms of identification, including one photo ID with signature.

[ ] Bring a watch to help you stay on schedule during the 4-hour test. A clock option is available on each computer, but some find it distracting and prefer to turn it off.

Food and drinks, dictionaries, cell phones and a host of other items are not permitted. Special permission is even required for bottled water.

WHAT HAPPENS AFTER THE EXAMINATION?

Test results are mailed approximately 4 weeks after the certification examination. Of the U.S. graduates taking the test for the first time in September 2000, about 83% passed. A score of 450 or higher is required to pass the certification examination. A grievance process is outlined in the Candidate Handbook. If you experience difficulty with the testing conditions or have any other complaints about your experience taking the exam, you must report it *immediately* to NBCOT.

Candidates can request that results be sent to the licensing agency of the state(s) in which they plan to practice. There is a fee for each report you request-no reports are sent free of charge. Almost all states require a copy of the report. It is recommended that the candidate complete an application for state licensure before taking the examination. Often, these applications require a notarized copy of transcripts from an accredited occupational therapy program, letters of reference, a picture identification, and so forth. Depending on the state licensure laws and facility requirements, OTRs may or may not be able to work with a temporary permit until examination results are received. Candidates should contact the licensing agency as soon as they know the state in which they plan to practice. Candidates should learn as early as possible what information will be necessary for licensure and when applications should be submitted.

Candidates who fail the examination must retake the entire examination. There is no longer a limit on how many times an individual may take the exam.

HOW TO USE THIS WORKBOOK

This workbook has five complete sample tests of 200 questions each that simulate the actual examination by asking questions in a four-option, multiple-choice format. Questions in the first three tests are organized to allow you to assess your performance in each of the seven categories. Questions in the fourth test are grouped by population, allowing you to assess your competence with various age groups and diagnostic categories. The sequence of questions in the fifth test is randomized, simulating the format of the NBCOT exam. This arrangement can be more difficult in that the topic and item areas change frequently. The final examination enables you to evaluate how well you have retained and been able to implement the techniques recommended in this book. The mix of questions in each test covers the range of entry-level occupational therapy practice, thus providing a general review of the profession.

A complete set of answers follows each examination. In order to help the test taker, the workbook provides a complete rationale for each answer, which explains both correct and incorrect answers. Hence, each question-answer unit is actually a mini-lesson on not one, but four concepts. In addition, each answer provides the test taker with a reference from which further information may be obtained on the subject matter. A complete reference list is located at the end of the workbook.

The section on test-taking tips will help you identify your strengths and weaknesses and organize and set priorities for study time. A guide for developing a study plan is provided at the end of this section.

WHERE TO BEGIN

Viewed as one task, preparing to take the examination can seem overwhelming. Breaking the process into smaller parts makes it more manageable. The first step is to identify your areas of strength and weakness. The personal study plan chart following this section can help you through this process. Once you have completed this step, the second step is to complete your study plan. The final step is to pull all of the information together and take the practice examinations. It may be helpful to review the test-taking tips occasionally.

TEST-TAKING TIPS

Test-Taking Tip 1

Visit the NBCOT web site periodically. You can access the candidate handbook and other vital information about the exam at the NBCOT web site (www.nbcot.org). It is essential that you read the Candidate Handbook thoroughly *and more than once*—you'll pick up something new each time. This web site has the most current information regarding test dates and locations and is updated frequently. It also has details about how the exam was developed and how it is scored.

Test-Taking Tip 2

Using this book to create a personal study plan. The question most frequently asked by occupational therapy students preparing for the examination is "How do I start?" This guide will help you put all your educational preparation together and organize your study time. It will also make you comfortable with multiple-choice questions. All students preparing for the examination should have their course work at their fingertips, including books, notes, handouts, etc. Once you have assembled the stacks of information accumulated over the years, the question arises: "Where do I start?"

One way to use this book is to develop a study plan based on your performance on the practice exams. Start by taking practice Exam 1 and record how many correct answers you score in each category compared to the number of questions that will be on the certification exam in this category.

This will give you some idea of the categories for which you need more concentrated review and study. The next step is to define your strengths and weaknesses. To do this, choose a category and then go through all the component parts of that category as well as the background knowledge areas suggested for review. Classify the areas in which you are weakest as "D," and those in which you are strongest as "A." Assign "B" or "C," with "B" being stronger than "C," to the remaining practice areas. Within each letter grouping, identify the weakest subject with a number 4 and sequentially number through to the strongest subject—the higher the number, the higher your study priority. Once this has been completed, your individualized studying needs have been organized and priorities set for accomplishment.

After completing practice Exams 2 and 3, record the numbers of your correct answers for each category. This will be further indication of areas for which you still need review.

Now that you have set your priorities for studying, set target dates for completing your review of each area or subject. For instance, you may choose to work on category #1 (evaluation) during the month of March. Another individual may choose to review evaluation the first week of March, treatment planning (category #2) the second week of March, and so forth. Design your study plan to meet your needs. Set target dates that are realistic and attainable.

When the planning is complete, it is time for the study to begin. Start with the area listed as "D4" (high priority and need) and work your way through to the last "D." Once this is finished, continue with the "C" and "B" and "A" items. When all areas have been reviewed you may choose to begin again at D4 or to reset priorities for your studying needs. The easiest part of this task will be defining the time frame in which to study specific topics. The toughest challenge will be implementing the examination review plan!

Table 1. STUDY PLAN OF CATEGORIES FOR CERTIFICATION EXAMINATION
1 - EVALUATION

	Self-Rating
Percentage of items on certification exam - 22% Number of questions in each review exam - 44	
Questions in this category test the ability to apply knowledge to the following kinds of tasks:	
• Methods for reviewing and using preliminary data from persons, records, charts • Performance of skilled clinical observations of persons and environments • Interview styles and formats used to gain information and related communication skills • Knowledge of the screening process including selection, administration, scoring and analysis of results • Standardized and non-standardized assessment selection, administration, and analysis of results • General evaluation procedures for sensory, motor, cognitive and psychosocial performance components • Assessment tools and methods for performance areas - ADL, work and productive activities, play and leisure • Assessment of developmental status • Interpretation of assessment findings to determine and prioritize needs for OT services • Development of documentation and reports based on assessment findings	
Background knowledge to review for the evaluation category:	
• Basic science knowledge, underlying performance; anatomy, kinesiology, psychology, neuroscience • Normal and abnormal human development • Progression of skill development in performance areas of ADL, work and productive activities, play and leisure • Pathological conditions and resulting sensorimotor, cognitive and psychosocial impairments • Impact of disability and injury in terms of the individual's roles and occupational performance • Impact of disability and injury on the individual's caregivers, family and sociocultural environment • Influence of the context such as physical and social environments, and temporal factors on human performance • Effects and side-effects of medications **Your score on practice exam 1** _____ /44_ **Your score on practice exam 2** _____ /44_ **Your score on practice exam 3** _____ /44_	

#2 - TREATMENT PLANNING

	Self-Rating
Percentage of questions from this category - 14% Number of questions in each exam - 28	
Questions in this category test the ability to apply knowledge to the following kinds of tasks:	
• Using principles of clinical reasoning • Utilizing collaborative skills with individuals, caregivers and team members in the treatment planning process • Selection of appropriate frames of reference and treatment approaches to address needs identified in evaluation • Development and documentation of measurable goals based on evaluation findings • Development and documentation of treatment plans reflecting intervention priorities	

• Selection of intervention methods and strategies from a wide range of restorative, compensatory, adaptive, preventive and education-based treatment options • Identification of relevant precautions and intervention contraindications • Recommendations for frequency, amount and duration of treatment • Analysis of individual potential based on clinical judgment	
Background knowledge to review for the treatment planning category:	
• Basic science knowledge, underlying performance; anatomy, kinesiology, psychology, neuroscience • Normal and abnormal human development • Progression of skill development in performance areas of ADL, work and productive activities, play and leisure • Pathological conditions and resulting sensorimotor, cognitive and psychosocial impairments • Impact of disability and injury in terms of the individual's roles and occupational performance • Impact of disability and injury on the individual's caregivers, family and sociocultural environment • Influence of the context such as physical and social environments, and temporal factors on human performance • Effects and side-effects of medications	
Specific areas to review:	
• Elements of a treatment plan, including construction of long- and short-term goals • Models of practice, theories and frames of reference underlying intervention for sensorimotor, cognitive and psychosocial performance components and for performance areas • Rationales for theory and intervention selection • Process of activity analysis and activity grading relative to performance areas, components and contexts • Adaptation possibilities for tasks, objects and environmental factors affecting performance **Your score on practice exam 1** _____ **/28** **Your score on practice exam 2** _____ **/28** **Your score on practice exam 3** _____ **/28**	

#3 - TREATMENT IMPLEMENTATION

Percentage of questions from this category - 37% Number of questions in each exam - 74	Self-Rating
Questions in this category test the ability to apply knowledge to the following kinds of tasks:	
• Communication and collaborative skills used in presenting treatment plans to individuals, family, team members and others • Selection and implementation of activities, modalities and media to achieve therapeutic goals • Adaptation and grading of activities • Selection and implementation of compensatory and adaptive methods to achieve therapeutic goals • Implementation of interventions to prevent or limit further impairment, disability or dysfunction • Training, teaching and instructional methods for use with adults and children of varying developmental and cognitive abilities • Revision of intervention based on continued monitoring of progress toward goal achievement	

Specific areas to review (in addition to background knowledge also noted for categories #1 and 2 above)	
• Interventions typically used with specific pathological conditions • Therapeutic use of self and motivational strategies to maximize treatment effectiveness • Interventions to address occupational performance deficits in ADL, work and productive activities and play and leisure • Principles and application of compensatory strategies including the use of assistive technologies, assistive and adaptive devices, environmental modification and assistance from others • Training, teaching and instructional methods for use with adults and children of varying developmental and cognitive abilities and for caregivers and supervised personnel • Specific approaches and techniques to address sensorimotor performance deficits including:	

• Specific approaches and techniques to address sensorimotor performance deficits including:

 use of physical agent modalities
 splinting, orthotics and prosthetics
 therapeutic exercise program and manual techniques
 sensory reeducation and sensory processing techniques
 motor learning, neurodevelopmental frames of reference and positioning strategies
 wheelchair selection and management
 adaptive device selection, adaptation and training
 occupation-based activities
 environment-based interventions

• Specific approaches to address cognitive performance deficits including:

 cognitive rehabilitation techniques such as dynamic interactional and functional approaches training techniques and methods of assisting and cueing compensatory methods used in dementia such as task-breakdown
 Allen's cognitive disabilities
 perceptual rehabilitation techniques

• Specific approaches to address psychosocial performance deficits including strategies for dealing with behavioral issues of specific psychiatric conditions, organic brain disorders and substance abuse, in children, adolescents and adults including:

 therapeutic use of self and individual treatment approaches
 group leadership skills and intervention techniques based on application of group process interventions which address living skills, coping skills and stress management, pre-vocational exploration and work readiness

• Knowledge of intervention possibilities in various settings and service delivery models and resources in the community and elsewhere that can support occupational performance
• Incorporation of relevant precautions and contraindications into treatment considerations
• Clinical problem solving related individual client/patient response to intervention and reassessment
• Recording of treatment process and documentation of progress
• Selection and implementation of methods to monitor outcome effectiveness of intervention

Your score on practice exam 1 _____ /74
Your score on practice exam 2 _____ /74
Your score on practice exam 3 _____ /74

#4 - EFFECTIVENESS OF TREATMENT AND DISCHARGE PLANNING

	Self-Rating
Percentage of questions from this category - 11% Number of questions in each exam - 22	
Questions in this category test the ability to apply knowledge to the following kinds of tasks:	
· Methods of reevaluation for monitoring treatment plan effectiveness and progress made by the individual · Revision of goals and modification of treatment plans on the basis of individual response to intervention · Planning for timely service termination · Initiating and completing the discharge planning process in collaboration with the individual · Prioritizing needs and making recommendations and referrals for follow-up services · Developing home programs and recommendations for strategies to maximize performance in expected discharge environment · Providing discharge related information and instruction to individuals, caregivers, team members and other professionals · Selecting and recommending adaptive devices, equipment and modifications · Documenting the OT services provided and writing discharge summaries and reports	
Background knowledge to review for the effectiveness of treatment and discharge planning category is similar to that of categories # 1, 2 and 3:	
· Basic science knowledge, underlying performance; anatomy, kinesiology, psychology, neuroscience · Normal and abnormal human development · Progression of skill development in performance areas of ADL, work and productive activities, play and leisure · Pathological conditions and resulting sensorimotor, cognitive and psychosocial impairments · Impact of disability and injury in terms of the individual's roles and occupational performance · Impact of disability and injury on the individual's caregivers, family and sociocultural environment. · Influence of the context such as physical and social environments, and temporal factors on human performance · Effects and side-effects of medications	
Specific areas to review:	
· Service delivery models available to individuals following discharge, such as home health, outpatient services and community resources · Factors which indicate the need for further services for children and adults in a variety of practice settings and performance contexts **Your score on practice exam 1** _____ /22 **Your score on practice exam 2** _____ /22 **Your score on practice exam 3** _____ /22	

#5 - OCCUPATIONAL THERAPY FOR POPULATIONS

	Self-Rating
Percentage of questions from this category - 4% Number of questions in each exam - 8	
Questions in this category test the ability to apply knowledge to the following kinds of tasks:	
• Identification and assessment of populations at risk for occupational performance deficits • Identification and assessment of under-served populations • Identification and assessment of well populations who may benefit from occupation-based services • Development of intervention recommendations for preventive, support-ive or remediative services • Implementation of programming for populations • Providing information, education and training to others to implement population-based programs	
Background knowledge to review for the effectiveness of treatment and discharge planning category is similar to that of categories # 1, 2, 3 and 4:	
Specific areas to review:	

• The significance of occupation in maintaining health and well being
• The role of occupation as intervention for chronic health problems and in prevention of disability
• Adaptation of tasks, objects and environments to enhance occupational performance and safety for groups
• Injury prevention methods and wellness strategies to promote health
• Strategies to support occupational performance at developmental stages throughout the life span
• Service delivery models benefiting from population-based programs including:
 	
     community settings such as senior centers and homeless shelters
     early intervention settings, schools and other training or educa-tional programs
     elderly care environments such as adult day programs and assisted living centers
     work and industrial environments
     wellness settings
 	
• The role of the consultant and consultation skills
• Methods of monitoring effectiveness of population-based interventions and programs
 	
Your score on practice exam 1 _____ /8
Your score on practice exam 2 _____ /8
Your score on practice exam 3 _____ /8	

#6 - SERVICE MANAGEMENT

	Self-Rating
Percentage of questions from this category - 9% Number of questions in each exam - 18	
Questions in this category test the ability to apply knowledge to the following kinds of tasks:	
• Planning and directing occupational therapy service operations • Management and coordination of resources and personnel • Promotion and marketing of occupational therapy services • Supervision of staff and students • Maintaining professional development and competence of staff • Identifying safety issues and implementing policies and procedures to minimize risk • Evaluation of service effectiveness, outcomes and quality through program evaluation methods	
Specific areas to review:	
• Provision of services in diverse systems and delivery models and how services vary in different settings • Standards of practice • Roles and expectations of various occupational therapy personnel • Principles of leadership, marketing, financial management and budgeting • Principles and standards of supervision and interpersonal management skills • Methods of service assessment and improvement, such as quality assurance, outcomes monitoring and utilization review **Your score on practice exam 1** _____ /18 **Your score on practice exam 2** _____ /18 **Your score on practice exam 3** _____ /18	

#7 - PROFESSIONAL PRACTICE

Percentage of questions from this category - 3% Number of questions in each exam - 6	Self-Rating
Questions in this category test the ability to apply knowledge to the following kinds of tasks:	
• Compliance with lawful regulations that govern the practice of occupational therapy • Adhering to ethical codes and applying ethical principles to the practice of occupational therapy • Engaging in presentations and publications that add to the professional knowledge base • Engaging in research activities and applying knowledge gained from research to practice • Contributing to the education of occupational therapy practitioners, students and others • Promotion and advancement of occupational therapy to the public • Maintaining professional competence through professional development activities	
Specific areas to review:	
• Standards of practice • OT Code of Ethics • Roles, responsibilities and scope of practice of OTRs and COTAs • The process of accreditation and certification for credentials • National requirements for credentialing and governing occupational therapy practice • National laws and policies which impact the practice of the profession • Basic elements in the design and implementation of research studies • Procedures of data collection for use in outcome and other evaluative studies • Methods for maintaining competence **Your score on practice exam 1** _____/6__ **Your score on practice exam 2** _____/6__ **Your score on practice exam 3** _____/6__	

Test-Taking Tip 3

Be prepared. The more prepared you are to take the examination, the more comfortable you will feel during the examination. Preparation includes studying the knowledge base of occupational therapy, getting a good night's sleep, and coming prepared to the exam. Although the exam is computerized, candidates do not necessarily need to have good computer skills. When studying is complete, most of the preparation is complete. However, when asked to identify the single most important thing in preparing for the examination, a graduating class of students agreed that the answer is getting a good night's sleep. Plan to arrive at the test site 20 to 30 minutes before the examination. Arriving early will give you time to register and acclimate yourself to the environment.

Test-Taking Tip 4

Prepare your body as well as your mind! Eating a well-balanced breakfast can actually help your performance on the examination. A breakfast high in carbohydrates and low in fat will increase your energy and will not produce a sluggish feeling. Avoid caffeine the day of the examination because caffeine will ultimately make you tired and drowsy. Finally, wear comfortable clothing in layers to allow you to adjust as necessary to the temperature of the room.

Test-Taking Tip 5

Pace yourself. The test is to be completed within 4 hours. Within this time frame, you have to answer 200 multiple-choice questions. Begin by familiarizing yourself with the computer test program. One technique for pacing the examination is to divide the test into four equivalent 50 question sections. You should aim to complete each of the four sections within 50 minutes to 1 hour. Understanding the format of the test and budgeting your time will help you work through the questions more efficiently and enable you to complete the examination in the time allotted. Another pacing technique is to use a watch or the clock provided by the computer test program. At the end of every 15 to 20 questions, briefly glance at the time to maintain a sense of your pace. If you have completed all the questions and have time left, go back to see if you can answer any of the questions you "flagged." If questions still remain incomplete within the last 10 minutes of the examination, select one letter and fill in all of the remaining questions with that letter. Remember, there is no penalty for guessing-only for leaving questions unanswered! Another method is to wear a watch that can be set to signal on the hour. When the examination begins, set the watch for 12:00. Between 12:00 and 4:00, the watch will signal each hour, so that you can check your pace without having to "watch the clock." The goal is to complete at least 25% of the examination, or 50 questions, within each hour. Avoid wasting time by looking frequently at your watch. If you find the computer test program clock too distracting, you have the option of turning it off.

Test-Taking Tip 6

When you use the same letter for more than three answers in a row, double check the questions to verify each answer. Test writers usually break up strings of four or more of the same letter or answer. The multiple-choice format is generally set so that three consecutive answers of the same letter is the maximum. If you have selected four or more of the same letters consecutively, it may be beneficial to recheck the answers. Save this task for the end of the examination!

Test-Taking Tip 7

Use key techniques to help select the correct answer.
1. *Follow your instincts when answering questions.* The first answer chosen is usually the correct one. Change an answer only if you later realize that it is absolutely correct.
2. *Ask, "What is this question about?"* Try to decipher what the question is testing by selecting the key terms in the questions and not being distracted by peripheral information. By sorting through the information provided to identify what the question is testing, you may be more likely to select the correct answer.
3. *Anticipate the answer.* Many times you may anticipate an answer while reading a question. If so, look for the anticipated answer among the options. However, it is important to read and consider all of the options to verify that the anticipated answer is the correct answer.
4. *Use logical reasoning.* A commonly used technique is the process of deduction-eliminating answers that are incorrect. Doing this allows you to concentrate on the options that remain.
   As you complete the questions on the exam, remember these techniques and practice using them when you have difficulty answering a question.

Test-Taking Tip 8

There are no trick questions. Questions are designed to test entry-level, not advanced, knowledge and reasoning. Be careful not to read too much into the questions. However, most questions will have two answers that appear to be correct. Many questions will ask for the "first" action the therapist should take, or the "best" or "most appropriate" choice. Make sure to note the qualifiers to help you determine the best answer.

Test-Taking Tip 9

Use the computer test program to your advantage. The computer test program allows you to "flag" a question so that you can go back to it later. It also allows you to identify unanswered questions and to change answers right up to the time you finally submit the test.

SIMULATION EXAMINATION 1

Directions: Circle the correct answer to the following questions. When you have completed this examination, check your answers against the answer key that follows. As you will see, an explanation is given for each answer along with a reference for further study. The book author is listed as well as the chapter author. See the bibliography for complete references. Study the areas in which your comprehension was low, then test yourself again by taking Simulation Examination 2.

Evaluation

1. **While performing a hand reassessment, the OT practitioner notices a deformity developing on the dorsal aspect of the client's second digit. The client's PIP joint appears flexed, and the DIP appears to be hyperextended. The OTR can BEST describe this condition as a:**
   A. mallet deformity.
   B. boutonniere deformity.
   C. subluxation deformity.
   D. swan neck deformity.

2. **An OTR is MOST likely to administer a test of visual motor integration to a child referred to OT for difficulty with:**
   A. copying letters.
   B. remembering letters.
   C. recognizing letters.
   D. sequencing letters.

3. **When performing a "naturalistic observation" of dressing skills with a young child diagnosed with developmental delay, an OT practitioner should FIRST:**
   A. provide oversized clothing to ensure success.
   B. have the child dress and undress in a distraction-free corner of the clinic.
   C. provide assistance as needed to minimize frustration.
   D. observe the child entering the clinic and taking off his coat and shoes.

4. **An OT student witnesses a seizure in a young client with hydrocephalus. The MOST relevant information to document and report to the supervising therapist is:**
   A. the child's positioning during the seizure.
   B. objective signs and duration of the seizure.
   C. responsiveness during the seizure.
   D. facial expression during and after the seizure.

5. **An OTR is evaluating an individual who has sustained a left-hemisphere cerebrovascular accident (CVA). After determining that the person was able to read before the CVA, the therapist presents a paper with typed letters of the alphabet randomly dispersed across the page. The individual is then asked to cross out all the M's. The OTR observes that the individual has missed letters in a random pattern throughout the page. This MOST likely indicates:**
   A. a left visual field cut.
   B. a right visual field cut.
   C. functional illiteracy.
   D. decreased attention.

6. **Which of the following assessment methods would an OT practitioner MOST likely choose to learn about a family's values and priorities?**
   A. Interview
   B. Skilled observation
   C. Inventory
   D. Standardized test

7. **An OT practitioner works on the trauma unit of a hospital and often sees patients**

with trauma and disease of the upper extremity musculoskeletal system that can impact their motor control function. Assessment of motor control **MOST** likely includes:

A. evaluation of developmental factors.

B. assessment of upper extremity function in ADL, work and leisure activities.

C. evaluation of pain, postural control, and alignment.

D. assessment of self-concept and self-awareness.

8. **A young client who will be using a wheelchair after discharge from the rehabilitation facility is going home. In determining accessibility of the interior home environment, the FIRST area of evaluation the OT will be concerned with is:**

A. location of telephones and appliances.

B. arrangement of furniture in bedrooms.

C. steps, width of doorways, and threshold heights.

D. presence of clutter in the environment.

9. **An OT practitioner is working on functional mobility skills with a child who has a pes varus deformity of the foot. The OT can BEST document this as a(n):**

A. enlarged great toe.

B. club foot.

C. pronated foot.

D. unstable heel.

10. **The OT practitioner is observing dressing skills in an individual with chronic obstructive pulmonary disease (COPD). While putting on his shirt, the individual becomes short of breath and stops to rest before finishing with the shirt and going on to his trousers. The OTR would recognize this as a deficit in:**

A. postural control.

B. muscle tone.

C. strength.

D. endurance.

11. **While assessing the motor skills of an 8-month-old child, the OT practitioner observes him assume a quadruped position and then begin to rock back and forth. This behavior MOST likely indicates:**

A. perseverative tendencies.

B. normal development.

C. low muscle tone.

D. limitation in movement repertoire.

12. **While standing and holding onto furniture, a 3-year-old boy with delayed motor development shifts his weight onto one leg and steps to the side with the other. This movement pattern is BEST described as:**

A. creeping.

B. crawling.

C. cruising.

D. clawing.

13. **An individual who works as a nurse reports difficulty squeezing the bulb of the sphygmomanometer when taking blood pressures and difficulty opening pill bottles. Which of the following instruments would be MOST appropriate for assessing this individual?**

A. Goniometer

B. Aesthesiometer

C. Volumeter

D. Dynamometer

14. **A computer programmer arrives at an OT clinic complaining of pain while on the job. Which of the following are MOST likely to be considered work-related injuries specifically linked to the age of technology?**

A. Systemic diseases

B. Edema and paresthesias

C. Burns and electrocution

D. Carpal tunnel and chronic cervical tension

15. **During an initial interview, parents describe their child as having severe difficulty in communicating and interacting with others. The OT practitioner also observes that the child exhibits many repetitive and ritualistic behaviors. The behaviors described are MOST likely to be associated with:**

A. attention-deficit hyperactivity disorder (ADHD)

B. childhood conduct disorder.

C. obsessive-compulsive disorder.

D. pervasive developmental disorder of childhood.

16. **In an acute mental health facility, an individual refuses to participate in OT activities, and the therapist notes the refusal in the subjective section of a documentation note. Which form of refusal would MOST likely reflect acute depression?**

A. "I had an argument with another group member and I'm too angry."

B. "I don't want to participate because I don't know how to do the activity."

C. "I'm just too tired."

D. "I'm waiting for my visitors to come."

17. **During evaluation, the OTR asks a client with rheumatoid arthritis to raise her arm. The client's range of motion is limited to 90 degrees and she can tolerate moderate resistance in this position. The OTR further observes that passive range of motion (PROM) is the same as active range of motion. The manual muscle test grade would MOST likely be documented as:**

A. normal (5).

B. good (4).

C. fair (3).

D. fair minus (3-).

18. **A child with spina bifida has a lesion at the lumbar level that causes her bladder to be flaccid. At what age should the OT practitioner consider lack of bladder control as a delay and institute a toilet training program?**

A. Never, because children with flaccid bladders typically cannot be toilet trained

B. At 3 years of age when normally developing children recognize the need to urinate

C. At 4 years of age because normally developing children tend to get toilet trained at this age

D. At 4 to 5 years of age

19. **An OT practitioner is working with a client who demonstrates motor limitations when swallowing. Which of the following represents a motor problem commonly associated with dysphagia?**

A. Coughing or choking

B. Disorientation or confusion

C. Pain while swallowing

D. Decreased smell and taste

20. **An individual with the goal of increasing attention span is frequently observed watching the person next to her instead of performing her assigned task. This behavior MOST likely indicates:**

A. memory deficits.

B. spatial operations.

C. generalization of learning.

D. distractibility.

21. **An OTR performing a motor skills evaluation observes that a child is awkward** at many gross motor tasks, particularly those which require relating the body to objects in space. Though able to skip rope in the regular forward pattern of movement, the child is unable to skip rope backwards, even after several attempts. This information would lead the therapist to be particularly observant for additional signs of:

A. delayed reflex integration.

B. inadequate bilateral integration.

C. developmental dyspraxia.

D. general incoordination.

22. **In administering an assessment of fingertip pinch strength, the OT practitioner would instruct the individual being tested to place the fingers in which position?**

A. Thumb against the tip of the index finger

B. Thumb against the side of the index finger

C. Thumb against the tips of the index and middle fingers

D. Thumb against the tips of all the fingers

23. **After assessing a client who had recently lost his spouse in a house fire, the psychiatrist classifies the client as having an anxiety disorder caused by the occurrence of a major life event. Which of the following BEST represents this disorder?**

A. Cyclothymic disorder

B. Dysthymia

C. Schizophrenia

D. Post-traumatic stress disorder

24. **The OT practitioner working with an infant observes the presence of the first stage of voluntary grasp. Which of the following would be the MOST appropriate statement for documenting this behavior?**

A. "The infant is exhibiting radial palmar grasp."

B. "The infant is exhibiting pincer grasp."

C. "The infant is exhibiting ulnar palmar grasp."

D. "The infant is exhibiting palmar grasp."

25. **An OT practitioner has planned to assess group interpersonal skills in an activity-based group of seven individuals. Shortly before the group is to begin, the therapist is asked to add two newly admitted clients to the group. Which of the following actions would yield the MOST efficient and effective result?**

A. Ask one or two of the original seven members to wait until later and include the two new clients in the group.

B. Add the two new clients and then divide the members into two groups.

C. Interview the two new clients separately and continue with the original evaluation group of seven.

D. Proceed with the group as planned, adding both new clients to the original seven.

26. **An OT practitioner is treating a client who demonstrates pain, progressive weakness of the thumb, atrophy of the thenar muscles and numbness and tingling in the thumb, index, long, and half of the ring fingers. The client is not experiencing proximal upper extremity limitations so the practitioner will MOST likely suspect problems with which of the following?**

A. Ulnar nerve

B. Median nerve

C. Radial nerve

D. Brachial plexus

27. **An OT practitioner is working on morning activities of daily living with a young adult who recently sustained a traumatic brain injury. The client requires prompting to apply shaving cream to his face and to pick up his razor. After these cues, the client is then able to complete the activity. This is MOST likely to be documented as a deficit in which of the following performance components?**

A. Impulsivity

B. Initiation

C. Memory

D. Attention

28. **Using the Model of Human Occupation as a frame of reference, evaluation of an individual should focus PRIMARILY on which of the following?**

A. Identification of problem behaviors that need to be extinguished

B. Clarification of thoughts, feelings, and experiences that influence behavior

C. Cognitive function, including assets and limitations

D. The effect of personal traits and the environment on role performance

29. **In screening a child who has been referred to occupational therapy, the PRI-**

MARY goal of the occupational therapist is to:

A. obtain necessary information for an occupational therapy consultation with teachers or parents.

B. test a wide variety of developmental behaviors.

C. establish an information base for the occupational therapy treatment plan.

D. determine the need for further evaluation.

30. **A method that an OT practitioner can use to document total finger flexion without recording the measurement in degrees would be to:**

A. measure the passive flexion at each joint and total the numbers.

B. measure the distance from the fingertip to the distal palmar crease with the hand in a fist.

C. measure the active flexion at each joint and total the measurements.

D. measure the distance between the tip of the thumb and the tip of the fourth finger.

31. **The BEST way for the OT practitioner to evaluate the presence of unilateral neglect is by using which of the following paper-and-pencil tests:**

A. six-block assembly.

B. line bisection.

C. proverb interpretation.

D. identification of the square in four overlapping figures.

32. **An individual with schizophrenia who is newly admitted to the hospital is asked by the therapist to tell about what brought the person to the hospital for admission. The individual responds by saying, "I took a cab." In the report, the therapist is MOST likely to identify this response is an example of:**

A. delusional thinking.

B. a distractible response.

C. a concrete response.

D. an insightful response.

33. **A child is observed grabbing toys from others, becoming easily frustrated, and is unable to sit still. This behavior MOST likely indicates:**

A. ADHD.

B. mood disorder; manic episode.

C. conduct disorder.

D. anxiety disorder.

34. **When measuring elbow range of motion with a goniometer, the OTR must position the axis of the goniometer:**
   A. at the lateral epicondyle of the humerus.
   B. at the medial epicondyle of the humerus.
   C. parallel to the longitudinal axis of the humerus on the lateral aspect.
   D. parallel to the longitudinal axis of the radius on the lateral aspect.

35. **A woman experienced repeated sexual abuse by her father as a child and now describes her father's abusive actions as being caused by his stress of being fired from a job because of new management. The defense mechanism she is MOST likely to be using is:**
   A. identification.
   B. projection.
   C. denial.
   D. rationalization.

36. **An OTR observes an individual having difficulty trying to find white socks on a bed with white sheets. The MOST appropriate performance component for the OT to address is:**
   A. figure-ground discrimination.
   B. unilateral neglect.
   C. position in space.
   D. cognitive mapping.

37. **An individual who had a myocardial infarction (MI) was transferred from the acute care unit to a rehabilitation unit. During the initial interview, he displays good memory of information processed before the MI but poor recall of the period spent in the acute care facility. He is able to recall information since the transfer. The OT practitioner would be MOST likely to document these behaviors as:**
   A. orientation problems.
   B. long-term memory deficits.
   C. anterograde amnesia.
   D. retrograde amnesia.

38. **An OTR requests that the COTA conduct a structured interview. During this type of interview, it is MOST important for the COTA to:**
   A. rephrase the interview questions in his or her own words.
   B. ask questions that he or she thinks are pertinent to this patient.
   C. ask the questions as they are stated on the interview sheet.
   D. ask additional questions (other than those listed) to gain further insight into the patient.

39. **The OT practitioner plans to use a checklist she has designed for evaluating a child's eating performance skills. Which term BEST describes the type of evaluation the OT practitioner will be using?**
   A. Norm referenced
   B. Criterion referenced
   C. Skilled observation
   D. Valid and reliable

40. **In the assessment of individuals in whom the early and middle stages of dementia are diagnosed, the functional ability that will MOST likely remain intact for the longest duration is:**
   A. the ability to read written information.
   B. the ability to write basic information.
   C. the ability to engage in superficial social conversation.
   D. the ability to dress and undress oneself.

41. **An OT practitioner is performing sensation testing on an individual with hemiplegia. The therapist should FIRST:**
   A. apply the stimuli distally to proximally.
   B. test the involved area then the uninvolved area.
   C. present test stimuli in an organized pattern to improve reliability during retesting.
   D. apply the stimuli to the uninvolved area proximally to distally in a random pattern.

42. **An OT practitioner observes a 5-year-old child with Down syndrome who has low muscle tone sitting on the floor exclusively using a "W" sitting position. This observation MOST likely indicates that the child is:**
   A. developing abnormally.
   B. using a noncompensatory position to achieve stability.
   C. demonstrating typical development for a child with Down syndrome.
   D. using a position normal for a younger child, not for a 5-year-old child.

43. **An individual who wears a hip brace is being measured for a wheelchair. The correct seat dimension for the OT practitioner to recommend would be:**
   A. 2 inches wider than the widest point across

the individual's hips while he or she wears the brace.

B. 2 inches wider than the widest point across the individual's hips.

C. 2 inches more than the distance from the back of the bent knee to the buttocks.

D. the same as the distance from the back of the bent knee to the buttocks.

44. **During morning self-care activities, a client is able to place his dentures in his mouth but has difficulty applying denture cream to the appropriate place on the dentures and attempts to place the cap on the tube backwards, then on the wrong end of the tube. This behavior would MOST accurately be reported as:**

A. constructional apraxia.

B. ideomotor apraxia.

C. visual agnosia.

D. unilateral neglect.

Treatment Planning

45. **A college student has been referred to a day treatment program following hospitalization for an acute schizophrenic episode. The individual is uncomfortable in social settings, has difficulty sustaining conversations, is unable to make eye contact, and responds with bizarre comments when spoken to. Which of the following would be the MOST effective treatment approach?**

A. Vestibular stimulation and gross-motor exercises

B. Modification of the environment

C. Pleasurable activities that don't require conscious attention to movement

D. Social skills training

46. **A flight attendant with a back injury is participating in a work hardening program. The client can successfully simulate distributing magazines to all passengers in a plane using proper body mechanics. To upgrade the program gradually, the OT practitioner should NEXT request that the client simulate:**

A. putting blankets in the overhead compartments.

B. distributing meals to the passengers.

C. distributing magazines to half of the passengers in the plane.

D. putting luggage in the overhead compartments.

47. **Which of the following interventions is MOST appropriate for an individual who has recently been diagnosed with rheumatoid arthritis and is in the acute stage of the disease:**

A. strengthening with resistive exercises.

B. positioning, adaptive equipment, and patient education.

C. discharge planning.

D. preparing the patient for surgical intervention.

48. **The occupational therapist is a member of the interdisciplinary team providing transition services for a 17-year-old male with moderate learning disabilities. The goal is to help the student engage in part-time work at a local stationery store. Which of the following interventions is MOST appropriate?**

A. Have student practice work tasks in the classroom with peers.

B. Observe performance at the job site and make recommendations to increase productivity.

C. Teach math and money management skills to help the student handle his pay check.

D. Teach the student interviewing skills to increase the likelihood of eventually obtaining full-time employment.

49. **A young child has just learned to sit independently on the floor. Which of the following is the NEXT step toward refining her postural reactions in sitting?**

A. Sit straddling a bolster with both feet on the floor

B. Maintain sitting balance on a scooter while being pulled

C. Ride a hippity-hop without falling off

D. Maintain floor-sitting position with the therapist providing pelvic support

50. **The treatment goal that BEST addresses the psychosocial skill of self-expression is:**

A. the client will identify and pursue activities that are pleasurable to the self.

B. the client will use facial expressions and gestures that are consistent with stated emotions during assertive, passive, and aggressive role-play situations.

C. the client will recognize his or her own behavior and possible negative and positive consequences.

D. the client will identify his or her own assets

and limitations after an art or movement group.

51. **The treatment goal for a 4-year-old child with hypotonia is to improve grasp. Which of the following activities would be BEST for preparing the child's hand for grasp activities?**
    A. Dropping blocks into a pail
    B. Placing pegs on a pegboard
    C. Weight-bearing on hands
    D. Holding and eating a cookie

52. **"The patient has taken a more active role in the task group, as evidenced by the patient's willingness to contribute ideas and offer to assist in designing the unit mural." This statement would MOST appropriately be documented in which portion of a SOAP note?**
    A. Subjective
    B. Objective
    C. Assessment
    D. Plan

53. **A client is working on prehension skills in order to return to work as a mechanic. Which of the following BEST resembles a prehension activity?**
    A. Loosening nuts and bolts
    B. Removing an air filter
    C. Cranking a car jack
    D. Grasping a hammer

54. **An OTR is about to begin working with a 2-year-old child with hypotonia and extremely poor head control who is unable to maintain a sitting position. The FIRST pre-sitting activity the OTR should introduce, while providing stability as needed, is:**
    A. forward and backward movement on a ball with the child in a prone position.
    B. forward and side-to-side movement with the child sitting on the therapist's lap.
    C. forward and side-to side movement on a tilting board with the child in a quadruped position.
    D. placing the child supine on a mat and pulling him or her into a sitting position.

55. **A sales executive is participating in a time management program. Which of the following would be the expected outcome for the client?**
    A. To control anxiety when arriving late for a meeting

B. To take responsibility when late with reports
C. To cope with feelings of inadequacy when missing a deadline
D. To arrive at work on time consistently

56. **A homemaker is learning how to perform transfers into a bathtub after a total knee replacement. Despite having surgery 2 weeks ago, the client is still unable to extend or flex the knee greater than 20 degrees. Which of the following would MOST likely allow for safe tub transfers?**
    A. Wait another 2-4 weeks, because showering and bathing are contraindicated for individuals with total knee replacements for four to six weeks after surgery
    B. Use of a hand rail attached to the side of the tub
    C. Use of a tub transfer bench and leg lifter
    D. Use of a beach chair in the tub

57. **Which of the following activities should be introduced FIRST when treating a child for tactile defensiveness?**
    A. Gently brush the child's face and neck.
    B. Rub lotion on the child's arms.
    C. Have the child roll around in a carpeted barrel.
    D. Swing the child in a hammock swing.

58. **A middle-aged client with a diagnosis of reactive depression is admitted to the hospital following an overdose of sleeping pills. The client was recently forced to retire from a job in public relations and his present goals are to increase his sense of competence and encourage development of enjoyable leisure activities. Based on the client's OT goals, what is an appropriate FIRST activity to recommend for this patient?**
    A. Pouring and glazing chess pieces.
    B. Designing and building a doll house.
    C. Copper tooling using a template.
    D. Learning how to play bridge.

59. **The therapist is performing UE activities for an individual with left hemiparesis following a CVA. She observes that active range of motion is limited throughout the LUE. In analyzing this client's performance, the therapist is MOST likely to consider the impact of which factors on range of motion:**

A. muscle tone, edema, sensation, and diadokinesis.

B. edema, proprioception, and muscle tone.

C. edema, contracture, muscle tone, and pain.

D. contracture, stereognosis, and sensation.

60. **Development of a treatment plan for a child with an underreactive vestibular system would MOST likely include specific activities to address:**

A. poor postural responses.

B. discomfort with motion activities.

C. anxiety when his or her feet are off the ground.

D. gravitational insecurity.

61. **An individual learning to use an augmentative communication system has mastered the task of understanding picture symbols and their use. The next step would be:**

A. sequencing of picture symbols.

B. recognizing letters of the alphabet.

C. recognizing whole words.

D. spelling letter by letter.

62. **Which of the following activities would BEST represent an expected outcome for an individual who completes an energy-conservation program?**

A. Getting dressed without becoming fatigued

B. Lifting heavy cookware without pain

C. Doing handicrafts without damaging his or her joints

D. Dusting and vacuuming more quickly

63. **An OT practitioner is working with a withdrawn child whose occupational therapy objectives include increasing the ability to express feelings and conflicts. Which of the following activities will MOST effectively promote this skill?**

A. Drawing a picture titled "This is me"

B. Playing adapted soccer with a large ball

C. Playing a structured board game, such as Monopoly

D. Singing folk songs in a group

64. **A therapist is planning a simple meal preparation activity that will result in success for a patient with cognitive deficits. The SIMPLEST activity would be preparing:**

A. a can of soup.

B. a casserole.

C. brownies from a box mix.

D. a meal with two side dishes and an entrée.

65. **An individual with a C6 spinal cord injury has been referred to OT two days post-injury. Immobilized with a Halo brace, the individual demonstrates fair plus wrist extension and poor minus finger flexion. Which of the following interventions should be implemented FIRST?**

A. Volar resting pan splints to prevent flexion contractures

B. Wrist support with universal cuff to promote independence

C. Wrist splints to promote development of tenodesis

D. Instruction in bed mobility techniques to prevent decubiti

66. **A preschooler has poor visual tracking skills, which affect her performance on tasks requiring eye–hand coordination. Which of the following activities is most appropriate for the OT practitioner to recommend to the child's parents in order to promote beginning visual tracking skills during summer vacation?**

A. Tossing and catching a water balloon

B. Catching and bursting soap bubbles

C. Throwing and catching a beach ball

D. Playing softball

67. **An OT practitioner is working with three individuals in a cooking group. The individuals demonstrate difficulty attending to task, frequently ask to leave the room, and do not interact with each other. Based on the developmental group concept, which of the following is the MOST appropriate goal for this group?**

A. Each member will take a leadership role within the session.

B. Members will share materials with at least one other group member.

C. Each member will express two positive feelings about themselves within the group session.

D. Each member will remain in the group without disrupting the work of others for 15 minutes.

68. **A person with peripheral neuropathy exhibits loss of pinprick, light touch, pressure, and temperature sensation resulting in an absence of protective sensation. The most appropriate form of intervention to address this type of sensory loss would be a program of:**

A. sensory reeducation.

B. sensory desensitization.

C. sensory bombardment.

D. sensory compensation.

69. **An infant born 15 weeks prematurely has a history of multiple medical issues including retinopathy of prematurity, mechanical ventilation for 5 weeks, and poor feeding skills. The infant is now a 43-week-old, medically stable and engaging infant, with a G-tube and oxygen supplement of 2 liters by nasal cannula. Which of the following is the MOST appropriate intervention to pursue at this time?**

A. Positioning and handling

B. PROM of all extremities

C. Multisensory input

D. Music therapy

70. **During an evaluation, you learn that a young child is easily aroused because of a sensory-processing disorder. Which environmental adaptation would be MOST effective in assisting this individual to fall asleep?**

A. A mini-trampoline in the bedroom to tire the child out before going to bed

B. A noise machine producing white noise at bedtime

C. A lightweight, fuzzy blanket providing light touch

D. Shutters on the windows to produce total darkness

71. **A deficit in visual memory is affecting a child's reading skills. Which would be the BEST game to promote visual memory?**

A. Dominoes

B. Concentration

C. Pickup sticks

D. Checkers

72. **An individual with weak grip strength and poor endurance wishes to bake something for a family member's birthday. The OTR wants to plan an activity during which the client can work on grasp/release for 5 minutes without becoming exhausted. The MOST appropriate activity for both purposes would be:**

A. mixing blueberry muffins from scratch using a hand-powered mixer and scooping them into muffin tins with a cup.

B. mixing an angel food cake from a box mix using an electric mixer and pouring the mix into a pan.

C. mixing cold chocolate chip cookie dough using a spatula with a built-up handle and dropping dollops onto a tray using an ice cream scoop.

D. slicing a prepared roll of sugar cookies at room temperature and placing them on a tray using a spatula.

Treatment Implementation

73. **In a home program to promote beginning symbolic play for a child with developmental delay, the OT practitioner would MOST likely recommend playing with:**

A. busy box, nesting toys, and blocks.

B. board games.

C. craft kits.

D. doll house and dress-up clothes.

74. **The home health OT practitioner is seeing a client in the middle stages of Alzheimer's disease. The family is very concerned that the client's memory loss is now interfering with performance of daily activities, even familiar self-care activities. The MOST relevant OT intervention at this point would be:**

A. memory retraining activities for the client.

B. ADL retraining program for the client.

C. instructing caregivers in task breakdown.

D. leisure activity planning.

75. **An OT practitioner is transferring a client with hemiplegia from a wheelchair to an elevated mat. The client is able to place both feet on the floor and move the buttocks to the edge of the wheelchair. The therapist then places one hand on the client's right anterior pelvis and the other hand on the client's left shoulder. The client is set up so the transfer can be performed toward the client's stronger side. The client then pushes to a standing position and pivots with the therapist's guidance. This is MOST likely an example of a(n):**

A. independent transfer from wheelchair to mat.

B. assisted stand pivot transfer.

C. pneumatic lift transfer.

D. dependent stand pivot transfer.

76. **An OT is applying PNF techniques for weight shifting during an activity that re-**

quires an individual to use the right hand to remove groceries from a bag on the floor to the right. The **MOST** benefit would be gained from this activity by then placing the groceries:

A. on the counter directly in front.

B. on the counter to the left side.

C. in the upper cabinet to the right side.

D. in the upper cabinet to the left side.

77. **The OT practitioner is treating a patient with a standard above-elbow amputation who is experiencing hypersensitivity of the residual limb. The OT would most likely perform which of the following interventions in the preprosthetic phase of treatment?**

A. Activities to strengthen the residual limb

B. Activities to increase the range of motion of the residual limb

C. Activities which provide tapping, application of textures, and weight bearing to the residual limb

D. Activities for practicing putting on and taking off the UE prosthesis

78. **A physician has informed an OTR that her client's headache problem at work is primarily caused by the increased neck and shoulder tension that the individual experiences while typing on a computer. The BEST stress management approach for the OTR to suggest in this situation is:**

A. assertiveness training focusing on increasing the individual's assertiveness with his or her boss.

B. progressive relaxation exercises and autogenic training.

C. training in cognitive reappraisal to decrease the frequency of the individual's tendency to generalize and exaggerate the negative side of work events.

D. teaching the individual more effective problem-solving strategies.

79. **During an infant's first OT session, the mother reports she has observed that the baby has difficulty with swallowing and frequently chokes. Which of the following feeding positions will MOST effectively reduce the risk of aspiration and facilitate swallowing?**

A. Head in neutral position

B. Head slightly flexed

C. Head slightly extended

D. Head rotated toward the feeder

80. **An individual with strong dependency needs is able to lace a leather wallet only with consistent verbal cueing. Which is the BEST way to grade this activity in order to decrease dependency?**

A. Provide written instructions on lacing techniques and ask the individual to continue on her own.

B. Ask the individual to try some lacing with distant supervision and praise her for what she has been able to do.

C. Ask the individual to take the lacing to her room and continue without the OT's assistance.

D. Tell the individual to complete a small amount of lacing while the OT assists another patient in the same room.

81. **An OTR is addressing concerns about sexual activity with a person who has left-sided hemiplegia with spasticity. The BEST recommendation for positioning during sexual intercourse for this person would be:**

A. lying on the left side while propped with pillows.

B. lying on the right side while propped with pillows.

C. lying in a supine position.

D. lying in a prone position.

82. **A woman with a head injury is impulsive during self-feeding and frequently attempts to place too much food in her mouth at one time. Which of the following methods would MOST effectively control her rate of intake during self-feeding?**

A. Cut her food into smaller pieces.

B. Have her count to 10 between bites of food.

C. Have her put the utensil down until she swallows.

D. Serve the various food items in separate containers on the meal tray.

83. **An OT practitioner is teaching a client who recently sustained an above-elbow amputation how to dress with one hand. Teaching a client to perform a familiar activity or skill is called the:**

A. problem-solving method.

B. retraining method.

C. altered task method.

D. compensation method.

84. **An OT practitioner is positioning a child with poor muscle tone and postural instability into a prone stander to develop head righting. The child rapidly shows fatigue and associated reactions. How can the therapist BEST adjust the stander to decrease these reactions while continuing to address the goal of head righting?**
   A. Place the child in prone on the floor.
   B. Position the stander at 45 degrees from the floor.
   C. Position the stander at 75 to 90 degrees from the floor.
   D. Position the child upright in a prone or supine stander.

85. **A new client exhibits no awareness of functional limitations resulting from his recent head injury, and he attempts to perform transfers without assistance. He also has expressed that he doesn't see the need for therapy. The BEST approach to promote awareness and insight is to:**
   A. have the patient explain why he believes he is not impaired.
   B. provide the client with a checklist of skills he must have to perform various activities and review these.
   C. have the client predict his performance before an activity, then have him self-evaluate the performance.
   D. disregard the client's perceptions and proceed with therapy.

86. **An individual with left upper extremity flaccidity is observed sitting in a wheelchair with his left arm dangling over the side. The FIRST positioning device that should be assessed for this individual is a(n):**
   A. lap tray.
   B. wheelchair armrest.
   C. arm sling.
   D. arm trough.

87. **An OT practitioner is working with a student on handwriting skills when she instructs the client to stabilize his forearm on the table when writing. The client is MOST likely to be demonstrating:**
   A. decreased vision.
   B. poor endurance.
   C. limited fine movement.
   D. incoordination.

88. **An OT practitioner is planning a group session in which the group members will be encouraged to participate in a game of chance. Which of the following would MOST likely be considered a game of chance?**
   A. Collecting baseball cards
   B. Bingo
   C. Charades
   D. Balloon volleyball

89. **Of the following, which would be the MOST effective strategy for increasing attention to the left for a person who has a diagnosis of unilateral neglect?**
   A. Encouraging participation in bilateral activities
   B. Encouraging any available hemiplegic limb movements before or during a task
   C. Participation in tasks that do not cross the midline
   D. Participation in tasks placed on the uninvolved side

90. **A school-age child has Duchenne muscular dystrophy. Although he is able to use a manual chair for distances between classes, he is tired on arrival. What would be the BEST recommendation the OTR could make for wheelchair use at school?**
   A. Retain the manual chair to build up strength.
   B. Change to an ultralight sports model because it requires less strength.
   C. Change to a power wheelchair to reduce effort.
   D. Encourage walking with a walker to alternate mobility methods.

91. **An individual with hand weakness has difficulty holding a fork. Using a biomechanical frame of reference, which of the following interventions would be MOST appropriate?**
   A. Elicit functional grasp using reflex inhibiting postures.
   B. Stimulate the hand flexors to promote a functional grasp.
   C. Repeatedly squeeze with the hand against increasing amounts of resistance.
   D. Build up utensil handles.

92. **A client with neurological deficits resulting from a head injury was performing the task of reaching for her brush on the shelf of her bathroom cabinet. During**

this task the OT practitioner observed that the client located the brush but became very distracted by the other items on the shelf. As a result of this observation, the OT is MOST likely to provide activities that will improve:

A. learning.
B. selective attention.
C. figure-ground perception.
D. problem solving.

93. **When working with a child who is at risk for shunt malfunction, it is MOST important for the therapist to observe for:**

A. increased tone.
B. headaches.
C. back pain.
D. unexplained sensory loss.

94. **An OT practitioner is planning a community living program for clients who are to be discharged after an average of 25 to 30 years of hospitalization. One of the goals of this program is to train the clients to effectively manage their money. Which of the following activities should be used FIRST?**

A. Provide each client with $25 to spend during a group trip to the local shopping center.
B. Provide samples of coins and paper money.
C. Use a board game to introduce the concept of receiving and spending money.
D. Establish a hospital-based community store where the clients can buy clothing.

95. **An OT practitioner is planning to demonstrate and then involve a group of individuals in practicing "broken record" behaviors. Which of the following interventions BEST encompasses the broken record technique?**

A. Music therapy activities
B. Self-awareness activities
C. Assertiveness training
D. Psychodrama approaches

96. **When instructing the parents of a toddler in the use and care of a hand splint, the OT practitioner should put MOST emphasis on:**

A. checking for irritation and pressure problems.
B. avoiding excessive heat exposure.
C. cleansing the splint regularly.
D. adhering strictly to the wearing schedule.

97. **When leading groups, OT practitioners should demonstrate consistency from day to day. Inconsistent behavior would MOST likely result in:**

A. overdependence of group members.
B. group members' knowing what to expect from the group leader.
C. anxiety and confusion among group members.
D. group members' receiving too much praise.

98. **An individual with a C6 spinal cord injury is unable to button his shirt. The OT would be MOST likely to select which type of adaptive equipment to assist this client with buttoning?**

A. A buttonhook with an extra-long, flexible handle
B. A buttonhook with a knob handle
C. A buttonhook on a 0.5 inch diameter, 5-inch long wooden handle
D. A buttonhook attached to a cuff that fits around the palm

99. **A child with a behavior disorder has an innately difficult temperament. Which of the following treatment approaches is MOST appropriate?**

A. Emphasize limit setting with the child during activities.
B. Help the child develop cognitive strategies for anxiety-producing activities.
C. Help care providers develop an unpredictable routine for activities that disorganize the child.
D. Provide a play environment in which the parent and child can demonstrate conflicts.

100. **Which of the following is the BEST method to use for encouraging problem solving during a craft media group?**

A. Begin with activities that have obvious solutions and a high probability of success and then gradually increase the level of complexity.
B. Begin with activities that require gross motor responses and then gradually progress to fine motor responses.
C. Select activities that require interaction with others and then provide opportunities to discuss and analyze how the group went.
D. Gradually increase the time used in the activity by 15-minute increments.

101. **An OT practitioner is planning a self-feeding session with an individual with a**

C5 spinal cord injury. Which piece of feeding equipment would be MOST appropriate for the OT practitioner to introduce to the client?

A. A wrist-driven flexor hinge splint
B. A mobile arm support
C. An electric self-feeder
D. Built-up utensils

102. An individual with emphysema reports recently "having an accident" when unable to "make it to the bathroom in time." When the home health OT practitioner recommends a bedside commode, the idea is immediately rejected. Which of the following actions should the OT practitioner take FIRST?

A. Identify options and the consequences of each option.
B. Document the individual's reasons for rejecting the bedside commode.
C. Practice with a "demo" bedside commode.
D. Allow time for the individual to think about the bedside commode.

103. When planning intervention for individuals in the acute phase of cardiac rehabilitation, it is MOST important for the OT practitioner to select activities that:

A. can be accomplished without causing fatigue.
B. decrease the effects of prolonged inactivity.
C. promote strength, range of motion and endurance.
D. can be carried out independently after discharge.

104. A young child has a diagnosis of spastic quadriplegia. The OT practitioner is teaching the child's parents how to effectively position the child in sitting so that participation in family games will be facilitated. What is the MOST important point the practitioner can make?

A. Make sure the child's head is upright.
B. Make sure the child's arms are on the armrests.
C. Make sure the child's back is straight.
D. Make sure the child's hips are secured against the back of the seat.

105. An OTR is working on sitting balance with an individual with C6 quadriplegia. The BEST position for the individual's hands to be in when using them for support is to have the fingers:

A. extended and adducted.

B. flexed at all joints.
C. extended and abducted.
D. adducted and flexed only at the metacarpal-phalangeal joints.

106. An OT practitioner, along with the assistive technology team, has made specific recommendations for electronic assistive technology for an adult with muscular dystrophy. After the devices are ordered, and modified as necessary, the NEXT step in the process of implementation is for the OT to:

A. evaluate how well the whole system works.
B. evaluate if the assistive technology devices match the needs of the client.
C. train the client in the operation of the assistive technology system and in strategies for its use.
D. determine if funding is available for the assistive technology recommended.

107. Which of the following is MOST important when using a remotivation approach with a group of elderly individuals?

A. Use pictures, music, and discussion to encourage discussion of memories.
B. Discuss an upcoming holiday and base an activity on that holiday.
C. Adapt the environment to maximize independent functioning.
D. Focus on group activities designed to enhance interpersonal skills.

108. A child with a diagnosis of ADHD also exhibits perceptual deficits. The activity that would be the MOST effective intervention for this child to train visual attention is:

A. playing a game of "Memory" in which images are matched by memory.
B. assembling a 200-piece puzzle.
C. finding "Waldo" against a complex visual background.
D. blowing cotton balls into a target.

109. An attractive unmarried patient with a spinal cord injury (SCI) is on a rehab unit and constantly flirts with the OT and PT staff. The staff should react by:

A. firmly rejecting his advances.
B. flirting back in order to promote his self-esteem.
C. selecting one team member to discuss the effects of SCI on sexual functioning with the patient.

D. setting personal boundaries appropriate to the therapist–patient relationship.

110. While running a nutrition awareness group, an **OT** practitioner observes that one member tends to monopolize the discussion by frequently interrupting. Which intervention would be **BEST** to implement after other, more conservative approaches have been unsuccessful?

A. Sit beside the person who is monopolizing and touch his or her hand or arm as a reminder not to interrupt others who are talking.

B. Confront the individual's behavior: "Are you aware that your frequent interruptions prevent others from having a chance to contribute?"

C. Redirect the individual: "Now let's hear what others have to say about this."

D. Restructure the task: Select a group activity that requires sequential turn taking.

111. In the middle of a wheelchair-to-bed transfer, an obese patient begins to slip from the grasp of an average-size **OT** practitioner. The **BEST** action for the **OT** practitioner to take is to:

A. ease the patient onto the floor, cushioning his fall.

B. reverse the transfer, getting the patient back in the wheelchair.

C. continue the transfer, getting the patient to the bed.

D. call next door for assistance.

112. A physical education teacher is being treated for osteoarthritis of the upper and lower extremities. Which of the following neuromuscular activities would the therapist **MOST LIKELY** suggest to prevent further complications?

A. Lifting weights three times a week for 1 hour

B. Listening to relaxation tapes three times a week before bedtime

C. Vocational retraining

D. Low-impact aerobics three times a week for 1 hour

113. Upon arrival to an infant's therapy session in the neonatal intensive care unit **(NICU)**, the **OT** finds the infant's parents present. Of the following, which is the **OPTIMAL** intervention to pursue?

A. Review the chart to complete birth history

information and speak to the infant's primary nurse.

B. Introduce yourself as their child's OT, explain your role in their child's developmental care and excuse yourself from the situation secondary to limited availability for intervention.

C. Issue written positioning and state regulation and readiness information for the parents to review.

D. Perform behavioral techniques and developmental positioning with parental observation and interaction.

114. A client is being seen by OT to promote independence in meal preparation and cleanup activities. The method of structuring activity practice that would **BEST** promote retention of learning and transfer of skills is to:

A. practice preparing a variety of foods, using different cooking methods and recipes.

B. practice cooking one meal from beginning to end in the same kitchen setting several times.

C. practice making a sandwich until that is mastered, then practice preparing another part of a meal until the person has mastered that skill, etc.

D. practice performing each step of the food preparation process, such as cutting vegetables.

115. A OT practitioner is working with a medically stable client who sustained bilateral upper extremity partial thickness burns 3 days ago while frying chicken. Which of the following **BEST** represents a typical ADL intervention?

A. Instruct the client to use all adapted equipment.

B. Encourage independent compression garment application.

C. Perform bilateral upper extremity PROM exercises twice a day.

D. Encourage independent self-feeding and dressing skills with minimal use of adapted utensils and tools.

116. A student has been working on learning to activate a switch for a communications device needed in the fourth grade classroom. The switch is mounted on the wheelchair tray, but the student is having difficulty operating it because of excessive muscle tone. Despite practicing for extended periods of time, the stu-

dent is not making any progress. The OTR decides to:

A. work on coordinated reach in sidelying position first and then transfer the skill to sitting position.

B. passively stretch the student's upper extremity to increase range of motion.

C. use a brightly colored switch to increase visibility.

D. use systematic behavioral reinforcement through shaping.

117. A patient diagnosed with Parkinson's disease is being seen by an OT practitioner to develop a routine for performing self-care activities. The therapist is MOST likely to begin this process by instructing the patient that self-care activities:

A. are more easily performed if coordinated with consistent timing of medications.

B. should be performed before medications are taken.

C. should be attempted only with the assistance of others.

D. should be performed at intervals throughout the day until completed.

118. The BEST method for handling a child who exhibits tactile defensiveness is to:

A. tickle him during play times.

B. play loud music when undressing him.

C. lightly stroke his arms and legs during baths.

D. hold him firmly when picking him up.

119. An individual with fine motor incoordination reports difficulty with self-care. Which of the following options would this individual find MOST beneficial?

A. Wash mitt

B. Spray deodorant

C. Toothpaste with a flip-open cap

D. Toothbrush with a built-up handle

120. The spouse of a patient with a progressive disease has come into the OT department to learn how to help the spouse perform functional activities at home. The FIRST focus of caregiver education for this person should be:

A. methods for motivating the patient to perform ADLs.

B. how to analyze activities to solve problems.

C. instruction in how to provide cues to the patient.

D. instruction in how to perform the activities safely.

121. An individual complains of perspiration which is causing his resting hand splint to be uncomfortable. The BEST action for the OT practitioner to take is to:

A. recommend putting talcum powder in the splint.

B. line the splint with moleskin.

C. fabricate a new resting hand splint with perforated material.

D. provide a stockinet for the individual to wear inside the splint.

122. A child with a diagnosis of mental retardation is currently learning to independently tie her shoes. To facilitate generalization of this skill, the OT practitioner should:

A. fit the child's shoes with Velcro closures.

B. have the child practice tying her shoes at home as well as in school.

C. use a backwards-chaining technique.

D. provide brightly colored shoelaces.

123. An OT practitioner is training an adult worker with a developmental disability to put a pencil in a box before putting the score pad in the box for a game packaging task in a sheltered workshop assembly line. The employee has not done this task before. The type of reinforcement schedule that will BEST achieve the goal of learning this task sequence is:

A. intermittent reinforcement with correct responses.

B. reinforcement every 10 minutes.

C. reinforcement for every fourth correct response.

D. continuous reinforcement of correct responses.

124. An OT practitioner receives a referral to fabricate a splint that will assist with the maintenance of a functional hand position while keeping the soft tissues of the hand in a midrange position. Which splint would the OTR MOST likely select to address these needs?

A. A bivalve cast

B. A resting pan splint

C. A dynamic extension splint

D. A wrist cock-up splint

125. An individual with Guillain-Barré syndrome was recently admitted to a reha-

bilitation unit and is expected to remain for 3 to 4 weeks. When should the OT practitioner order adaptive equipment for this individual?

A. After the patient and family have accepted the individual's disability

B. As soon as the insurance provider approves it

C. Within the first week of therapy

D. Just before discharge

126. An OT practitioner is working with a client who has severe cognitive deficits. Using a functional skill training approach, the MOST appropriate method to teach the client to brush his or her teeth is based on:

A. rote repetition of the task substeps with gradually fading cues.

B. practice of fine-motor activities that incorporate motions needed in tooth brushing.

C. teaching the caregiver how to set up the task and guide the client's performance.

D. use of instructional cards, which the client will learn to use to remind him of how to perform the task.

127. Prevention of cumulative trauma disorders (CTD) in the workplace is the primary focus of an OT practitioner who is working as an industry consultant. The MOST appropriate way to reduce risk of CTD in an industry where there is heavy keyboard use is to:

A. teach employees to identify the symptoms of cumulative trauma disorder early.

B. educate employees about ergonomic adaptations including correct typing techniques, posture, hand positioning, and equipment modification.

C. provide inexpensive resting splints to employees to rest hands and wrists at night if symptoms appear.

D. instruct employees in exercise routines to increase strength in weak upper extremities.

128. While participating in activities to improve strength, an individual with multiple sclerosis (MS) who was recently admitted to the hospital complains of fatigue. Which of the following actions is the most appropriate for the OT practitioner to take?

A. Instruct the individual to work through the fatigue to complete the session.

B. Instruct the individual to work through the fatigue for another 5 to 10 minutes.

C. Discontinue strengthening activities.

D. Give the individual a rest break.

129. An OT practitioner is showing a parent how to bathe a child with hypertonic muscle tone. Which of the following approaches is MOST appropriate to use?

A. Avoid the use of adaptive equipment.

B. Avoid explanations of the procedure.

C. Handle the child slowly and gently.

D. Stand and lean over the tub to support and wash the child.

130. An individual with amyotrophic lateral sclerosis (ALS) has asked an OT practitioner how to maintain strength in weak (fair plus) wrist extensors. Which is the MOST appropriate intervention for the OT practitioner to recommend?

A. A cock-up wrist support

B. Playing Velcro checkers to tolerance

C. Active range of motion for wrist daily without resistance

D. Wrist extension exercises several times a day against maximal resistance

131. An individual with low endurance complains of becoming too fatigued during sexual activity to enjoy it. The BEST strategy for the therapist to recommend is for the individual to:

A. time sex for the end of the day.

B. take the top, prone position.

C. take the bottom, supine position.

D. experiment with a variety of positions.

132. An OT practitioner working in a sheltered workshop with adult clients with developmental disabilities is preparing for a group of clients functioning at Allen's Cognitive Level 4. Which of the following is the BEST method for introducing an assembly activity?

A. Provide repetitive, one-step activities.

B. Demonstrate a three-step assembly process.

C. Provide project samples for clients to duplicate.

D. Provide written directions for the individuals to follow.

133. An OT practitioner is working with a client who complains of pain while completing kitchen cleaning tasks. Which of the following positions would be MOST

effective in alleviating low back pain when the patient is loading the dishwasher?

A. Place dishes next to dishwasher and load from a standing position.
B. Wash dishes in the sink.
C. Place dishes next to dishwasher and load from the front of the dishwasher.
D. Place dishes near the dishwasher, bend down on one or both knees, and load.

134. An OT practitioner requests that an OT student treat a client with a condition involving the upper extremity. The OTR suggests the use of contrast baths, retrograde massage, and pressure wraps. The OT student can consider these interventions as **PRIMARY** techniques to address:

A. heterotopic ossification.
B. edema.
C. wound healing.
D. scar management.

135. The **PRIMARY** functions of an OTR leading a therapeutic group in the beginning stages of group development will be to:

A. set the climate, provide structure, and offer support.
B. leave members to set the climate, provide structure, and offer support to each other.
C. aid group members in separation and reinforce gains made in the group.
D. work individually with group members until each is ready to join group activity.

136. An OT practitioner is performing discharge teaching with a client who sustained a deep laceration of the median and ulnar nerves. The practitioner informs the client that the two tactile senses that are the earliest to recover after a peripheral nerve injury are:

A. vibration and pain.
B. temperature and pain.
C. light touch and proprioception.
D. tactile localization and proprioception.

137. A toddler has feeding difficulties because of deficient oral-motor control and oral defensiveness. The child's parents would like to eat family meals together and include such foods as meats (cut up), sandwiches, and vegetables. The OT practitioner explains to the parents that they can start to introduce these foods

when their child is able to tolerate which foods?

A. Apple sauce and mashed bananas
B. Dry cereals with milk
C. Strained fruits and vegetables
D. Scrambled eggs

138. A mother of four teenage children who was diagnosed with a right **CVA** is receiving home care **OT** services. The treatment plan includes "activities to improve left upper extremity function" and "activities to improve balance in sitting and standing." Which of the following activities would be most appropriate?

A. Stacking cones
B. Door pulley
C. Folding laundry
D. Throwing a ball

139. An OT practitioner is instructing a client with a total hip replacement how to perform a passenger side car transfer. Which of the following **BEST** represents the initial steps of this transfer?

A. Stand the body parallel to the car, hold onto a stable section of the car, lift and place the left leg into the car, and slowly sit and follow with opposite leg.
B. Back up the body to the passenger seat, hold onto a stable section of the car, extend the involved leg, and slowly sit in the car.
C. Back up the body to the passenger seat, hold onto a stable section of the car, flex both legs simultaneously, and slowly sit in the car.
D. Back up the body to the passenger seat, hold onto a stable section of the car, flex the involved leg, and slowly sit in the car.

140. An OT practitioner is working on hand function with a school-age child diagnosed with juvenile rheumatoid arthritis. Which of the following devices will **MOST** effectively prevent hand fatigue?

A. Reacher
B. Jar opener
C. Pencil gripper
D. Plate guard

141. An individual with quadriplegia complains of frequently slumping to the side when sitting in a wheelchair. The wheelchair adaptation that would **BEST** enable this individual to maintain an optimal position is:

A. a reclining wheelchair.

B. an arm trough.
C. lateral trunk supports.
D. lateral pelvic supports.

142. An OT practitioner is fabricating a splint for a client who sustained a low-level ulnar nerve injury. The OTR explains that the PRIMARY purpose of an ulnar nerve splint is to:

A. block hyperextension of the PIP joints and allow PIP flexion.
B. block hyperextension of the MCP joints and allow MCP flexion.
C. block PIP flexion and allow for PIP hyperextension.
D. block MCP flexion and allow for MP hyperextension.

143. A nursing home resident with Alzheimer's disease also has limitations in shoulder range of motion. The OT goal for this patient is to improve shoulder motion so that the person can resume self-care activities. Which strategy which would be MOST effective in getting the client actively engaged?

A. Telling the resident to perform repetitions of active UE range of motion exercises independently.
B. Training the resident to use long-handled adaptive devices to compensate for decreased shoulder motion.
C. Incorporating simple, familiar activities such as hanging up clothing or catching a ball.
D. Performing PROM exercises on the resident.

144. An OT practitioner is working with a confused patient who is having difficulty placing both feet into his pants legs. An example of a prefunctional treatment activity would MOST likely be:

A. pulling up pants during toileting activities.
B. teaching the individual to use a reacher to pull up his pants to knee level.
C. pulling off socks using a dressing stick.
D. having him place his feet through loops of therapeutic band.

145. An OT practitioner is instructing a patient with left hemiplegia and unilateral neglect to put on a t-shirt. The BEST sequence to teach the patient would be:

A. (1) place left hand into sleeve and pull up sleeve past elbow; (2) place right hand into

sleeve and pull up sleeve; (3) pull shirt up over head; (4) pull shirt down over trunk.
B. (1) position shirt on lap; (2) place left hand into sleeve and pull up sleeve past elbow; (3) place right hand into sleeve and pull up sleeve; (4) pull shirt up over head.
C. (1) position shirt on lap; (2) place right hand into sleeve and pull up sleeve past elbow; (3) place left hand into sleeve and pull up sleeve; (4) pull shirt up over head.
D. (1) pull shirt up over head; (2) place left arm into sleeve; (3) place right arm into sleeve; (4) pull down shirt over trunk.

146. An OT practitioner has conducted a home evaluation for a client with Parkinson's disease whose primary functional problems are caused by a shuffling gait. The MOST relevant environmental recommendation the OT could make to address a potential safety hazard is to:

A. increase illumination in hallways.
B. screen out distracting stimuli in the environment.
C. place door locks higher or lower than eye level.
D. remove scatter rugs throughout the house.

Effectiveness of Treatment and Discharge Planning

147. A child with developmental delays has just developed the strength and stability in his right hand to hold scissors properly and make snips in the paper. Which of the following would be the NEXT scissors skill to develop?

A. Cut cardboard and cloth
B. Cut along curved lines to cut out a circle
C. Cut along straight lines to cut a triangle
D. Cut the paper in two following a straight line

148. The husband of an individual who is being treated for bipolar disorder describes his frustration with the ups and downs of his wife's condition. Which of the following is the BEST support group to recommend to this husband?

A. Al-Anon
B. Family therapy
C. National Alliance for the Mentally Ill
D. Recovery, Inc.

149. An individual with lower extremity paralysis uses a standard manual wheelchair and is ready to be discharged to home.

During the home evaluation, the **OT** practitioner notes that the entrance to the bathroom is 32 inches wide and the toilet is 15 inches high. Which of the following recommendations will **MOST** facilitate use of the bathroom for this individual?

A. Widen the doorway
B. Raise the toilet
C. Widen the doorway and raise the toilet
D. Widen the doorway and lower the toilet

150. **An occupational therapist is discharging a 4-year-old child with athetoid cerebral palsy from a rehabilitation setting to home. The MOST appropriate instructions for the OTR to provide to the family for maintaining correct jaw control while feeding the child from the side are:**

A. "Jaw opening and closing are controlled with your index and middle fingers; place your thumb on the child's cheek."
B. "Jaw opening and closing are controlled with your index and middle fingers; place your thumb on the child's larynx for stability."
C. "Jaw opening and closing are controlled with your whole hand on the child's jaw."
D. "Jaw opening and closing are controlled with your index and middle fingers; place your thumb on the child's ear for stability."

151. **An OT practitioner in an acute care hospital is using the SOAP note format to document information about an individual with dementia. Which statement is the BEST example of subjective information?**

A. The therapist will establish a daily self-feeding routine using verbal and physical cues to encourage the individual to open containers on the lunch tray.
B. The individual has been able to identify closed liquid-beverage containers on the meal tray for four of six presentations.
C. The individual is able to identify and drink liquids presented in cups without lids but leaves beverages in closed containers untouched.
D. The individual asks for more beverages during meals, but appears surprised when the therapist indicates beverages in closed containers are on the meal tray.

152. **An OT practitioner is educating the parents of a high school age patient who is being discharged from the burn center**

to his home environment after an 8-month inpatient stay for severe burns. The therapist is reviewing common psychological reactions that occur in burn victims. The therapist will **MOST** likely educate the client and family about:

A. the possibility of decreased range of motion and sensation.
B. the potential for depression and low self-esteem.
C. the likelihood of violent behavior and sexual acting out.
D. the potential for delirium and fatigue.

153. **An individual being evaluated for meal preparation skills demonstrates minimal to moderate difficulty when asked to prepare a macaroni and cheese dish. Which of the following is the MOST appropriate cooking activity to use for the next OT session?**

A. Making baked chicken and mashed potatoes
B. Making a peanut butter and jelly sandwich
C. Preparing a can of soup
D. Making instant pudding

154. **An OT practitioner is determining a third-grader's readiness for discharge from direct OT as a related service. The essential criteria which the practitioner needs to assess is:**

A. whether the areas of concern to the OT interfere with the child's education.
B. the degree of functional skills possessed by the child.
C. the level of independence in ADL.
D. the degree of accessibility of the learning environment.

155. **An OT practitioner is working in an acute care inpatient psychiatric facility. Upon admission, the FIRST step in planning for the discharge of a socially isolated individual is to:**

A. provide community reentry activities to introduce the individual to community resources to use after discharge.
B. evaluate the individual's occupational performance.
C. educate the family about the individual's ability to return home.
D. make a referral to an outpatient socialization program.

156. **An individual with ALS swims three times a week to maximize strength and**

endurance. Initially able to swim for only 10 minutes, the individual is now able to swim 20 minutes without becoming fatigued. The **NEXT** step is:

A. continue the program of swimming 20 minutes three times a week.

B. decrease swimming frequency to two times a week.

C. increase swimming time to 25 minutes or to tolerance.

D. provide adaptive equipment that will enable the individual to swim using less energy.

157. **A child who has difficulty with visual perception of "position in space" will soon be discharged from an outpatient occupational therapy program and the OT practitioner will be meeting with the classroom teacher and parents. Of the following, which would be the BEST activity to promote this type of visual perception?**

A. Identifying letters on a distracting page.

B. Finding geometric shapes scattered in a box.

C. Following directions about objects located in front, in back, and to the side.

D. Making judgments about moving through space.

158. **A child with limited upper-extremity range of motion is being readied for discharge. The MOST important home adaptation for the OT practitioner to recommend concerning use of the toilet is:**

A. installation of safety bars next to the toilet seat.

B. mounting of a wide-base toilet seat.

C. placement of a skidproof stepping stool next to the toilet.

D. installation of a bidet with a spray wash and air-drying mechanism.

159. **A long-term goal for a 60-year-old client with back pain is to be able to return to work as an illustrator. The client has achieved the short-term goal of sitting at a work table for 20 minutes. The BEST example of a revised short-term goal for this client is:**

A. "Client will draw sitting at work table."

B. "Client will draw for 1 hour, taking stretch breaks every 20 minutes."

C. "Instruct client in stretching techniques to be performed every 20 minutes."

D. "Instruct client in the use of proper body mechanics that apply to prolonged sitting."

160. **A child with a swallowing dysfunction is being discharged with a home-feeding program that includes eliminating foods with consistencies that are difficult to swallow. The OT would MOST likely recommend that the following type of food texture be AVOIDED:**

A. smooth semisolids (pureed bananas).

B. lumpy semisolids (cottage cheese).

C. liquids and solids combined (minestrone soup).

D. thickened liquids (malted milk).

161. **The therapist is reevaluating an individual's PROM for elbow flexion by completing three consecutive measurements. A 10-degree discrepancy exists between the first two measurements and the third. The MOST likely response of the therapist would be to:**

A. check the alignment of the goniometer.

B. use a larger goniometer.

C. use a smaller goniometer.

D. attempt to force the individual's arm further into flexion.

162. **Which of the following is the BEST example of "objective" information as written by an OT practitioner for the objective section of a discharge summary?**

A. "Pt. reports he can work at the computer much longer and more comfortably than he could initially."

B. "Pt. was initially able to work at the computer for only 10 minutes. Upon discharge, he can work at the computer for 3 hours with stretch breaks every 30 minutes."

C. "Pt. has improved significantly in his ability to work at the computer."

D. "Pt. reports he is now able to work at the computer for 3 hours, where initially he was only able to tolerate 10 minutes."

163. **An OTR and COTA are collaborating on a discharge summary. Which of the following is the MOST appropriate contribution for the COTA to make?**

A. Describe the treatment received

B. Make the referral for community-based services

C. Compare the initial and final status

D. Formulate the OT follow-up plans

164. **An individual is about to be discharged to home following a hip arthroplasty. He is able to ambulate with a quad cane, but his balance remains slightly impaired.**

During the home evaluation, which is the MOST important safety recommendation for the OT practitioner to make?

A. Remove all throw or scatter rugs
B. Place lever handles on faucets
C. Install a ramp if steps exist
D. Install a handheld shower

165. An OT practitioner is treating a client who has demonstrated a decrease in paranoid behavior. The BEST way to document this change is:

A. "The patient is no longer as afraid of men."
B. "The patient has not accused any men of attacking her this week."
C. "The patient is participating more actively in beauty group."
D. "The patient will tolerate sitting next to a man in group one time this week."

166. An individual has made gains in fine-motor coordination in the past week. Which of the following statements belongs in the assessment section of a SOAP note?

A. "Patient performed the Nine Hole Peg Test in 20 seconds."
B. "Patient reports being able to button the buttons on most items of clothing."
C. "Patient is demonstrating gradual improvement in fine-motor coordination."
D. "Family reports patient is performing more fine-motor activities independently."

167. An OT practitioner has been asked to work on laundry skills with an adult with cognitive disabilities. Initially, the OT practitioner recommended that the staff in the group home work with the individual for 2 months on how to recognize when clothing is dirty and needs to be laundered. After 2 months, however, the individual continues to wear soiled garments. The OT practitioner determines that the individual is unable to recognize or judge when clothing is dirty. What is the NEXT step the OT practitioner should take to maximize the individual's independence in doing laundry?

A. Instruct the individual to wear clothes for 2 days and to then launder those items.
B. Assess the individual's ability to recognize dirty clothing.
C. Recommend that the individual take clothes for dry cleaning rather than wash them at home.
D. Recommend to the staff that they do the individual's laundry from now on.

168. A COTA and OTR are planning for the discharge of a child from an early intervention program. What advice to the parents will MOST likely result in effective carryover of a therapeutic home program?

A. Set aside a certain time daily to focus on therapeutic activities.
B. Incorporate therapeutic activities into family routines.
C. Provide therapeutic activities on an as-needed basis.
D. Do therapeutic activities daily, but vary the time of day.

Occupational Therapy for Populations

169. An OT practitioner functioning in the role of a consultant in an adult day care facility would be MOST likely to provide which of the following services:

A. evaluating clients to determine OT needs.
B. implementing recreational activity groups.
C. serving as a personal advocate for the client and family liaison.
D. providing OT expertise to run the program and solve problems.

170. An OT who is employed by a community health center has determined that there is a need to provide group activities for groups of clients with specific diagnoses. One group the therapist is recommending starts with the clients engaging in a game of rhythmic exercises performed to music. The group activity also includes teaching the clients strategies to get up from a chair and start walking and specially adapted handwriting activities. This is MOST likely an OT group for people with the diagnosis of:

A. Parkinson's disease.
B. Guillain-Barré.
C. COPD.
D. spinal cord injury.

171. An OT practitioner working in a sheltered workshop with individuals with mental retardation must be aware of how the agency that provides services to the developmentally disabled population is accredited. Which of the following is responsible for accrediting these workshops?

A. JCAHO

B. CARF

C. AC MRDD

D. NLN/APHA

172. **An OT practitioner is providing accessibility consultation services to a local library. In the back of the library there is a reference room with a doorway that has a threshold of 1-inch height. Concerning the threshold and accessibility according to the ADA guidelines, the BEST recommendation would be:**

 A. keeping the threshold as is, place a sign near the door alerting people to the threshold.

 B. providing a throw rug which covers the threshold.

 C. removing the threshold altogether.

 D. ramp the threshold.

173. **An OT practitioner working in an acute psychiatric facility is meeting with a client who has mental health issues. The client is preparing for discharge and is ready for the least restrictive level of care. The facility that BEST represents the least restrictive level of care is:**

 A. a quarterway house.

 B. a halfway house.

 C. a supervised apartment.

 D. outpatient counseling.

174. **Which of the following components is MOST essential to include when designing a work-hardening program?**

 A. Pain management techniques

 B. Achieving a balance between work and leisure

 C. Energy conservation techniques

 D. Vocational counseling

175. **An OT wishes to assess the results of a life-skills training program provided to individuals at a shelter for abused women. Which of the following methods would be BEST for obtaining this information?**

 A. Final evaluation of each client involved

 B. Client satisfaction survey

 C. Program evaluation

 D. Utilization review

176. **An OT consults to a vocational instructor in a high school program for students with moderate mental disabilities. Which of the following activities would**

be MOST appropriately provided by the OT?

 A. Developing an in-house prevocational work program

 B. Bringing in outside speakers from different job settings

 C. Teaching the vocational instructor different assessment tools and scoring procedures

 D. Meeting the vocational instructor weekly to discuss adaptations to work tasks

Service Management

177. **An OTR and COTA share and coordinate therapy for a caseload. Which of the following jobs would be MOST appropriate for the COTA to perform:**

 A. completing the chart reviews.

 B. completing the nonstandardized portions of the evaluation.

 C. interpreting the results of the nonstandardized portion of the evaluation.

 D. independently designing a treatment plan for the individual.

178. **As health care changes through the next century, the focus will move more toward health status and away from health care. This trend focuses on enhancing wellness and health through activities using various strategies, including education and behavioral change efforts. The OT practitioner's role in this trend is BEST described as:**

 A. occupational behavior.

 B. intervention.

 C. self-efficacy.

 D. health promotion.

179. **The OT is working with a patient on an acute care floor when the patient's IV equipment disengages, splashing the therapist in the eye with the medication and IV "backwash" fluid. The therapist's FIRST response should be to:**

 A. rub the eye and continue treatment.

 B. rinse the eye with an eye wash or water immediately.

 C. write an incident report.

 D. cover the eye with a bandage and contact the immediate supervisor.

180. **An OT practitioner is supervising an OT aide. The MOST appropriate kinds of activities and level of supervision for the aide include:**

A. selected tasks in which aides have been trained, with intense close supervision.

B. various intervention activities with routine supervision.

C. completing ADL training with a patient without supervision.

D. selecting adaptive equipment from a catalog with general supervision.

181. A patient who has had surgery for a malignant tumor was seen once in OT and is being discharged home, though the patient is weak and needs to continue receiving IV chemotherapy with a home health nurse. The MOST appropriate recommendation the OT practitioner could make for this patient to receive OT services would be:

A. from a home health OTR or COTA.

B. staying in the hospital a little longer.

C. going to a rehabilitation center.

D. coming back for outpatient OT.

182. During a routine transfer, a patient's legs buckle, causing him and the OT practitioner to fall to the floor. The most appropriate way for the OT practitioner to document this accident is in a(n):

A. incident report.

B. daily progress note.

C. letter to the department head.

D. verbal report to the department head.

183. While documenting the week's OT sessions in an individual's chart, an OT practitioner notices that a progress note from 2 weeks ago was not completed. The therapist recalls providing treatment that week and how the patient responded. The ONLY appropriate action for the OTR to take is to:

A. complete the note using the original date.

B. document services provided and date the note as a late entry.

C. leave the chart as is without documenting services provided.

D. write a brief note stating that documentation was not completed for the specified dates.

184. A hospital-based multidisciplinary team meets bimonthly to monitor their services in regard to the creation of an environment that meets or exceeds consumer needs. This model is MOST appropriately called:

A. total quality management.

B. cost accounting.

C. employee empowerment.

D. horizontal structuring.

185. An OT practitioner completing a home assessment has recommended a hospital bed, lightweight wheelchair, bedside commode, reachers long-handled sponge, shower chair, and hand-held shower. The family states they can only afford the items that can be billed as durable medical equipment. Which of the following can be billed as durable medical equipment?

A. Lightweight wheelchair and reachers

B. Shower chair, hand-held shower and bedside commode

C. Hospital bed, shower chair and hand-held shower

D. Lightweight wheelchair and hospital bed

186. An OTR is working with a patient that has Medicare part B. The OTR informs the patient that Medicare part B will MOST likely reimburse for assistive devices, such as a wheelchair, if it meets the criteria of:

A. increasing functional independence.

B. medical necessity.

C. maintaining patient function.

D. reducing deformity.

187. An OT practitioner working in a school-based setting is interested in training students in level-II fieldwork. Before accepting level-II students, the OT practitioner should have at least:

A. 6 months experience.

B. 1 year experience.

C. 2 years experience.

D. 3 years experience.

188. According to the Joint Commission on Accreditation of Hospital Organizations (JCAHO) an OT managing delivery of therapy services in a hospital setting would have to review and update occupational therapy policies and procedures as follows:

A. review and update annually.

B. review and update on years in which JCAHO surveys are performed.

C. review and update when new occupational therapy managers take over a department.

D. review every other year.

189. A home health OT has received a referral for a Medicare patient. Which one of the following items is MOST necessary to have before the therapist can initiate evaluation or treatment?

A. Identification of the deficits that impair functional abilities.

B. Established short-term and long-term goals.

C. A physician's order identifying services to be provided.

D. The individual's history of the current illness.

190. OT practitioners should PRIMARILY wear gloves when working with:

A. individuals with open wounds who have been diagnosed with human immunodeficiency virus.

B. individuals with third-degree burns.

C. individuals with open wounds who have been diagnosed with hepatitis.

D. all individuals with open wounds.

191. At the beginning of fieldwork, a student asks an OTR who is the clinical supervisor about student objectives. The MOST accurate statement about student objectives for fieldwork is:

A. objectives vary in each facility.

B. objectives are standardized for all facilities.

C. are written by the NBCOT.

D. must meet state licensure requirements.

192. An OT providing services to a community mental health program has been asked to examine the effectiveness of the OT groups that have been provided over the past 6 months. Which of the following procedures should be used to accomplish this goal?

A. Quality assurance

B. Peer review

C. Utilization review

D. Program evaluation

193. A new, inexperienced COTA has joined the staff of a rehabilitation facility and the OTR is required to provide "close supervision" for the first few months. As specified by AOTA, the amount of supervisory contact the OTR should provide to the COTA is:

A. contact with supervisor once a day.

B. contact with supervisor once a week.

C. contact with supervisor once a month.

D. contact with supervisor as needed.

194. Many COTAs are employed in long-term care facilities and perform many functions. The function which the OTR MUST perform in this setting is:

A. activity programming, environmental adaptations, and caregiver and staff education.

B. ADL training, and running feeding and leisure activity groups.

C. interpreting results of assessments for the purposes of treatment planning.

D. positioning, providing adaptive devices, and instructing in use of splints.

Professional Practice

195. An OT practitioner evaluating a child notices a bruise on the child's shoulder that looks like an adult's hand and fingerprint. Which of the following actions is it MOST critical for the OT practitioner to take?

A. Discuss this with the family member who picks up the child.

B. Observe for additional injuries.

C. Make a report to appropriate authorities.

D. Avoid becoming involved in personal family matters.

196. An OT practitioner is asked, "What is the primary emphasis of occupational therapy services?" by another health professional. The MOST accurate response for the OT to give is that the emphasis is on:

A. skill acquisition.

B. compensation for deficits.

C. environmental adaptation.

D. reinforcement and enhancement of performance.

197. An OT practitioner is conducting a research study on the effects of using a sling with individuals who sustained a stroke with resultant hemiplegia. If the researcher were to chose a sample population for his research, he would MOST likely use:

A. the entire population of the facility's stroke patients.

B. all patients who have had a CVA with resulting deficits in upper extremity function.

C. a numbers table to select the population.

D. a small group of patients who are representative of the population, with each individual meeting criteria which validate that they are a representative subset of the population.

198. One OT practitioner witnesses another OT practitioner under the influence of alcohol treating patients. The practitioner decides to take action to prevent this practitioner from practicing in the United States. Which of the following would be the MOST appropriate organization to contact?

A. AOTA

B. State regulatory board

C. NBCOT

D. Administration of the facility

199. Upon completion of a level-II fieldwork placement on a rehabilitation unit, a student is functioning slightly below minimal entry-level competence. The supervising fieldwork educator should:

A. fail the student.

B. pass the student with the requirement that the student not practice in a rehabilitation setting.

C. pass the student and recommend addition-

al training or volunteer work in a rehabilitation setting.

D. pass the student.

200. An OT practitioner spends 15 minutes reviewing a new patient's chart and talking to the nurse, who indicates that the patient is preoccupied with finances. As the OT practitioner enters the room, the patient states that he does not want to be seen by any of the therapists because his insurance has run out and he cannot afford to pay for the treatment. Which of the following actions would be MOST appropriate for the OT practitioner to take?

A. Treat the individual per the physician's order and notify the nurse that the man's preoccupation with finances continues.

B. Do not treat the individual based on his refusal and document the interaction in the chart.

C. Treat the individual but do not charge or document the services.

D. Do not treat the individual and only charge for the time spent completing the chart review.

ANSWERS FOR SIMULATION EXAMINATION 1

1. (B) boutonniere deformity. A boutonniere deformity is typically characterized by PIP joint flexion and DIP joint hyperextension. Answer A, a mallet deformity, is characterized by DIP joint flexion and a loss of active extension. Answer C is not a typical description used to describe a deformity. Answer D, a swan neck deformity, is characterized by PIP joint hyperextension and DIP joint flexion. See reference: Pedretti (ed): Belkin, J, and English, CB: Orthotics.

2. (A) copying letters. A test of visual motor integration usually consists of design-copying tasks that can yield information on the child's ability to translate a visual image into a motor output. Visual motor integration is defined as "the ability to integrate the visual image of letters and shapes with the appropriate motor response necessary" (p. 396). Remembering (answer B), recognizing (answer C), and sequencing (answer D) are cognitive and perceptual skills, which do not require a motor response and therefore are not considered visual motor skills. See reference: Case-Smith (ed): Schneck, CM: Visual perception.

3. (D) observe the child entering the clinic and taking off his coat and shoes. "In a naturalistic observation, the therapist gathers information in the typical or natural setting [in which] the activity occurs" (p. 494). The most reliable information can be

gained by observing the child as he or she normally does the activity; this is especially true of children with developmental delay, who may have difficulty generalizing learning from one situation to another. Therefore, answer B may not provide a sample of the child's true skill level. Answers A and C describe situations in which the practitioner is providing assistance, therefore not allowing the child to demonstrate his skill in independent dressing. See reference: Case-Smith (ed): Shepherd, J: Self care and adaptations for independent living.

4. (B) objective signs and duration of the seizure. In order to assess the efficacy of antileptic medication or during periods of gradual withdrawal, staff members are often asked to monitor the child for seizure activity. Type and duration of seizures should be documented carefully. Observations about the child's position (answer A), responsiveness (answer C), and facial expression (answer D) are somewhat less important than isolated observations. See reference: Case-Smith (ed): Rogers, SL, Gordon, CY, Schanzenbacher, KE, and Case-Smith, J: Common diagnosis in pediatric occupational therapy practice.

5. (D) decreased attention. An attention deficit is indicated if the individual recognizes the letter and marks it accurately on both the right and left sides of the paper but misses letters in a random pattern. A visual field cut (answers A and B) is evidenced by the missed letters appearing close together in one area, on either the left or right side of the page. The OTR previously determined that the client was literate (answer C) before the test, either during the interview or from the chart review, so this answer is incorrect. See reference: Trombly (ed): Quintana, LA: Remediating perceptual impairments.

6. (A) interview Interviews provide "an opportunity for the parents to identify their values and priorities about the skills being evaluated by the therapist" (p. 207). Open-ended questions are best for eliciting information about the family's feelings about the intervention. Answers B, C, and D are structured observation methods, through which information on specific skills or functional levels is collected. See reference: Case-Smith (ed): Stewart, KB: Purposes, processes, and methods of evaluation.

7. (B) assessment of upper extremity function in ADL, work and leisure activities. Assessment of upper extremity function in ADL, work, and leisure activities is evaluated both through the involved and uninvolved extremity. Answer C, evaluation of pain, postural control, and alignment, is associated with neuromuscular performance. Answer D, assessment of self-concept and self-awareness, is related to the psychological impact of trauma. Answer A, developmental factors, pertains to an individual's life experiences and how those experiences relate to coping with the musculoskeletal disorder. See reference: Neistadt and Crepeau (eds): Atkins, J: Orthopedic and musculoskeletal problems in children.

8. (C) steps, width of doorways, and threshold heights. The first area of evaluation would be the steps, width of doorways, and presence and height of door thresholds to determine whether the wheelchair user will be able to enter or exit interior spaces in the wheelchair or whether structural modifications are required. Answers A, B, and D reflect areas that will also need to be evaluated; however, they are not as critical to initial interior access. See reference: Pedretti (ed): Foti, D, Pedretti, LW: Activities of daily living.

9. (B) club foot. Pes varus or equinovarus is also called club foot. This deformity involves forefoot inversion and supination, heel varus, equinus through the ankle, and medial deviation of the foot in relationship to the knee. See reference: Smith, Weiss, and Lehmkuhl: Ankle and foot.

10. (D) endurance. A deficit in endurance is demonstrated by the person's inability to sustain cardiac, pulmonary, and musculoskeletal exertion for the duration of the activity. Answer A, a deficit in postural control, would be correct if the client had been unable to maintain his balance while putting on the shirt. A deficit in muscle tone (answer B) would have

been evident if the client had demonstrated spasticity while putting on the shirt. Inability to push his arms through the resistance created by the shirt sleeve would demonstrate a deficit in strength (answer C). See reference: AOTA: Uniform Terminology for Occupational Therapy, third edition.

11. (B) normal development. Proximal movement on a fixed distal limb component—that is, on hands and knees—is an example of the development of mobility superimposed on stability. This stage is essential in the development of coordinated antigravity movement. The development of this type of movement in the quadruped position occurs between the ages of 7 and 12 months. This pattern is typical of normal development and does not indicate answers A, C, or D. See reference: Case-Smith (ed): Nichols, DS: Development of postural control.

12. (C) cruising. The described pattern is cruising. Cruising occurs at approximately 12 months of age and directly precedes walking. Creeping (answer A) refers to four-point mobility in prone position with only hands and knees on the floor, a pattern that occurs at between 7 to 12 months. Crawling (answer B) is the term for the ability to move forward while in a prone position; this pattern occurs at about 7 months of age. Clawing (answer D), also called "fanning," is the ability to spread the toes to maintain balance in standing. See reference: Case-Smith (ed): Wright-Ott, C and Egilson, S: Mobility.

13. (D) Dynamometer This individual exhibits difficulty in the area of strength. A dynamometer measures grip strength through gross hand grasp. A volumeter (answer C) is a container used to measure edema in the hand by measuring the amount of water displaced when the hand is placed into the container. A goniometer (answer A) is a tool with two arms used to measure movement at a joint. One arm is held stationary while the other arm moves around an axis of 360 degrees. An aesthesiometer (answer B) measures two-point discrimination with a moveable point attached to a ruler that has a stationary point at one end. See reference: Trombly (ed): Trombly, CA: Evaluation of biomechanical and physiological aspects of motor performance.

14. (D) Carpal tunnel and chronic cervical tension Carpal tunnel syndrome and chronic cervical tension are just some of the work-related occurrences secondary to the arrival of visual display terminals and specialized technology that require repetition and unusual body positioning. Answers A and C are injuries typically not associated with repetitive motion or cumulative trauma disorders. Answer B, edema and paresthesias, are typical symptoms (not injuries) of repetitive motion and cumulative trauma disorders. See reference: Neistadt and Crepeau (eds): Fenton, S, and Gagnon, P: Treatment of work and productive activities: Functional restoration, an industrial approach.

15. (D) pervasive developmental disorder of childhood. This disorder "is characterized by severe and complex impairments in social interaction, communication and behavior" (p. 164). Children with ADHD display behaviors of inattention, hyperactivity, and impulsivity; therefore, answer A is incorrect. Children with childhood conduct disorder (answer B) would display repetitive and persistent antisocial behavior. Obsessive-compulsive disorder (answer C) is characterized by obsessive thoughts and displayed in compulsive behaviors such as handwashing. See reference: Case-Smith (ed): Rogers, SL, Gordon, CY, Schanzenbacher, KE, and Case-Smith, J: Common diagnosis in pediatric occupational therapy practice.

16. (C) "I'm just too tired." One of the main symptoms of severe depression is decreased energy; therefore, the response of "I'm too tired" indicates fatigue. Answer A reflects a level of feeling that is higher than the usual subdued feelings associated with depression. Answer B reflects the individual's perceptions of his or her ability or competence. Answer D is a response reflecting interests or values that conflict with the proposed activity. See reference: Bonder: Mental disorders.

17. (B) good (4). The individual's "available" range is the range through which the joint may be moved passively. Therefore, if an individual is able to move the joint actively through the entire movement that is completed passively and then take maximum resistance, the grade is normal (5). Good (4) is the grade given when an individual is able to move a part through the available range against gravity and is able to sustain moderate resistance. Fair (3) is the grade given when an individual is able to move a part through the full range against gravity but lacks the strength for any resistance. Fair minus (3-) is the grade given when an individual moves a part against gravity through less than the full range of motion. Fair minus is the last graded range for movement against gravity. Grades poor and trace are for gravity-eliminated movements. See reference: Trombly (ed): Evaluation of biomechanical and physiological aspects of motor performance.

18. (A) Never, because children with flaccid bladders typically cannot be toilet trained Answer (A) is correct because, "when the lesion is in the lumbar region or below, the bladder is flaccid (lower motor neuron bladder)... the reflex arc is not intact, and the bladder has lost all tone... children with a flaccid bladder cannot be trained because the bladder has no tone to empty" (p. 508). These children are commonly provided with some type of catheterization technique after medical testing is performed. Typically, nighttime bowel and bladder control may not be accomplished until the normally developing child is 4 or 5 years of age. Other developmental trends in toilet training are that daytime control is usually attained by 30 months and that

girls may precede boys by 2.5 months. See reference: Case-Smith (ed): Shepherd, J: Self-care and adaptations for independent living.

19. (A) Coughing or choking Coughing and choking are motor problems that are commonly noted in patients with dysphagia. Disorientation and confusion (answer B) are related to cognitive problems, and pain and decreased smell and taste (answer C and D, respectively), are related to sensory problems in patients with dysphagia. See reference: Pedretti (ed): Nelson, KL: Dysphagia: Evaluation and treatment.

20. (D) distractibility. Distractibility involves losing one's focus because of other stimuli. Memory (answer A) is the ability to recall knowledge and past events. Problems with spatial operations (answer B) are generally observed when individuals attempt to fit objects into specific spaces. Generalization of learning (answer C) may be observed by asking the client to use existing knowledge in a new situation. See reference: Early: Responding to symptoms and behaviors.

21. (C) developmental dyspraxia. The motor problem described as it occurs during the evaluation is characteristic of developmental dyspraxia. Children with dyspraxia often learn tasks such as jumping rope with great difficulty, effort, and considerable practice. However, when the task is altered, such as in this case by asking the child to skip backwards, the child is unable to adapt the task for a long while. Answer A is incorrect because the child with delayed reflex integration would have difficulty with all aspects of the task. Answer B is incorrect because a problem of bilateral integration would affect both aspects of this task, jumping rope forward and backward. Answer D is also incorrect because general incoordination would probably affect performance of both forward and backward rope jumping. See reference: Case-Smith (ed): Parham, LD, and Maillous, Z: Sensory integration.

22. (A) Thumb against the tip of the index finger The correct position for tip pinch is the thumb against the tip of the index finger. The thumb against the side of the index finger describes the position for lateral pinch. The thumb against the tips of the index and middle fingers describes the test position for three-jaw chuck, or palmar pinch. The thumb against the tips of all the fingers is not a standard test position. See reference: Trombly (ed): Trombly, CA: Evaluation of biomechanical and physiological aspects of motor performance.

23. (D) Post-traumatic stress disorder Posttraumatic stress disorder is an anxiety disorder that follows a traumatic event in a person's life. Answers A and B are mood disorders, and answer C is a psychotic disorder. See reference: Neistadt and Crepeau (eds): Giles, GM, and Neistadt, ME: Treatment for psychosocial components: Stress management.

24. (C) "The infant is exhibiting ulnar palmar grasp." Ulnar palmar grasp precedes the other types of grasp. The infant first grasps on the ulnar side of the hand against the palm, then with all four fingers against the palm (palmar grasp), and finally the grasp moves to the radial side of the hand (radial grasp). The highest level of grasp is pincer grasp, in which the pad of the index finger meets the opposed thumb. See reference: Case-Smith (ed): Exner, CE: Development of hand skills.

25. (B) Add the two new clients and then divide the members into two groups. It is generally not cost-effective to run groups of less than three individuals, and it is not effective to have more than eight in a group. Maintaining an appropriate group size enables the OT practitioner to adequately observe the interpersonal skills of the members. Using interviews or groups with three or fewer members (answer C) will provide dyadic interaction information but not information about group interpersonal skills. Asking those originally asked to wait (answer A) is countertherapeutic to those individuals. A group of nine (answer D) would be too large to be effective. See reference: Cole: Writing a group treatment protocol.

26. (B) Median nerve The median nerve passes through the carpal tunnel at the wrist. Impingement in this region causes sensory changes in the thumb, index finger, long and half of the ring finger. Prolonged impingement in the carpal tunnel results in atrophy of the thenar eminence and weakness of the opponens pollicis. Injury to the radial nerve in the wrist area causes sensory damage only. Damage to the ulnar nerve at the wrist causes decreased grip strength and complete or partial loss of sensation over half of the fourth digit (ring finger) and all of the fifth digit (little finger) plus the proximal hypothenar region. A brachial plexus injury may result in damage to any or all of the UE peripheral nerves. This may cause motor and/or sensory impairments. See reference: Pedretti (ed): Kasch, MC: Hand injuries.

27. (B) Initiation The inability to perform the first step of an activity without prompting indicates that the individual has initiation problems. A problem with impulsiveness (answer A) during self-care would be evidenced by the individual's attempting to complete several steps of an activity rapidly, which would probably result in him cutting himself or doing a poor job of shaving. Memory or attention deficits (answers C and D) are demonstrated by the individual's skipping steps of the activity, either because he does not remember the steps or is distracted by internal or external stimuli. Memory deficits could also be evidenced by the performance of task steps out of correct sequence. The individual with initiation problems may be able to plan or carry out activities but

be unable to begin until prompted by someone else. An individual who has difficulty with impulsivity, memory, or attention would have no difficulty with beginning the activity but would have difficulty in completing the task successfully. See reference: Zoltan: Executive functions.

28. (D) The effect of personal traits and the environment on role performance Evaluation according to the Model of Human Occupation would focus on the effect of personal traits and the environment on role performance. Evaluation according to the Behavioral frame of reference identifies problem behaviors that need to be extinguished (answer A). The Object Relations frame of reference seeks to clarify thoughts, feelings, and experiences that influence behavior (answer B). An OT using the Cognitive Disability frame of reference should evaluate cognitive function, including assets and limitations (answer C). See reference: Bruce and Borg: Model of human occupation.

29. (D) determine the need for further evaluation. The purpose of screening is to determine whether further assessments are needed and, if so, which tests would be appropriate for that child. A screening test is not designed for planning programs (answer C) or consultation (answer A), and they do not test any skills (answer B) in a comprehensive way. See reference: Solomon (ed): Peralta, AM, and Kramer, P: General treatment considerations.

30. (B) measure the distance from the fingertip to the distal palmar crease with the hand in a fist. The distance from the fingertip to the distal palmar crease with the hand fisted may be measured in either inches or centimeters. This measures how close the fingertip comes to the palm. A person who has full flexion would have a measurement of O. Answers A and C are incorrect as actively or passively measuring the flexion at each joint and totaling them are measurements taken with a goniometer and recorded in degrees. Answer D, measuring the distance between the tip of the thumb and the fourth phalanx, is incorrect because it is a measurement of opposition. See reference: Hunter, Schneider, Mackin, and Bell (eds): Cambridge, C: Range of motion measurements of the hand.

31. (B) line bisection. Line bisection is used as a method of determining unilateral neglect. The block assembly (used for constructional apraxia) is not a paper-and-pencil task, and the other tests may be performed with or without the individual writing. Proverb interpretation (abstraction) may be performed verbally, and overlapping figures (figure-ground discrimination) testing may be performed by pointing. See reference: Unsworth (ed): Corben, L. and Unsworth, C: Evaluation and intervention with unilateral neglect.

32. (C) a concrete response. Literal and concrete responses to general inquiries indicate the difficulty that people with schizophrenia have in understanding questions with several possible meanings. Delusional responses (answer A) would most likely be completely off topic. A distractible response (answer B) would change the topic or stop in the middle of responding. An insightful response (answer D) would include reasons that led up to being hospitalized. See reference: Hemphill (ed): Shaw, C: The interviewing process in occupational therapy.

33. (A) ADHD. This behavior exemplifies the excessive fidgeting and restlessness, inattention, and impulsiveness characteristic of ADHD. Although some of the symptoms of overactivity and impulsiveness are part of a mood disorder of the manic type (answer B), there usually are also symptoms of grandiosity and inflated self-esteem. A child with a conduct disorder (answer C) would exhibit interference with the basic rights of other children or societal rules. A child with anxiety disorder(answer D) would show signs of uneasiness, apprehension, or dread associated with anticipation of danger. See reference: Neistadt and Crepeau (eds): Florey, L: Psychosocial dysfunction in childhood and adolescence.

34. (A) at the lateral epicondyle of the humerus. The lateral epicondyle of the humerus is the bony prominence on the lateral side of the elbow. The medial epicondyle (answer B) is the bony prominence on the medial side of the elbow. The stationary arm of the goniometer should be positioned parallel to the longitudinal axis of the humerus on the lateral aspect (answer C). The movable arm of the goniometer should be positioned parallel to the longitudinal axis of the radius on the lateral aspect (answer D). See reference: Trombly (ed): Trombly, CA: Evaluation of biomechanical and physiological aspects of motor performance.

35. (D) rationalization. Making excuses for or justifying others' behaviors that are generally considered to be unacceptable is called rationalization. Identification (answer A) occurs when one takes on the characteristics of another person. Projection (answer B) is the blaming of other people for performing the behaviors. Denial (answer C) is refusing to acknowledge that the behavior occurred. See reference: Christiansen and Baum (eds): Bonder, B: Coping with psychological and emotional challenges.

36. (A) figure-ground discrimination. Figure-ground discrimination is the ability to distinguish an object from the background. A person with impaired figure-ground discrimination would have difficulty finding the sock despite its position on the bed. Other deficits that may be demonstrated by the person would be an inability to see the sock on one side of the bed (unilateral neglect), to find it in relation to the bed (position in space), and to know how to get back to the bed to look for the sock (cognitive mapping).

See reference: Trombly (ed): Quintana, LA: Evaluation of perception and cognition.

37. (C) anterograde amnesia. Anterograde amnesia is the inability to recall events after a trauma. Retrograde amnesia (answer D) is the inability to recall events prior to trauma. Long-term memory (answer B) is the storage of information for recall at a later time. Orientation (answer A) is the awareness of person, place, and time. See reference: Trombly (ed): Quintana, LA: Evaluation of perception and cognition.

38. (C) ask the questions as they are stated on the interview sheet. A structured interview requires following the procedure, order, and wording of the questions to be asked. Answers A, B, and D are appropriate for semi-structured interviews (e.g., in pursuit of more details and information). See reference: Early: Data collection and evaluation.

39. (C) Skilled observation Checklists are simple lists of factors or behaviors that a therapist thinks are important to observe as a support for referral or screening of a child. Although checklists may appear in a standard format, they are not well developed enough to include establishment of normative data and other attributes of tests, such as validity and reliability. See reference: Case-Smith (ed): Stewart, KB: Purposes, processes, and methods of evaluation.

40. (C) the ability to engage in superficial social conversation. The onset of most dementias is slow and progressive. Cognitive abilities such as reading and writing are most often initially affected. Sensorimotor abilities such as dressing tend to follow. Superficial social abilities are often preserved until the last stages of dementia and may often hide the earlier cognitive and sensorimotor changes. See reference: Neistadt and Crepeau (eds): Ward, JD: Psychosocial dysfunction in adults.

41. (D) apply the stimuli to the uninvolved area proximally to distally in a random pattern. The general guidelines for sensation testing are that the person's vision should be occluded, the stimuli should be randomly applied with false stimuli intermingled, a practice trial should be performed before the test, and the unaffected side or area should be tested before the affected side or area. Also, the amount of time a person has to respond should be established. See reference: Trombly (ed): Bentzel, K: Evaluation of sensation.

42. (C) demonstrating typical development for a child with Down syndrome. Answer C is correct because exclusive "W" sitting is commonly seen in children with low muscle tone. The child is compensating for an inability to achieve stability in a variety of positions that require dynamic postural control, depending on skeletal rather than neuromuscular structures for stability. Answers A and D are not correct because exclusive "W" sitting would be considered both normal and age appropriate for a 5-year-old child with Down syndrome. Answer B is not correct because exclusive "W" sitting is considered to be a compensatory position. See reference: Kramer and Hinojosa (eds): Schoen, SA, and Anderson, J: Neurodevelopmental treatment frame of reference.

43. (A) 2 inches wider than the widest point across the individual's hips while he or she wears the brace. Measuring the individual with the brace on and adding 2 inches, as in answer A, allows the individual to easily get in and out of the chair, while preventing pressure to the individual's sides. Answer B measures only the hips and would not allow enough room for the individual to sit or move easily in the chair while wearing the brace. Answers C and D are both incorrect measurements for seat length because both would have the seat too deep for the individual's leg length. The correct length of the seat should be 2 inches shorter than the distance from the back of the bent knee to the back of the buttocks. See reference: Pedretti (ed): Pedretti, L, and Stone, G: Wheelchairs and wheelchair transfers.

44. (A) constructional apraxia. An individual with constructional apraxia may have full sensory awareness of the affected side of the body but be unable to perform the construction of one or more objects onto each other to carry out a verbal command or put on clothing in the proper sequence or position. Ideomotor apraxia (answer B) is the "inability to imitate gestures or perform a purposeful motor task on command even though the patient fully understands the idea or concept of the task" (p. 54). Visual agnosia (answer C) is an inability to recognize familiar objects. Unilateral neglect (answer D) occurs when the individual neglects the affected side of the body and performs activities toward or with the unaffected side. See reference: Zoltan: Apraxia.

45. (D) Social skills training Social skills training can be used to develop the ability to relate appropriately and effectively with others. The sensory integration treatment approach, which aims to improve the reception and processing of sensory information within the central nervous system, uses vestibular stimulation and gross-motor exercise (answer A). This approach involves the use of pleasurable activities that don't require conscious attention to movement (answer C), and is best suited to individuals with chronic schizophrenia who have proprioceptive deficits. Environmental modification (answer B) is most appropriate for individuals with cognitive disabilities. See reference: Early: Some practice models for occupational therapy in mental health.

46. (A) putting blankets in the overhead compartments. When distributing magazines, the flight attendant uses negligible reaching and bending. Up-grading the activity increases the degree of reaching and bending and adds more resistance than that provided by magazines. Handling meal trays (answer B), which are significantly heavier than magazines, especially extending them to passengers in window seats, is more than a gradual increase or upgrade. Putting luggage into the overhead compartments (answer D) would be the final step in the work hardening process because it involves the most weight and the riskiest back position. Distributing magazines to half of the passengers (answer C) is an example of downgrading the activity. See reference: Pedretti (ed): Smithline, J: Low back pain.

47. (B) positioning, adaptive equipment, and patient education. Positioning and adaptive equipment are necessary to maintain the integrity of the musculoskeletal system and prevent deformity; patient education about the disease and ways of dealing with its effects can also be started at this point. Resistive exercises (answer A) are not appropriate if there is joint swelling and inflammation and are always used cautiously with individuals with RA because of the potential for tissue damage. Discharge planning would be more relevant at a later time (answer C). Surgical intervention (answer D) would not be needed in the early stages of rheumatoid arthritis. It may be offered as a corrective measure for long-standing deformities. See reference: Pedretti (ed): Hittle, JM, Pedretti, LW, and Kasch, MC: Rheumatoid arthritis.

48. (B) Observe performance at the job site and make recommendations to increase productivity. One of the roles of the OT in transition services includes consulting with the employer on adaptation to the job activities to accommodate individuals with disabilities. The other members of the educational team can provide classroom-based instruction as in answers A, C, and D. See reference: Case-Smith (ed): Spencer, K: Transition services: From school to adult life.

49. (A) Sit straddling a bolster with both feet on the floor Once the child has learned to sit independently on the floor, external stabilizing support is no longer necessary (answer D). After having developed independent postural reactions on a stable surface, that is, the floor, the child can now further refine sitting skills by learning to maintain posture when placed on an unstable surface. At first, the child should be left in control of the movement on this surface, and she should have both feet on the floor for maximal stability. Later, these skills can be refined by placing the child on more challenging surfaces, such as on the hippity-hop (answer C) or on a scooter pulled by another person (answer B). See reference: Case-Smith (ed): Nichols, DS: The development of postural control.

50. (B) the client will use facial expressions and gestures that are consistent with stated emo-

tions during assertive, passive, and aggressive role-play situations. Self-expression is the use of a variety of styles and skills to express thoughts, feelings, and needs. It is also the ability to vary one's expressions, thoughts, feelings, and needs. Being able to vary one's expression during three different styles of expressing feelings is an example of this. Identifying pleasurable activities (answer A) will help to develop interests. Recognition of one's behaviors and consequences (answer C) relates to self-control. Identifying one's own assets and limitations (answer D) is related to self-concept. See reference: AOTA: Uniform Terminology for Occupational Therapy, third edition.

51. (C) Weight-bearing on hands This is the only activity that will facilitate hand function in the preparation phase. Weight-bearing on the hands gives deep pressure to the surface of the hand and facilitates wrist and arm extension, as well as shoulder cocontraction, to prepare the arm for reach and stabilization of the hand for grasping. The other answers all provide different types of grasp activities that could be used as therapy. See reference: Case-Smith (ed): Exner, CE: Development of hand skills.

52. (B) Objective The objective portion of the SOAP note (answer B) focuses on measurable or observable data obtained by the OT practitioner through specific evaluations, observations, or use of therapeutic activities. The subjective portion of a SOAP note (answer A) should feature relevant patient reports or comments. The assessment part of a SOAP note addresses the effectiveness of treatment and any changes needed, the status of the goals, and the justification for continuing OT treatment. The plan section of a SOAP note includes statements related to continuing treatment; the frequency and duration of the treatment; suggestions for additional activities or treatment techniques; the need for further evaluations; and, when needed, recommendations for new goals. See reference: Ryan (ed): Practice Issues in Occupational Therapy: Backhaus, H: Documentation.

53. (A) Loosening nuts and bolts Loosening nuts and bolts is the activity that most closely resembles a tip or lateral prehension activity. Prehension is a hand position that permits finger and thumb contact while facilitating the manipulation of objects. Answers B, C, and D are more closely related to grasping activities, which encourage contact of an object against the palm and the flexed digits. See reference: Pedretti (ed): Belkin, J, and English, CB: Orthotics.

54. (B) forward and side-to-side movement with the child sitting on the therapist's lap. Answer B is correct because the position of the child requires the least resistance to gravity. By tilting the child in this position, the practitioner controls how much the child will work against gravitational pull and assures

that the child is well supported. Answers A and D are incorrect because they would require the child to lift his or her head directly against gravity. Answer C is also incorrect because the child's head is positioned against gravity in the quadruped position and a child with extremely poor head control probably could not hold this position. See reference: Case-Smith (ed): Nichols, DS: Development of postural control.

55. (D) To arrive at work on time consistently Time management mandates that one "recognize one's values and priorities, structure a daily routine, schedule one's time, and organize tasks efficiently" (p. 467). Answers A, B, and C are ways of coping with being late, not strategies for the time management goal of being on time. See reference: Early: Psychosocial skills and psychological components.

56. (C) Use of a tub transfer bench and leg lifter The use of a tub transfer bench would allow the client to back up to the tub bench, sit, and manually lift the leg over the side of the tub, either by using her own hands or a leg lifter. Answer A, the prohibiting of showering and bathing, is not considered to be a standard course of treatment. Answer B, use of a hand rail, would assist with transfers but would not address the knee motion limitation. Answer D, using a beach chair, would not be considered a safe or stable selection for transfer training in the tub. See reference: Pedretti (ed): Adler, C, and Tipton-Burton, M: Wheelchair assessment and transfers.

57. (C) Have the child roll around in a carpeted barrel. Because tactile defensiveness is an area of sensory integration treatment that should be approached cautiously, the child-controlled rolling on a textured surface is less intrusive to the nervous system than gentle brushing or rubbing lotion (answers A and B), when the therapist is providing sensory stimulation to the MOST sensitive areas of the body. Swinging activities (answer D) generally do not address the problem of tactile defensiveness. See reference: Case-Smith (ed): Parham, LD, and Mailloux, Z: Sensory integration.

58. (C) Copper tooling using a template. When choosing activities to address self-competence and self-confidence, it is important first to choose activities that are relatively simple, structured, of short duration, and guaranteed to provide a successful experience to the patient. Answers A and B are fairly complex projects that require decision making and several sessions to complete and that have the potential for problems in any of the many stages of construction. Although they may be appropriate later in the treatment program, they are contraindicated at the beginning of treatment. Learning to play bridge (answer D) may be a good choice when addressing development of leisure activities, but it also involves learning a series of steps and interacting with others, requirements that are premature at this stage in treatment. See reference: Early: Responding to symptoms and behaviors.

59. (C) edema, contracture, muscle tone, and pain. Edema limits range of motion because of the increase of fluid in the extremity. A contracture can result when joint motion is limited by a prolonged spasticity or change in the tissues, causing resistance to passive stretch. Muscle tone may also be a limiting factor in one's ability to complete range of motion. If an individual is unable to move a part through full range against gravity, the therapist may put the individual in a gravity-eliminated position to attempt the same movement. Finally, pain may be a limiting factor. This may particularly be seen in individuals with arthritis or changes in joint structure. Pain generally occurs in the end ranges of motion. Other options listed (proprioception and diadokinesis) may affect the quality of active movement or coordination but do not limit active or PROM. See reference: Trombly (ed): Trombly, CA: Evaluation of biomechanical and physiological aspects of motor performance.

60. (A) poor postural responses. Poor postural responses, such as poor balance and postural control against gravity, are often symptoms of an underreactive vestibular system. Possible symptoms of an overreactive vestibular system are answers B, C, and D, which are problems of intolerance for motion and gravitational insecurity. See reference: Fisher, Murray, and Bundy (eds): Fisher, AG: Vestibular-proprioceptive processing and bilateral integration and sequencing deficits.

61. (A) sequencing of picture symbols. A person needs to use picture symbols to indicate a two- or more part thought or sequence of activities. For example, pointing to pictures of a shoe and a closet would indicate the place to find a shoe in response to a question. Understanding letters or words (answers B and C) and then sequencing them (answer D) are significantly higher level skills than recognizing and sequencing pictures. See reference: Angelo and Lane (eds): Written and spoken augmentative communication.

62. (A) Getting dressed without becoming fatigued Prevention of fatigue is the primary purpose of energy conservation. Energy conservation techniques may often result in slower, not faster (answer D), performance. Using proper body mechanics may enable an individual with back pain to lift heavy cookware without pain (answer B). Using joint protection techniques may prevent further joint damage to arthritic hands when the patient is doing handicrafts (answer C). See reference: Pedretti (ed): Hittle, JM, Pedretti, LW, and Kasch, MC: Rheumatoid arthritis.

63. (A) Drawing a picture titled "This is me" Children who have trouble expressing their emotions verbally are sometimes able to express their feelings in open-ended drawing activities. Among the answers given, answer A is the only projective activity. Answers B, C, and D are highly structured activities with minimal potential for open-ended expression. See reference: Case-Smith (ed): Cronin, AS: Psychosocial and emotional domains.

64. (A) a can of soup. Grading activities according to complexity is an important part of the therapist's selection of appropriate activities for each individual. Complexity increases as the number of steps, number of different ingredients or tools used, and time to complete the task increases. Answers B, C, and D all require more steps, materials, and time than preparing a can of soup. See reference: Bruce and Borg: Appendix.

65. (C) Wrist splints to promote development of tenodesis Hand splinting to promote tenodesis is implemented in the acute phase of rehabilitation. A tenodesis grasp is developed by allowing the finger flexors to shorten. The person is then able to achieve a functional grasp by extending the wrist. This improves the ability of an individual with a C6 or C7 spinal cord injury to grasp and hold objects. A volar pan splint (answer A) would not allow finger flexors to shorten, and would interfere with the development of tenodesis. Interventions related to promoting independent performance (answer B) should begin as soon as possible, but issues related to positioning must be addressed first. An individual would not be instructed in bed mobility (answer D) until after the acute phase. See reference: Pedretti (ed): Adler, C: Spinal cord injury.

66. (B) Catching and bursting soap bubbles This activity involves visually tracking a slow-moving target and requires minimal fine motor precision to accomplish a successful "hit." Answers A, C, and D also require visual tracking and eye–hand coordination, but they involve more fast-moving targets and require immediate, more precise movements. These activities can therefore be used to promote more advanced skills. See reference: Case-Smith (ed): Dubois, SA: Preschool services.

67. (D) Each member will remain in the group without disrupting the work of others for 15 minutes. Parallel groups are most appropriate for people who do not have the ability to interact successfully with other group members. Participants in parallel groups are involved in individual tasks that require minimal, if any, interaction. Therefore, appropriate expectations for parallel groups focus on remaining in the group and working alongside others. Taking leadership roles (answer A) is a goal consistent with egocentric–cooperative groups. Sharing materials with some of the other group members (answer B) is a project group goal. Expressing feelings within a group (answer C) is consistent with a cooperative group. See reference: Cole: Appendix B.

68. (D) sensory compensation. When protective sensation is severely decreased or absent, the primary focus of intervention becomes protection of the insensate part through educational methods to increase awareness of potential injury dangers, teach safety procedures, and train in the use of vision to compensate for sensory loss. Sensory reeducation (answer A) is a remedial retraining technique which focuses on helping the patient correctly interpret sensory impulses through a program of graded sensory stimuli. Sensory desensitization (answer B) involves a program of graded sensory stimuli to gradually decrease hypersensitivity to sensory stimuli. Sensory bombardment (answer C) is a sensory retraining method of stimulating many senses. See reference: Pedretti (ed): Pedretti, LW: Evaluation of sensation and treatment of sensory dysfunction.

69. (C) Multisensory input Each of the possible four answers describes appropriate treatment interventions for infants in the NICU. However, an infant approaching full term or post term is now equipped with a maturing sensory system tolerant and in demand of a multisensory diet including oral stimulation, vestibular input, and auditory and visual orientation, to assist with age-appropriate motor and behavioral skill acquisition. It is often found that these very premature infants are limited in the amount of social interaction and appropriate sensory stimuli because of necessary medical equipment and procedures: e.g., ventilators, IV catheters, isolettes, warmers, bililights, and nasogastric tubing. Therefore, stable, growing post-term premature infants would most benefit from a multisensory diet, answer C, to best meet the demands of their maturing sensory system and capitalize on their socialization skills. Answers A, B, and D are all possible treatments for the 32 to 35-week-old infant who responds best to unimodal sensory input and minimal direct intervention, e.g., range of motion and positioning, because of immature sensory systems and compromised respiratory systems. See reference: Case-Smith (ed): Hunter, JG: Neonatal Intensive Care Unit.

70. (B) A noise machine producing white noise at bedtime For a child who is easily aroused, a constant, monotonous auditory input can be calming to the degree of inducing sleep. The other answers may actually increase arousal. Quick repetitive proprioceptive input, as experienced when jumping on a trampoline (answer A), and light touch provided by a fuzzy blanket (answer C) are types of sensory input that have direct arousing effects on the nervous system. Blocking out all light (answer D) may produce arousal as a result of fear generated by total darkness. See reference: Case-Smith (ed): Cronin, AF: Psychosocial and emotional domains of behavior.

71. (B) Concentration This game requires the player to remember visual cues. Answers A, C, and D re-

quire visual skills, but not memory. See reference: Case-Smith (ed): Schneck, CM: Visual perception.

72. (D) slicing a prepared roll of sugar cookies at room temperature and placing them on a tray using a spatula. This answer describes the lowest level of physical exertion and may be completed within the time frame designated by the therapist. The sugar cookie dough would be soft enough to provide minimal resistance without causing immediate fatigue. In addition, the activity provides for isotonic contractions during the repetitive grasp and release of the knife and the spatula. While muffin and cake batter provide the least amount of resistance, the hand is using sustained isometric grasp on the electric or hand-powered mixer, which combined with the minimal resistance of the batter and mixer weight is fatiguing. The chocolate chip cookie dough is resistive whether it is warm or cold and to maintain an isometric grasp while mixing with a spatula or scooping with an ice cream scooper would cause the individual to fatigue before the activity is finished. If the individual becomes fatigued while performing any of the activities, only the sugar cookies or the chocolate chip cookies would allow the individual time to rest without affecting the final product. See reference: Trombly (ed): Stewart, C: Retraining housekeeping and child care skills.

73. (D) doll house and dress-up clothes. To encourage symbolic play, the child should be exposed to toys offering imaginative, open-ended play opportunities, encouraging formulation of ideas and feelings. Answers A, B, and C are not only representative of the younger (answer A) or older child (answers B and C), but they also offer more defined, closed-ended play opportunities with predictable results. See reference: Case-Smith (ed): Morrison, CD, Metzger, P: Play.

74. (C) instructing caregivers in task breakdown. Instructing the caregivers in task breakdown, or breaking down tasks into simple steps and then providing step-by-step instructions, will allow the client to perform activities as capabilities decline. At this stage of the disease, memory retraining (answer A) and ADL retraining (answer B) will probably not be effective. Leisure activities (answer D) structured to meet the needs of the client with Alzheimer's disease could be helpful but will not address the primary problem of performance of self-care activities. See reference: Pedretti (ed): Atchison, P, Pedretti, LW, McCormack, GL: Alzheimer's disease.

75. (B) assisted stand pivot transfer. An assisted stand pivot transfer is implemented when the client assists with the transfer. Answer A, an independent transfer from a wheelchair to an elevated mat or plinth, is done independently without the assistance of the practitioner. Answer C, a pneumatic lift, is a device that may be used when the client is larger than the therapist. Answer D, a dependent stand pivot transfer, is one in which the therapist assists with more than 50% of the transfer. See reference: Pedretti (ed): Adler, C, and Tipton-Burton, M: Wheelchair assessment and transfers.

76. (D) in the upper cabinet to the left side. This pattern of movement promotes the greatest degree of weight shift to the affected side. Putting groceries on the counter directly in front of the person (answer A) or in the upper cabinet to the right side (answer C) would not cause enough weight to be shifted to the affected side and would even shift weight away from that side. When placing groceries on the counter to the left side (answer B), minimal weight shift occurs. See reference: Pedretti (ed): Pope-Davis, SA: The proprioceptive neuromuscular facilitation approach.

77. (C) Activities which provide tapping, application of textures, and weight bearing to the residual limb Massage, tapping, use of textures and weight bearing on the distal end of the residual limb are techniques used to develop tolerance to touch and pressure in the hypersensitive limb. Answers A and B will not affect hypersensitivity and answer D is incorrect because the patient is in the preprosthetic phase and does not have access to the prosthesis. See reference: Trombly (ed): Celikol, F: Amputation and prosthetics.

78. (B) progressive relaxation exercises and autogenic training. Progressive relaxation exercises, answer B, is the answer most relevant to the client's shoulder tension. This technique "involves tensing and relaxing muscle groups, one group at a time, from head to foot" (p. 462), while autogenic training utilizes the concept of mental imagery in order to "achieve muscle relaxation and vasodilation" (p. 462). Answer A is for individuals who are unable to distinguish between assertive and aggressive behaviors and therefore do not respond assertively when necessary. Answer C is useful for individuals whose irrational beliefs and thought processes lead to maladaptive behaviors. Answer D applies to individuals who have difficulty selecting effective solutions or identifying the source of their problems. See reference: Neistadt and Crepeau (eds): Giles, GM, and Neistadt, ME: Treatment for psychosocial components: Stress management.

79. (B) Head slightly flexed Postural alignment is important in promoting oral motor function. The spine and pelvis should be in a neutral position. Normally, the head should be neutral or slightly flexed (answer A). When a child has difficulty swallowing, however, tucking the chin slightly can reduce the risk of aspiration and facilitate swallowing. Positioning the child with the head in extension (answer C) can increase the risk of choking. Rotating the head (answer D) does not facilitate swallowing. See reference: Case-Smith (ed): Case-Smith, J, and Humphry, R: Feeding intervention.

80. (B) Ask the individual to try some lacing with distant supervision and praise her for what she has been able to do. All of the responses are increments of approaches used for decreasing dependency needs, but answer B is the best next step in this case because it allows the individual to attempt some lacing in the presence of the OT, who in turn offers reassurance that the individual is actually able to do the activity. The step in answer B would be followed by the step in answer D. Here the individual is required to attempt some lacing without benefit of the OT at her side; the OT is nearby, but working with another client. As the individual is able to do more of the activity independently, written instructions (answer A) replace the OT as instructor. Finally, when the individual is feeling comfortable with self-instruction, asking her to work on the project out of the presence of the OT (answer C) heightens the level of self-responsibility. See reference: Early: Analyzing, adapting, and grading activities.

81. (A) lying on the left side while propped with pillows. This positioning allows the unaffected right extremities to remain free and provides weight bearing to the affected side to assist with tone reduction. The pillows behind the individual allow support, and the individual may lean against the pillows to also provide pressure relief as needed to the affected side because sensation may be reduced on that side along with movement. Sidelying on the right (answer B) would not provide any tone reduction, which is needed during a stressful activity such as sexual intercourse and also impairs the movement of the unaffected extremities, which would be needed for activities involving foreplay or applying contraceptive devices. Lying in a supine (answer C) or prone (answer D) position would not provide tone reduction to an individual with spasticity and may be uncomfortable without many pillows to assist with positioning comfortably. Also, an individual lying prone has less mobility than when he or she is lying on the right side. See reference: Griffith and Lemberg: Neurological impairments relating to sexuality.

82. (C) Have her put the utensil down until she swallows. The individual needs to learn to pace herself during feeding. An individual with problems relating to the rate of intake tends to put too much food in her mouth in spite of the size of the pieces (answer A). An impulsive person who eats too fast will also have difficulty counting slowly enough (answer B) to clear her mouth by the time she reaches the count of 10. Putting the various items of food in separate containers (answer D) would slow the meal down if items were presented one at a time, but would not necessarily slow the rate of food intake. See reference: Neistadt and Crepeau (eds): Holm, MB, Rogers, JC, and James, AB: Treatment of activities of daily living.

83. (C) altered task method. "When the task method is altered, the same task objects are used in the same environment, but the method of performing the task is altered to make the task feasible given the performance deficits" (p. 338). An example would be substituting one-handed techniques for someone who previously used both hands (i.e., one-handed shoe tying for an individual who recently had an above-elbow amputation). Problem solving is the ability to organize information from several levels to generate a solution to a problem. Retraining teaches the same skills of an activity to the person who previously had mastery of those skills. (e.g., having a person with hand weakness practice tying knots). Compensation would be avoiding performance of the activity entirely by using an alternative piece of equipment or method. See reference: Neistadt and Crepeau (eds): Holm, MB, Rogers, JC, and James, AB: Treatment of activities of daily living.

84. (C) Position stander at 75 to 90 degrees from the floor. Answer C is most correct because by adjusting the prone stander nearer to vertical (the least effect of gravity on the head or posture), the child will be able to tolerate working on head righting. Answer A is not correct because while working on the floor in prone, the head and neck are doing the most work against gravity. Answer D is not correct because the head, neck, and postural work against gravity are the least in the standing position. See reference: Kramer and Hinojosa (eds): Colangelo, CA: Biomechanical frame of reference.

85. (C) have client predict his performance before an activity, then have him self-evaluate the performance. Having the client predict his performance before an activity (self-estimation) and comparing his predicted performance with a self-evaluation of the actual performance can provide meaningful self-initiated feedback and would be the best way to increase awareness. Simply discussing the client's perceptions (answer A) would not provide concrete immediate feedback about performance. Reviewing a checklist of necessary skills, answer B, would probably not be effective in increasing awareness, since the patient feels he already possesses these skills. Answer D, ignoring the patient's perceptions, would not address the patient's therapeutic need to increase awareness and could lead to increased resistance. See reference: Pedretti (ed): Wheatley, CJ: Evaluation and treatment of cognitive dysfunction.

86. (D) arm trough. An arm trough would provide a stable surface that would keep the individual's arm in a safe and appropriate position. In addition, the arm trough approximates the humeral head into the glenoid fossa at a natural angle. If the individual has edema in his hand, a foam wedge may be placed in the trough to elevate the hand. A lap tray (answer A) would provide support but is more restrictive than an arm trough, which should be attempted first. The fact that the individual's arm was seen dangling by the side of the wheelchair indicates that the wheel-

chair armrest alone (answer B) is inadequate. Answer C, an arm sling, would provide support for his arm but would immobilize it in adduction and internal rotation, an undesirable position. Current literature supports the use of slings only when necessary, such as during ambulation when a flaccid upper extremity may sublux or cause loss of balance. See reference: Pedretti (ed): Pedretti, LW, Smith, JA, and Pendelton, HM: Cerebral vascular accident.

87. (D) incoordination. A person with tremors or poor coordination can reduce instability by stabilizing the limb proximally before working distally. Stabilization adds a secure base of support from which to work. Reduced vision, poor endurance, and limited fine movement (answers A, B, and C) do not require stabilization when writing; the effects of these deficits can be reduced by the use of paper with high-contrast guiding lines, more frequent rests, or built-up writing tools. See reference: Trombly (ed): Retraining basic and instrumental activities of daily living.

88. (B) Bingo Luck is the key element in games of chance. Bingo is a game whose outcome depends on the calling out of random numbers. Collecting baseball cards (answer A) is a hobby. Charades and balloon volleyball (answers C and D) are games based on strategy and skill. See reference: Early: Leisure skills.

89. (B) Encouraging any available hemiplegic limb movements before or during a task Any contralesional limb movement (even shoulder elevation) will activate additional motor units which will then increase attention to the left. Bilateral activities (answer A) may reduce attention to the left by inhibiting function of the affected hemisphere. Activities that do not cross the midline (answer C), and activities that focus on the uninvolved side of the body (answer D) only reinforce neglect of the involved side of the body. See reference: Unsworth (ed): Evaluation and intervention with unilateral neglect.

90. (C) Change to a power wheelchair to reduce effort. Considering the progressive nature of the child's disease, as well as strength and endurance, the best recommendation would be to change to a power wheelchair. The child would be better able to participate in the cognitive tasks of school if less effort was required for mobility. Answer A, retaining the manual chair, would be counterproductive to functioning well at school, and strength will not be improved with this child's condition. Answer B might make mobility a little easier but will not solve the long-term problem of decreasing strength and endurance. Answer D would still make demands on strength and energy that would appear unwise considering the nature of Duchenne muscular dystrophy. The team's recommendation should also be integrated with the family's needs and resources. See reference: Case-Smith (ed): Case-Smith, J, Rogers,

J, and Johnson, JH: School-based occupational therapy.

91. (C) Repeatedly squeeze with the hand against increasing amounts of resistance. The biomechanical approach is a treatment approach used when a person has a deficit in strength, endurance, or range of motion but has voluntary muscle control during performance of activities. The biomechanical approach focuses on decreasing the deficit area to improve the person's performance of daily activities. Eliciting functional grasp using reflex inhibiting postures (answer A) is an example of a neurophysiologic approach, which emphasizes an understanding of the nervous system in a person with brain damage and how to elicit a desired response from that person. Muscles can be stimulated through a variety of neurodevelopmental techniques (answer B), using an understanding of the nervous system to elicit a response in a developmental sequence. Building up utensils (answer D) is an example of the rehabilitative approach, which teaches a person how to compensate for a deficit on either a temporary or permanent basis. See reference: Trombly (ed): Zemke: Remediating biomechanical and physiological impairments of motor performance.

92. (B) selective attention. The client demonstrated difficulty in attending to the activity because the presence of other environmental stimuli was distracting. This suggests a deficit in selective or focused attention. The client's performance of the activity provides no observable information about learning (answer A) or problem solving skill (answer D). Since the client visually located the brush initially, the problem would not be perceptual in nature, so answer C, figure-ground perception is not correct. See reference: Unsworth (ed): Unsworth, C: Evaluation and intervention with concentration impairment.

93. (D) unexplained sensory loss. The major signs of shunt malfunction in children are irritability, nausea and vomiting, irritability, changes in behavior or school performance, fever, pallor, visual perceptual difficulties, and headaches. Answers A, B and C are incorrect. See reference: Solomon (ed): Parker, GE: Other common pediatric disorders.

94. (C) Use a board game to introduce the concept of receiving and spending money. This activity provides an opportunity for the individuals to experience the value and purpose of money. Although it is important to introduce the actual value of coins and paper money, it is essential to combine this with concrete applications. Answers A, B, and D are examples of graded activities to be used after the initial introduction of money concepts. See reference: Early: Activities of daily living.

95. (C) Assertiveness training Broken record is a specific assertiveness skill concerned with repeating your position without losing control. Music therapy (answer A) is a creative arts discipline. Psychodrama (answer D) is a group technique for expressing catharsis. Self-awareness groups (answer B) tend to focus on feeling identification and expression versus skill building. See reference: Posthuma: Process and leadership.

96. (A) checking for irritation and pressure problems. Because a toddler cannot communicate discomfort effectively, skin irritation may go unnoticed for too long. A young child, therefore, is at higher risk for developing skin and pressure problems than an older, more verbal one. Although answers B, C, and D describe important factors in splint care, for the young child, primary emphasis should be placed on answer A. See reference: Case-Smith (ed): Exner, CE: Development of hand skills.

97. (C) anxiety and confusion among group members. It is important for group leaders to demonstrate consistency by showing the same degree of respect, interest, and authority toward every group member. Overdependence (answer A) would be a result of the group leader's not giving group members enough autonomy. Group members know what to expect from the group leader (answer B) when the group leader demonstrates consistent behavior. Too much (answer D), too little, or inappropriate praise are aspects of nurturing behavior, which support growth and development of group members. See reference: Early: Group concepts and techniques.

98. (D) A buttonhook attached to a cuff that fits around the palm Individuals with C6 quadriplegia may have a tenodesis grasp or no grasp at all available to them. Therefore, a buttonhook that fits onto the palm or a buttonhook with a built-up handle are the only appropriate choices. A buttonhook with a knob handle (answer B) or on a 5-inch dowel (answer C) is appropriate for an individual with a functional grasp but limited dexterity. A buttonhook with an extra-long, flexible handle benefits an individual with limited range of motion. See reference: Trombly (ed): Trombly, CA: Retraining basic and instrumental activities of daily living.

99. (B) Help the child develop cognitive strategies for anxiety-producing activities. Children with innate temperament problems need cognitive strategies to help them to overcome anxiety in order to approach and participate in activities. Parents need to understand the innate temperament problem and the discomfort the child feels during activities, and limit setting (answer A) will not promote understanding. Children find a predictable routine helpful when activities are disorganized, so answer C is not correct. Answer D is not correct because the parent and child need to learn mutual play in an environment that promotes positive engagement. See reference: Kramer and Hinojosa (eds): Olson, LJ: Psychosocial frame of reference.

100. (A) Begin with activities that have obvious solutions and a high probability of success and then gradually increase the level of complexity. Beginning with activities that have obvious solutions and are successful and gradually increase in complexity is an effective method for developing problem-solving skills. Sensorimotor activities (answer B) in a group can facilitate self-awareness. Increasing the time (answer D) facilitates attention span improvement. Activities that require interactions with others (answer C) are useful for developing social conduct and interpersonal skills See reference: Early: Analyzing, adapting and grading activities.

101. (B) A mobile arm support A C5 quadriplegic with fair shoulder flexors and abductors and at least poor minus biceps, upper trapezius, and external rotators will be able to operate a mobile arm support for self-feeding and facial hygiene activities. A wrist-driven flexor hinge splint would be used for a lower level spinal cord injury (C6-C8) in which the individual had functional use of the shoulder and arm muscles and has fair plus or better wrist extension strength. This splint is indicated for individuals who lack prehension power. An electric feeder is indicated for individuals with a higher level of involvement (C4) and who demonstrate poor plus or weaker shoulder strength. Built-up utensils may be indicated for individuals with C8 or T1 injuries because they may lack the strength to tightly grasp regular utensils. See reference: Trombly (ed): Hollar, LD: Spinal cord injury.

102. (A) Identify options and the consequences of each option. Individuals are frequently resistive to changes that will affect the familiar home environment, such as moving furniture or adding medically necessary equipment. For them to accept change, their feelings and cultural attitudes and beliefs must be recognized. Then the following steps can be implemented to encourage acceptance of change: (1) identify options and the consequences of each option; (2) allow time for reflection and consideration of options (answer B); (3) practice with a "demo" device (answer C); (4) reassess the decision; (5) if acceptable, order the equipment; and (6) if rejected, document the steps taken and the reasons for rejection (answer D). See reference: Bonder and Wagner (eds): Hunt, LA: Home health care.

103. (B) decrease the effects of prolonged inactivity. Some of the main objectives of inpatient cardiac rehabilitation include decreasing the effects of prolonged inactivity, such as thromboembolism, orthostatic hypotension, and muscle atrophy; safely providing a program of monitored activity performance to maximize function; reinforcing cardiac precautions; and providing instruction in energy conservation techniques. It is acceptable and expected to

encounter fatigue (answer A) in this population after activity; however, activities that produce cardiac symptoms should be avoided. Activities that promote endurance and strength are beneficial, but range of motion (answer C) is not usually an area of concern. Most individuals do not need to relearn activities, other than applying energy conservation techniques; therefore, independent performance (answer D) is not a primary concern. See reference: Pedretti (ed): Matthews, MM, Foderaro, D, and O'Leary, S: Cardiac dysfunction.

104. (D) Make sure the child's hips are secured against the back of the seat. The hips are one of the key points of control when positioning a child. Positioning the hips securely against the back of the seat with a seat belt or an abductor wedge (or both) in the correct angle serves to break up the extensor pattern and facilitate the positioning of the other body parts (answers A, B, and C), so that the child can participate in family games. See reference: Case-Smith (ed): Wright-Ott, C, and Egilson, S: Mobility.

105. (B) flexed at all joints. When weight bearing, the fingers should be flexed at all joints (the fisted position). This preserves the tenodesis function by protecting the finger flexors from overstretching. Another reason for this position is to prevent claw-hand deformity by protecting the intrinsic hand muscles from overstretching. See reference: Pedretti (ed): Adler, C: Spinal cord injury.

106. (C) train the client in the operation of the AT system and in strategies for its use. Training activities in the use of the assistive devices are the next critical step after setup of the system, and are essential because the complex nature of assistive technologies can require many hours of practice to master. Evaluating how well the whole system works (answer A) usually occurs after training is completed during the follow-up phase. Evaluating the match between the client and the technology (answer B) is done earlier in the process to ensure maximum success and because expensive technological devices may only be ordered once. Funding sources (answer C) are also determined before ordering equipment. See reference: Pedretti (ed): Cook, AM, and Hussey, SM: Electronic assistive technologies in occupational therapy practice.

107. (A) Use pictures, music, and discussion to encourage discussion of memories. Remotivation approaches are used to encourage the expression of thoughts and feelings related to intact long-term memories. The topic should be linked to the group's past experiences and be easy to understand. The reality orientation approach is designed to maintain or improve awareness of time, situation, and place and often uses activities related to holidays and other temporal concepts (answer B). The environmental adaptation approach (answer C) promotes independence but has no relevance to remotivation. Inter-personal skills (answer D) are most effectively addressed through role-playing and discussion groups. See reference: Early: Cognitive and sensorimotor activities.

108. (D) blowing cotton balls into a target. Children with ADHD have difficulty with sustained attention and effort. Answers A, B, and C require sustained visual vigilance and involve delayed gratification. By contrast, blowing cotton balls into a target is a short-term activity with immediate reward for successful completion. This activity is therefore the most appropriate one, responding to the child's dual needs. See reference: Neistadt and Crepeau (eds): Florey, L: Psychosocial dysfunction in childhood and adolescence.

109. (D) setting personal boundaries appropriate to the therapist–patient relationship. It is important to acknowledge the individual's need for sexual expression while supporting the sense of self and identifying acceptable relationships and behaviors. Setting boundaries while accepting the individual is the most appropriate therapeutic response. Outright rejection (answer A) may cause an individual to believe he or she is sexually undesirable or unlovable. Flirting back (answer B) may imply that a sexual relationship between therapist and patient is being encouraged. Although the individual may need to know how SCI affects sexual functioning (answer C), the behavior that requires a response is not about a lack of knowledge but rather about how to appropriately express sexual interest and the need for reinforcement of a sexual identity. See reference: Pedretti (ed): Burton, GU: Issues of sexuality with physical dysfunction.

110. (B) Confront the individual's behavior: "Are you aware that your frequent interruptions prevent others from having a chance to contribute?" In general, the group leader should try answers A, C, or D before confronting the individual who is monopolizing the conversation. Answer B, confronting the behavior, is the approach that would most likely be taken after more conservative attempts have failed the practitioner. See reference: Posthuma: What to do if....

111. (A) ease the patient onto the floor, cushioning his fall. Proper body mechanics must be used when transferring patients. No one should "attempt a transfer that seems unmanageable because of the discrepancy between the patient's size and her own or because of the patient's level of dependency" (p. 294). Attempting to continue or reverse the transfer of an obese patient who has already begun to slip (answers B and C) is likely to result in injury to the OT practitioner and perhaps to the patient as well. Once the patient has started to slip, the OT practitioner should begin easing him to the floor immediately. Although calling for assis-

tance is an appropriate action, the higher-priority action is to begin easing the patient to the floor to prevent injury to the individuals involved. See reference: Trombly (ed): Trombly, CA: Retraining basic and instrumental activities of daily living.

112. (D) Low-impact aerobics three times a week for 1 hour The avoidance of activities that promote hyperextension and resistance to the joints best addresses the neuromuscular aspect of preventing further damage to arthritic joints. Answer B would be an appropriate selection for assisting an individual to cope with the potential psychosocial aspects of arthritis. Answer C, vocational retraining, would not address the neuromuscular aspect, but rather the developmental consequences of the disease. Answer A, lifting weights, is considered to be an activity that promotes hyperextension and resistance, possibly leading to increased pain, immobility, and further damage to the joints, in addition to joint pain and fatigue. See reference: Pedretti (ed): Spencer, EA: Musculoskeletal dysfunction in adults.

113. (D) Perform behavioral techniques and developmental positioning with parental observation and interaction. The NICU environment can often undermine the importance of the family. Therefore, implementing and integrating parental involvement with daily neonatal care becomes of primary importance for the carryover of learned techniques to best promote developmental acquisition. Answers B, C, and D are all family-centered strategies and are recommended for NICU intervention. However, D is clearly the optimal strategy for fostering parental observation skills, building positional and handling skills, and developing their ability to interpret and respond to their infant's behaviors. Initial chart review and updating with nursing staff (answer A) are essential assessment steps made prior to initial contact with the infant and family and is the least optimal intervention strategy to pursue with the family present. See reference: Case-Smith (ed): Hunter, JG: Neonatal Intensive Care Unit.

114. (A) practice preparing a variety of foods, using different cooking methods and recipes. Recent findings in motor learning suggest that practicing a variety of tasks in a nonsystematic but repetitive way (variable practice) can enhance learning retention and transfer of skills because the novelty introduced into the task engages more cognitive effort. The practice methods identified in answers B, C, and D focus more on systematic practice. This type of practice may result in better performance of different parts of the task, or of one task, but not in improved learning retention and skill transfer. See reference: Neistadt and Crepeau (eds): Neistadt, ME: Theories derived from learning perspectives.

115. (D) Encourage independent self-feeding and dressing skills with minimal use of adapted utensils and tools. Encouraging independent self-feeding and dressing skills with minimal use of adapted utensils and tools is the most significant ADL intervention. It is important to avoid an overreliance on adapted equipment so the client can experience full active range of motion when engaged in ADL. Answer B, instructing the client to use all forms of adaptive equipment, may interfere with the achievement of reaching full active range of motion when engaging in ADL. Answer C, the use of compression garments, is typically contraindicated with open wounds and is not implemented until wound closure. Answer D, PROM, is not considered an ADL intervention. See reference: Neistadt and Crepeau (eds): Rivers, EA, and Jordan, CL: Skin system dysfunction: Burns.

116. (A) work on coordinated reach in sidelying position first and then transfer the skill to sitting position. The OT practitioner should teach the skill with the child in the position in which the child can most easily learn the skill and then teach the child to transfer the skill to a more functional position. Answer B addresses a limitation in range of motion; answer C is a strategy for dealing with a visual impairment; and answer D pertains to behavioral and cognitive issues, none of which were mentioned as concerns for this child. See reference: Case-Smith (ed): Exner, CE: Development of hand skills.

117. (A) are more easily performed if coordinated with consistent timing of medications. A patient with Parkinson's needs to learn to use the period of reduced symptoms and improved mobility resulting from medication use to best advantage for performing ADL. Medications taken regularly and consistently aid the establishment of routines for self-care. Performance of self-care activities before medications (answer B) and stretched out throughout the day (answer D) would not make best use of the medication's positive effects. Answer C is incorrect because it discourages attempts at independent functioning. See reference: Pedretti (ed): Hooks, ME: Parkinson's disease.

118. (D) hold him firmly when picking him up. Holding the child firmly inhibits responses to light touch, which are usually uncomfortable for children with tactile defensiveness. Tickling (answer A) and light stroking (answer C) are also uncomfortable or intolerable for a child with tactile defensiveness. A strong stimulus such as loud music causes further startling and discomfort during a time when the child is MOST vulnerable to the sensation of light touch (i.e., when clothing is being removed). See reference: Case-Smith (ed): Parham, LD, and Mailloux, Z: Sensory integration.

119. (C) Toothpaste with a flip-open cap An individual with fine motor incoordination would be able to manage a toothpaste cap that flips open much more easily than a cap that must be removed completely from the tube. Also, toothpaste tubes with flip-open caps are larger in diameter, which make them easier to manage. A wash mitt (answer A) and a toothbrush with a built-up handle (answer D) are good options for those with weak grasp. Spray deodorant (answer B) has a small button to push, which would be difficult to operate for someone with incoordination. See reference: Pedretti (ed): Foti, D, Pedretti, LW, and Lillie, SM: Activities of daily living.

120. (D) instruction in how to perform the activities safely. Instructing caregivers in methods that promote safe performance of functional activities, such as locking wheelchair brakes before standing up, is the first focus for caregiver training. Answers A, B, and C are also useful areas of caregiver instruction, however, safety is the first priority. See reference: Neistadt and Crepeau (eds): Hom, MB, Rogers, JC, and James, AB: Treatment of activities of daily living.

121. (D) provide a stockinet for the individual to wear inside the splint. A stockinet liner worn inside the splint keeps the perspiration from irritating the skin by absorbing the perspiration and keeping the skin away from the damp plastic. A stockinet liner is inexpensive enough to have several, so the individual can always have a clean one available. Answer A, putting talcum powder in a splint, works well with a small splint, but in a large splint would require a larger amount, and feel muddy when an individual perspires. Answer B, moleskin as a liner, does not clean well after wearing for a short time, and although it may be comfortable, it usually is discarded because of the soiled appearance and smell. Answer C, an individual using a splint made with perforated material, will continue to have perspiration and will need to use another method to keep the damp plastic from irritating the skin. See reference: Ryan (ed): The Certified Occupational Therapy Assistant: Schober-Branigan, P: Thermoplastic splinting of the hand.

122. (B) have the child practice tying her shoes at home as well as in school. Children with mental retardation often have difficulty generalizing learning from one setting to another. For instance, they learn to tie their shoes in the OT clinic but are unable to perform the same skill at home or at school. The ability to generalize is essential in making the new skill functional in this child's daily life. Answers A, C, and D are adaptations or teaching techniques that do not address generalization. See reference: Logigian and Ward (eds): Ward, JD: Mental retardation.

123. (D) continuous reinforcement of correct responses. Continuous reinforcement is provided every time the correct behavior occurs. Continuous reinforcement is helpful with learning of new behaviors. Time-based and intermittent reinforcement (answers A, B, and C) are best for maintaining behaviors. See reference: Pedretti (ed): Pedretti, LW, and Umphred, DA: Motor learning and teaching activities in occupational therapy.

124. (B) A resting pan splint A resting pan splint is the most appropriate splint to fabricate for the maintenance of a functional hand position. Answers A, C, and D are all inappropriate for the requests made by the referral. See reference: Pedretti (ed): Belkin, J, and English, CB: Orthotics.

125. (D) Just before discharge Because the prognosis for patients with Guillain-Barré syndrome is usually good, equipment should be ordered just before discharge to accurately determine the individual's needs. Equipment ordered during the first week of therapy or as soon as approved (answers B and C) may not be necessary by the time the individual is discharged. Although collaborating with the patient and family on decisions about ordering equipment is essential, acceptance of the disability (answer A) may not necessarily correspond with the appropriate time for ordering equipment. See reference: Pedretti (ed): McCormack, GL, and Pedretti, LW: Motor unit dysfunction.

126. (A) rote repetition of the task substeps with gradually fading cues. Functional skill training focuses on mastery of a specific task. It requires the client to repeatedly practice the substeps of a task with the number of cues given for each step gradually decreased or faded. Answer B, fine-motor activities, is incorrect because the functional training approach does not emphasize underlying performance components. Answer C, caregiver training, and answer D, use of instructional cards, represent adaptation and compensation approaches, rather than actual skill training. See reference: Neistadt and Crepeau (eds): Toglia, JP: Cognitive-perceptual retraining and rehabilitation.

127. (B) educate employees about ergonomic adaptations including correct typing techniques, posture, hand positioning, and equipment modification. Educating employees on correct positioning and equipment modification would be an effective way to introduce this population to a change in task methods related to keyboarding which may prevent CTD. Answers A, C, and D are incorrect because they represent interventions that might occur at some point following the onset of CTD. See reference: Pedretti (ed): Kasch, MC: Hand injuries.

128. (D) Give the individual a rest break. Fatigue may cause additional structural damage in the acute stage of MS and should be avoided. Rest breaks need to be scheduled to avoid fatigue. Strengthening activities (answer C) do not need to be discontinued but should be designed to benefit the patient without causing undue fatigue. See reference: Dutton: Biomechanical postulates regarding intervention.

129. (C) Handle the child slowly and gently. Answer C is correct because the child with hypertonicity will be most relaxed and easier to handle if tone is inhibited by the OT practitioner's slow and gentle handling of the body. Answer A is incorrect because adaptive equipment is frequently needed to provide a child with a sense of security during bathing. Answer B is not correct because an explanation of the procedures also increases a parent and child's sense of security during bathing. Answer D is not correct because it provides the parent with a poor model of good body mechanics; rather, the practitioner should kneel or sit on a stool. See reference: Case-Smith (ed): Shepherd, J: Self-care and adaptations for independent living.

130. (B) Playing Velcro checkers to tolerance Gentle, repetitive, resistive exercises help maintain strength and endurance in weakened muscles. A wrist support (answer A) compensates for loss of muscle strength but does not help to maintain strength. Exercising without resistance once a day (answer C) will not help maintain strength either. Exercising against maximal resistance (answer D) is contraindicated for individuals with ALS. See reference: Dutton: Biomechanical postulates regarding intervention.

131. (C) take the bottom, supine position. This position requires the least amount of energy expenditure and should be recommended. In addition, the therapist may encourage experimentation with a variety of positions (answer D). Timing sex for times when there is most energy would also be beneficial, but the individual will most likely be more fatigued at the end of the day (answer A). See reference: Pedretti (ed): Burton, GU: Issues of sexuality with physical dysfunction.

132. (C) Provide project samples for clients to duplicate. Individuals functioning at cognitive level 4 are able to copy demonstrated directions presented one step at a time. They find it easier to copy a sample than to follow directions or diagrams. Individuals functioning at cognitive level 3 are capable of using their hands for simple, repetitive tasks (answer A) but are unlikely to produce a consistent end product. Those functioning at cognitive level 5 can generally perform a task involving three familiar steps and one new one (answer B). Individuals functioning at cognitive level 6 can anticipate errors and plan ways to avoid them. These individual would be capable of following written directions (answer D). See reference: Early: Some practice models for occupational therapy in mental health.

133. (D) Place dishes near the dishwasher, bend down on one or both knees, and load. Bending down on one or both knees increases balance while reducing the need to bend at the waist. Answer A, loading from a standing position, is the traditional method of loading a dishwasher, and it increases bending at the waist. Answer B, washing the dishes in the sink, does not address the most effective way to alleviate back pain when actually loading the dishwasher. Answer C, standing in front of the dishwasher and loading, is similar to answer A in that trunk rotation and flexion are required to effectively perform the activity. See reference: Pedretti (ed): Smithline, J: Low back pain.

134. (B) edema. Contrast baths cause vasodilation and vasoconstriction, which facilitate a pumping out of the edema. Retrograde massage assists with the facilitation of blood and lymph movement. Pressure wraps (coban) are applied distal to proximal to address edema issues. Answers C and D, wound healing and scar management, may be contraindicated for these techniques because of possible inadequate wound closure and the potential for skin breakdown. Answer A, heterotopic ossification, is typically treated with gentle active range of motion within the pain free range and is often treated surgically. See reference: Pedretti (ed): Kasch, MC: Hand injuries.

135. (A) set the climate, provide structure, and offer support. Answer A reflects typical leadership involvement in OT groups. Answer B is incorrect because it reflects minimal direction from the leader that is not characteristic of OT groups. Answer C is incorrect because the group leader performs these functions but at the termination stage, rather than the initial stages of the group. Working individually with group members (answer D) is incongruous with current OT group treatment formats that use properties of the group to achieve therapeutic goals. See reference: Neistadt and Crepeau (eds): Schwartzberg, SL: Group process.

136. (B) temperature and pain. The sensations of pain and temperature are carried along small, unmyelinated nerve fibers, which recover more rapidly than senses carried by larger, myelinated fibers. The sensations of pain and temperature are also part of the protective or primary sensory systems, which are the receivers of simple information. More complex information is carried through the discriminative or epicritic system. The senses carried on this system are vibration, light touch, proprioception, and tactile localization. See reference: Trombly (ed): Bentzel, K: Evaluation of sensation.

137. (B) Dry cereals with milk Foods selected for this child's diet should reflect the current skill level. To increase oral tolerance and control of food, textures are gradually modified from smooth and consistent (answer C) to smooth and slightly varied (answers A and D), to increasingly resistive foods and a combination of contrasts, for example, hard and crunchy mixed with soft or liquid (answer B). After the child has mastered this level of control and tolerance, he or she can safely proceed to an even greater variety of textures, tastes, and temperatures offered at family meals. See reference: Case-Smith (ed): Case-Smith, J, and Humphry, R: Feeding intervention.

138. (C) Folding laundry Sorting and folding laundry (answer C) challenges balance and upper extremity function in ways that are more functional than stacking cones or throwing a ball. Rather than seeking contrived activities (answers A, B, C) that challenge single-component deficits, the focus of home care is to find ways for the patient to actually perform the daily activities that are presenting the challenges. Because this patient is the mother of four, it is presumed that her occupational role includes homemaking activities. See reference: Piersol and Ehrlich (eds): Seibert, C: The clinic called home.

139. (B) Back up the body to the passenger seat, hold onto a stable section of the car, extend the involved leg, and slowly sit in the car. This is the safest way to perform a car transfer after surgery for a total hip replacement. Answers A, C, and D would all be contraindicated and are not representative of total hip precautions. See reference: Pedretti (ed): Adler, C, and Tipton-Burton, M: Wheelchair assessment and transfers.

140. (C) Pencil gripper These are all adaptive devices that can be used with a child who has JRA for various reasons. However, the correct answer is C because the pencil gripper will probably make grasping the pencil easier and reduce hand grasp fatigue. Because of hand weakness and because printing and handwriting are common tasks for children this age, it is important that fatigue be reduced. The reacher (answer A) frequently requires grasp strength and is useful for children who have problems with extended reach. The jar opener (answer B) is a useful tool for individuals with hand weakness, but opening jars is not a task frequently performed by school-age children. The plate guard (answer D) is a useful device for those with incoordination or one-handedness but is not particularly necessary when hand strength is decreased (adapting the utensil would be more reasonable). See reference: Case-Smith (ed): Rogers, SL, Gordon, CY, Schanzenbacher, KE, and Case-Smith, J: Common diagnoses is pediatric occupational therapy practice.

141. (C) lateral trunk supports. Lateral trunk supports would help maintain correct alignment of the pelvis and trunk in the wheelchair. Answer A, a reclining wheelchair, would shift the individual's weight posteriorly but would not prevent lateral shifting of the trunk. One arm trough (answer B) would probably contribute to lateral shifting, although bilateral arm troughs or a lapboard could help maintain a more centered trunk position. Lateral pelvic supports (answer D) would stabilize the pelvis and prevent it from shifting sideways but would be too low to prevent the trunk from moving laterally. See reference: Pedretti (ed): Adler, C, and Tipton-Burton, M: Wheelchair assessment and transfers.

142. (B) block hyperextension of the MCP joints and allow MCP flexion. An ulnar nerve splint's primary purpose is to support the hand secondary to ulnar intrinsic muscle paralysis. This splint also allows for MCP flexion. Answers A, C, and D are all inappropriate techniques for fabricating an ulnar nerve splint. See reference: Pedretti (ed): Kasch, MC: Hand injuries.

143. (C) Incorporating simple, familiar activities such as hanging up clothing or catching a ball. Incorporating simple activities would be most effective for gaining active cooperation participation from a person with Alzheimer's. Telling the person to perform repetitions of active exercises (answer A) might not be effective because the patient may not be able to remember to perform repetitions of exercises or may not understand the purpose and become confused. Training in the use of adaptive devices would not increase active shoulder motion and could be confusing if cognitive deficits were present (answer B). PROM exercises (answer D) would not lead to improvement of active range of motion. See reference: Hellen: Communication: Understanding and being understood.

144. (D) having him place his feet through loops of therapeutic band. A prefunctional activity is when an individual is unable to perform a specific task, so an activity is used that practices the same movement as placing his feet into his pants legs. Activities that teach him to pull his pants up (answers A and B) do not practice the same skill, and removing socks (answer C) is an activity that practices the opposite skill, removing feet from something. The other choices are also functional tasks that practice a specific skill. A prefunctional activity provides a base to improve a functional activity and may be practiced before or at the same time as a functional task. See reference: Neistadt and Crepeau (eds): Holm, MB, Rogers, JC, and James, AB: Treatment of activities of daily living.

145. (B) (1) position shirt on lap; (2) place left hand into sleeve and pull up sleeve past elbow; (3) place right hand into sleeve and pull up sleeve; (4) pull shirt up over head. Answer B would be the best sequence because positioning the shirt first on the lap may provide cues for patients with unilateral neglect. Starting with the left side allows the unaffected right hand to perform the first part of the task successfully and requires the eyes to then scan to the left to locate the left arm. Answers A, C, and D are all examples of sequences that are less likely to be successful. See reference: Pedretti (ed): Foti, D, Pedretti, LW, and Lillie, S: Activities of daily living.

146. (D) remove scatter rugs throughout the house. The client would face the greatest safety hazard from the presence of scatter rugs in the house, which could cause the client with shuffling gait to trip and fall. Persons with Parkinson's disease are at high risk for falls. Answer A, increasing illumination

in hallways, would be more important if the client had low vision. Answer B, screening out distracting stimuli, and answer C, placing door locks higher or lower than eye level, are safety adaptations made for persons with cognitive deficits, rather than motor deficits. See reference: Neistadt and Crepeau (eds): Griswold, LA: Community-based practice area.

147. (D) Cut the paper in two following a straight line Scissors skills develop from first cutting snips to cutting a single straight line. The ability to cut heavier materials such as cardboard and cloth (answer A) develops last in the sequence of scissors skills. The ability to cut along curved lines (answer B) develops after the ability to cut a straight line. The ability to cut along straight lines with enough control to cut a triangle (answer C) develops after the ability to cut a single straight line and before the ability to cut a curved line. See reference: Case-Smith (ed): Exner, CE: Development of hand skills.

148. (C) National Alliance for the Mentally Ill This is a support group that is open to clients and families and focuses on education and support related to all mental illnesses. Al-Anon (answer A) is a support group for alcohol use among family members. Family therapy (answer B) is not a support group. Recovery, Inc. (answer D) is a self-help support group for clients with mental disorders. See reference: Early: Who is the consumer?.

149. (B) Raise the toilet The minimum doorway width that allows a standard wheelchair to pass through easily is 32 inches. A standard toilet is 15 inches, which is 3 inches lower than the standard wheelchair seat. Raising the toilet 18 inches would make transfers easier for this individual. See reference: Neistadt and Crepeau (eds): Holm, MB, Rogers, JC, and Stone, RG: Person-task-environment intervention: a decision-making guide.

150. (A) "Jaw opening and closing are controlled with your index and middle fingers; place your thumb on the child's cheek." The correct position of the adult's hand for jaw control is as described in answer A when the child is fed from the side. Answers B and D are incorrect because the thumb should be placed on the cheek to provide joint stability. Answer C is incorrect because controlling the child's jaw movement with the adult's whole hand provides less control of the child's jaw than the recommended method. Placing the adult's thumb on the ear (answer D) is also incorrect because of discomfort for the child and because thumb placement should be near the fulcrum of jaw movement (at the temporomandibular joint). If the child is fed from the front, the adult's thumb is placed on the chin, with middle finger under the chin to control opening and closing of the jaw. The index finger then rests on the side of the child's face to provide stability. See reference: Case-Smith (ed): Case-Smith, J, and Humphry, R: Feeding intervention.

151. (D) The individual asks for more beverages during meals, but appears surprised when the therapist indicates beverages in closed containers are on the meal tray. The subjective portion of the SOAP note should contain information that is gained through a chart review, or communication with the patient, his or her family, or staff. This information is not measurable and therefore is considered subjective. Answer A would be in the program plan. Answers B and C would be in the objective portion because they are either measurable or based on specific observations. See reference: Trombly (ed): Trombly, CA: Planning, guiding, and documenting therapy.

152. (B) the potential for depression and low self-esteem. The potential for depression and low self-esteem is commonly associated with the long-term psychological mode of recovery. Answer A, the possibility of decreased range of motion and sensation, is a physical response to a burn. Answers C and D are psychological reactions typically associated with the early and intermediate stages of recovery. See reference: Richard and Staley (eds): Moss, BF, Everett, JJ, and Patterson, DR: Psychologic support and pain management of the burn patient.

153. (C) Preparing a can of soup The Rehabilitation Institute of Chicago identified five levels of complexity for meal preparation ranging from easiest (level one) to hardest (level five). Preparing macaroni and cheese, a hot one-dish meal, falls into the fourth level. Because the individual is unable to successfully perform at this level, the task must be downgraded to the next lowest level, three, which includes preparation of hot beverages, soups, or frozen dinners. Having the individual prepare a multicourse meal such as chicken and mashed potatoes (answer A) would be upgrading the activity to level five. Cold meals and foods such as instant pudding and peanut butter and jelly sandwiches (answers B and D) are at level two; downgrading to this level would be appropriate if the individual had experienced significant difficulty. See reference: Neistadt and Crepeau (eds): Culler, KH. Treatment for work and productive activities: home and family management.

154. (A) whether the areas of concern to the OT interfere with the child's education. Related services are defined as services needed to help a student benefit from education. If the student's disability no longer interferes with education, OT as a related service can be discontinued. Functional skills (answer B) and ADL (answer C) may be ongoing goals in therapy as provided in a rehab setting or hospital but would not be provided as a related service in the schools. Accessibility of the learning environment (answer D) is an important concern, but it would be covered in consultation with the school or teacher, not through direct service provision. See reference: Case-Smith (ed): Case-Smith, J, Rogers, J, and Johnson, JH: School-based occupational therapy.

155. (B) evaluate the individual's occupational performance. Discharge planning in short-term hospitalizations should begin at admission. The OT practitioner's evaluation of occupational performance is the first step in the OT discharge planning. Answers A, C, and D would all occur later in the treatment process. See reference: Early: Treatment settings.

156. (C) increase swimming time to 25 minutes or to tolerance. This individual's goal is to maximize strength and endurance. Although ALS is a progressive degenerative disease, improvements in strength and endurance are possible if the individual was not previously functioning at maximum capacity. This individual's performance indicates potential for further improvement. The program should therefore be upgraded, not downgraded (answer B). Methods for improving endurance include increasing the frequency, intensity, or duration of the activity. The correct answer (C) increases the duration of the activity while recognizing the importance of avoiding fatigue. Answer A continues the program at a maintenance level. Using adaptive equipment (answer D), such as a flotation belt, is an energy-saving strategy that would be appropriate if the individual were experiencing fatigue during swimming. See reference: Dutton: Biomechanical postulates regarding intervention.

157. (C) Following directions about objects located in front, in back, and to the side. Answer C is correct because a deficit in position in space refers to difficulty in perceiving the relationship of an object to the self. Answer A, identifying letters on a distracting page, is not correct because it refers to a problem of size and shape (form) constancy. Answer D, making judgments about moving through space, is incorrect because it refers to a problem in perceiving spatial relationships. See reference: Case-Smith (ed): Schneck, CM: Visual perception.

158. (D) installation of a bidet with a spray wash and air-drying mechanism. Use of a bidet for hygiene after use of the toilet eliminates any upper-extremity reach requirement. Answers A, B, and C describe adaptations appropriate for a child with poor postural control in need of external stability devices; these devices would not reduce reach requirements. See reference: Case-Smith (ed): Shepherd, J: Self-care and adaptations for independent living.

159. (B) "Client will draw for 1 hour, taking stretch breaks every 20 minutes." Goals should be functional, measurable, and objective. This answer meets those criteria. Answer A is not measurable. "Goals need to be written to show what the patient will accomplish, not what the [OT practitioner] will do" (p. 94). Answers C and D describe what the OT practitioner will do. See reference: AOTA: Effective documentation for occupational therapy.

160. (C) liquid and solids combined (minestrone

soup). Answer C is correct because it combines two food consistencies. Liquids are very difficult for children with poor oral motor organization to manage in eating. When solids are added to the liquid, the child will have difficulty managing two different forms of food. Answers A, B, and D, depending on the child's oral motor skills, are easier to move and manage within the mouth. See reference: Case-Smith (ed): Case-Smith, J, and Humphry, R: Feeding intervention.

161. (A) check the alignment of the goniometer. If the goniometer is not aligned correctly, any joint measurements will demonstrate a discrepancy. A variability of 5 degrees is normal between two different evaluators, and may be that much less on a retest by the same therapist. Changing the size of the goniometer to larger (answer B) or smaller (answer C) during measurements could make the discrepancy greater, because it could make aligning the arms of the goniometer with the landmarks more difficult. It is much faster to check the alignment of the goniometer first when using one of the proper length for the job. Forcing the individual's arm further into flexion (answer D) would be painful to the individual because measurements are taken at the end of the individual's full range of motion and the joint would be unable to go further. See reference: Norkin and White: Procedures.

162. (B) "Pt. was initially able to work at the computer for only 10 minutes. Upon discharge, he can work at the computer for 3 hours with stretch breaks every 30 minutes." The objective section of the discharge summary should summarize the patient's condition upon discharge from the facility and "summarize the patient's stay" (p. 49). Some facilities compare initial and final evaluations while others only address progress from the time of the previous note. Answers A and D are subjective reports. Answer C is an example of a statement that belongs in the assessment section of a discharge summary. See reference: Borcherding: Writing the "O"—objective.

163. (A) Describe the treatment received According to the 1991 *Role Delineations for OTRs and COTAs*, COTAs can record factual information at the time of discharge. Making referrals to outside agencies, comparing initial and final status, and independently making follow-up plans are not within the entry-level COTAs responsibilities. See reference: Early: Medical records and documentation.

164. (A) Remove all throw or scatter rugs Regardless of whether an individual with instability walks with the help of a walker, cane, or no equipment, the floor should be cleared of any obstacles that could cause him or her to slip or trip. Scatter or throw rugs may catch on a person's foot or on the tip of an assistive device. Rugs also may not be firmly taped down or secured with nonskid backing, causing a safety hazard. Installing lever handles, a ramp, or a handheld shower would make certain tasks easier for a patient, but they would not be necessary for safety. See reference: Ryan (ed): Practice Issues in Occupational Therapy: Gower, D, and Bowker, M: The elderly with a hip arthroplasty.

165. (B) "The patient has not accused any men of attacking her this week." The number of times the patient demonstrates one aspect of paranoid behavior (fear of men) is objectively stated in the correct answer. Answer A indicates improvement, but does not provide substantiation for the statement. Answer C may be indicative of improved interpersonal skills and self-esteem but does not reflect decreased paranoid behavior. Answer D is a statement of a goal, not of improvement. See reference: Early: Medical records and documentation.

166. (C) "Patient is demonstrating gradual improvement in fine-motor coordination." The assessment portion of the note "contains the analysis of plans and goals for the patient ... and involves the professional judgment of the therapists" (p. 110). It is also where the OT practitioner draws conclusions and justifies decisions. The objective portion of the SOAP note should contain information that is measurable or based on specific observations (answer A). The subjective portion contains information gained from communication with the patient, his or her family (answers B and D), or other staff members. This information is not measurable and therefore is considered subjective. See reference: Kettenbach: Writing assessment (A).

167. (A) Instruct the individual to wear clothes for 2 days and to then launder those items. Teaching the individual to recognize and judge when clothing needs to be laundered has been unsuccessful, indicating that the individual may not have the capacity to learn this skill. If the OT practitioner determines that the individual can usually wear clothes for 2 days before they need to be laundered, then providing a rigid schedule based on this average removes the need for judgment and provides a schedule that will result in the individual's wearing clean clothes at least most of the time, if not always. Assessment of the individual's clothing management capabilities (answer B) would have been performed before the implementation of the initial intervention. Taking the clothes to the dry cleaner (answer C) would be cost prohibitive and would still require judgment to determine when they needed to be cleaned. Turning the responsibility over to the staff (answer D) would not promote independence in clothing management for the individual. See reference: Bruce and Borg: Cognitive disability frame of reference.

168. (B) Incorporate therapeutic activities into family routines. "Suggestions that the family can incorporate into the daily routine are the most successful" (p. 722). Separate "therapeutic activities" (answers A and D) can take up an excessive amount of time and energy and may interfere with family life; therefore long-term follow-through may not be as effective as when activities can be made to fit the existing daily routines and developed into habits. Activities provided on an as-needed basis (answer C) will never become habits, and therefore follow-through is less effective. See reference: Case-Smith (ed): Stephens LC, and Tauber, SK: Early intervention.

169. (D) providing OT expertise to run the program and solve problems. An OT practitioner could perform all of the functions identified. The OT consultant in this setting typically offers information and skill knowledge to both OT and non-OT staff and administration to help plan programs that meet the needs of the clients. Answer A, evaluating clients, would be the function of the OT direct-care clinician. Implementing activity groups would be the role of the activity program director, which could be performed by an OT practitioner. Answer C is the function of the case manager, which is one of the newer roles that an OT practitioner may perform in this setting. See reference: Larson, Stevens-Ratchford, Pedretti, and Crabtree (eds): Conyers, KH: Adult day care.

170. (A) Parkinson's disease. People with Parkinson's disease can benefit from rhythmic exercises, movement strategies, and handwriting activities. Providing these interventions in a group format is of particular benefit to this population because of the added advantage of social interaction. From a planning point of view, group treatment for this condition is also cost efficient. See reference: Neistadt and Crepeau (eds): Schwartzberg, SL: Group process.

171. (C) AC MRDD The AC MRDD stands for Accreditation Council for services for the Mentally Retarded and other Developmentally Disabled persons. JCAHO (answer A) stands for the Joint Commission of Accreditation of Hospital Organizations. The JCAHO is an agency that reviews medical care of hospitals, psychiatric facilities, hospices, long-term care agencies, and MR/DD programs seeking accreditation. CARF (answer B) stands for the Commission on Accreditation of Rehabilitation Facilities; CARF reviews programs in free-standing facilities as well as those that are part of a hospital system. The NLN/APHA stands for the National League for Nursing, American Public Health Association; the NLN/APHA surveys nursing homes. See reference: AOTA: The Occupational Therapy Manager: MacRae, N: Accreditation council on services for people with disabilities.

172. (C) Removing the threshold altogether. Removing the threshold altogether would be the simplest and safest solution. Door thresholds may have a maximum height of a half inch and these must be beveled; keeping it as it is (answer A) would provide a barrier to wheelchair accessibility and a safety hazard for people with visual deficits. Placing a throw rug to cover the threshold (answer B) would not improve accessibility and would present a slipping hazard. Because the threshold height is over a half inch, placing a ramp over the threshold (answer D) would be required if the threshold could not be removed. But the best solution would still be to remove the threshold altogether to provide the most accessible surface. See reference: Americans with Disabilities Act: ADA Accessibility Guidelines.

173. (D) outpatient counseling. Transitional programs after hospitalization offer a range or continuum of support to mental health consumers. Outpatient counseling is the least restrictive situation because it provides support through counseling but does not require any residential treatment. Answers A, B, and C are all residential programs with varying amounts of supervision. See reference: Neistadt and Crepeau (eds): Griswold, LS: Community-based practice settings.

174. (A) Pain management techniques Work-hardening programs focus on returning individuals to work in physically appropriate settings as quickly as feasible through reconditioning. As part of that program, pain management techniques (answer A) are included to assist the person with managing and coping with pain during work-related activities. A work-hardening program teaches proper body mechanics to prevent further injury rather than focusing on energy conservation (answer C), which is emphasized with individuals who need to minimize or avoid fatigue. Vocational counseling (answer D) helps individuals enhance their vocational potential and addresses skills necessary for job seeking and job acquisition. See reference: Pedretti (ed): Burt, CM, and Smith, P: Work evaluation and work hardening.

175. (C) Program evaluation Program evaluation is the compilation of the intervention results for a population of individuals. Final evaluations of clients involved in the program and client satisfaction surveys (answers A and B) may both be components of the program evaluation. Utilization review (answer D) evaluates the care that is provided to ensure that services were appropriate and not overutilized or underutilized. Utilization review also analyzes the services to ensure that the interventions were provided in an economical manner. See reference: Neistadt and Crepeau (eds): Perinchief, JM: Management of occupational therapy services.

176. (D) Meeting the vocational instructor weekly to discuss adaptations to work tasks Effective consultation involves ongoing communication that helps team members problem solve more effectively. Answers A and B are activities typically done by the vocational teacher. A vocational instructor should be able to perform assessments (answer C). See reference: Case-Smith (ed): Spencer, K: Transition services: From school to adult life.

177. (A) completing the chart reviews. An identified role of the COTA is to complete data collection records such as a record review, general observation checklist, or behavior checklist. Answers B and C suggest that the COTA is independently collecting nonstandardized data and interpreting the data. These roles are not appropriate for an assistant. A COTA can contribute to the development of a treatment plan, but it is not within the COTA scope of practice to develop treatment plans independently. See reference: AOTA: Occupational therapy roles.

178. (D) health promotion. Health promotion is the advancement of healthy lifestyles, which may include education, behavioral change, and cultural support. Answer A, occupational behavior, is the developmental continuum of play to work. Answer B, intervention, is actually the provision of treatment. Answer C, self-efficacy, would be promoting the positive effects of OT services. See reference: Christiansen and Baum (eds): Kneipmann, K: Prevention of disability and maintenance of health.

179. (B) rinse the eye with an eye wash or water immediately. It is necessary to immediately wash the eye because the "backwash" fluid in the IV is unidentifiable body fluid and universal precautions should be followed. It is recommended to flush an exposed area with warm water or normal saline immediately. Therefore, answers A, C, and D are incorrect. Following the cleansing of the eye, it is recommended to contact the immediate supervisor and report the exposure through the facility reporting system. See reference: Occupational Safety and Health Administration: Standard #1910. 1030, 1 FR 5507, February 13, 1996.

180. (A) selected tasks in which aides have been trained, with intense close supervision. To maximize efficiency and cost-effectiveness of therapy services, there has been increasing use of occupational therapy aides. Such aides must be very closely supervised and are expected to receive site specific training in selected activities determined by the supervising OT practitioner and must be utilized in accordance with state regulations. Activities and levels of supervision in answers B, C, and D are all beyond the scope of the OT aide. See reference: Neistadt and Crepeau (eds): Cohn, ES: Interdisciplinary communication and supervision of personnel.

181. (A) from a home health OTR or COTA. Home health services, which may include nursing, OT, PT and speech therapy are provided in the patient's home. Individuals who require continued care following discharge from the hospital may be appropriate for home health services if they are unable to travel to the hospital for outpatient services. If the decision to discharge the person has already been made, recommendations for a continued stay in the acute care hospital or transfer to a rehabilitation center (answer B and C) are not appropriate. The persons's

weakness and continuing requirement for intravenous drug therapy would make it extremely difficult for the patient to return to the hospital for outpatient therapy (answer D). See reference: Neistadt and Crepeau (eds): Griswold, LS: Community-based practice arenas.

182. (A) incident report. Facilities use incident reports to document incidents such as this. Although the incident may be referred to in a daily progress note (answer B), an incident report must also be filed. An incident report form includes a level of detail that may not be achieved in a letter (answer C), and a verbal report (answer D) is not a form of documentation. See reference: Ryan (ed): Practice Issues in Occupational Therapy: Jones, RA: Service operations.

183. (B) document services provided and date the note as a late entry. It is the responsibility of the OT practitioners to document services provided. After the error was found, the therapist should document the services as she recalled. Therefore, answers C and D are incorrect because they do not provide for documentation of services. Answer A is unethical in that it is not appropriate for the therapist to document the note and backdate it. See reference: AOTA: Effective documentation for occupational therapy.

184. (A) total quality management. This model "encourages health care institutions to move away from a focus on compliance to standards and refocus on improvement goals in an effort to deliver high quality care" (p. 121). Answers B, C, and D, are all concepts that contribute to the model of total quality management and include finance, marketing, and operations. See reference: Jacobs and Logigian (eds): Logigan, MK: Quality management.

185. (D) Lightweight wheelchair and hospital bed Durable medical equipment is defined by Medicare as "that which can withstand repeated use, is primarily and customarily used to serve a medical purpose, and generally is not useful to a person in the absence of illness or injury." Answers A, B, and C are incorrect because they include items that are not considered "durable medical equipment" (e.g., reachers, a shower chair, or a hand-held shower). Depending on the patient's medical condition, a bedside commode may be covered. See reference: AOTA: The Occupational Therapy Manager: Thomas, VJ: Evolving health care systems: payment for occupational therapy services.

186. (B) medical necessity. Medicare defines medical necessity as "necessary and reasonable to treat an illness or an injury or to improve the functioning of a malformed body member" (p. 583). Medicare part B does not typically cover items such as elevated toilet seats, grab bars, or adaptive equipment because they are not considered to be medically necessary. Answers A, C, and D may all be a part of the broader statement of medical necessity not pertaining to Medicare part B. See reference: AOTA: The Occupational Therapy Manager: Thomas, VJ: Evolving health care systems: Payment for occupational therapy services.

187. (B) 1 year experience. Fieldwork educators, or supervisors, may be COTAs or OTRs with a minimum of 1 year of experience. These individuals should be competent and knowledgeable and able to function as good role models. There is no similar guideline indicating the amount of experience needed to supervise level-I students. See reference: AOTA: Occupational therapy roles.

188. (A) review and update annually. The JCAHO supports a long-term ongoing emphasis on quality and therefore recommends that policies and procedures be reviewed and updated annually. Facilities that attempt to update their manual specifically for JCAHO surveys will not be able to demonstrate a program of continual process assessment and improvement. Therefore, answers B and C are incorrect. Answer D is incorrect as well in that it does not allow for the manuals to be updated every year. See reference: Neistadt and Crepeau (eds): Perinchief, JM: Management of occupational therapy services.

189. (C) A physician's order identifying services to be provided. Within the home-care setting, the therapist must have a physician's order, which identifies the services that are to be provided. Following the OT's assessment, identification of deficits as well as short-term and long-term goals (answers A and B) can be established. The individual's history of the current illness (answer D) is contained within the initial assessment. See reference: Piersol and Ehrlich (eds): Zahoransky, M: The system and its players.

190. (D) all individuals with open wounds. Treating blood and body substances of all individuals as though they are contaminated is the concept of universal precautions. There are several strategies to protect employees from potential exposure. Engineering controls modify the work environment to reduce risk of exposure; for example, using sharps containers, eyewash stations, and biohazard waste containers. Work practice controls are policies that require a procedure be performed a certain way so that potential for exposure is minimized. Examples of work practice controls include the technique for disposal of sharps using only one hand and frequent handwashing during and after patient contact. Personal protective equipment, another strategy, is the use of appropriate gear to prevent contact with blood or identified bodily substances. Equipment may include goggles, masks, gowns, and gloves. Answers A, B, and C are all examples of individuals with open wounds, where exposure to blood is likely. Both the health-care provider and the patient could be placed at risk unless gloves are worn. See refer-

ence: Occupational Safety and Health Administration: Standard #1910. 1030, 1 FR 5507, February 13, 1996.

191. (A) objectives vary in each facility. Objectives are behavioral descriptors of the expectations the student will be required to achieve. Each fieldwork site is unique in the provision of OT and, therefore, the objectives may vary from site to site. Therefore, answers B, C, and D are incorrect. See reference: Neistadt and Crepeau (eds): Cohn, ES: Interdisciplinary communication and supervision of personnel.

192. (D) Program evaluation Program evaluation is a systematic collection and reporting of outcomes data to document program effectiveness and cost-efficiency. Quality assurance (answer A) identifies problems and implements corrective actions. Peer review (answer B) is the system of other service providers' assessing the provision of care to ensure appropriate interventions and documentation practices. Answer C, utilization review, is the process of analyzing the provision of services to promote the MOST economical delivery of service. See reference: Neistadt and Crepeau (eds): Perinchief, JM: Management of occupational therapy services.

193. (A) contact with supervisor once a day. The Guide for Supervision of Occupational Therapy Personnel document provides definitions for levels of supervision. Close supervision is defined as "daily, direct contact at the site of work." Other levels of supervision are routine, general, and minimal. Routine supervision is provided when direct contact is made every 2 weeks with "interim supervision occurring by other methods such as telephone or written communication." Under general supervision, contact is made monthly, answer C. Minimal supervision is provided on an "as needed" basis as in answer D. It is possible that this may be less than once a month. See reference: AOTA: Guide To Occupational Therapy Practice.

194. (C) interpreting results of assessments for the purposes of treatment planning. Interpretation of assessment results for purposes of treatment planning must be performed by the OTR. The functions noted in answers A, B, and D may all be performed by the COTA in a long-term care facility. See reference: AOTA: Occupational therapy roles.

195. (C) Make a report to appropriate authorities. In many states, the OT practitioner, as a health professional, is in the position of being a "mandated reporter" who must make a report if there is reason to believe a child has been abused. A report of the injury should be made to appropriate authorities. Answers A, B, and D delay or prevent proper assistance to a family involved in the occurrence of child abuse. All agencies serving children have policies and procedures for reporting injury in these situations. See reference: Neistadt and Crepeau (eds): Davidson, DA: Child abuse and neglect.

196. (D) reinforcement and enhancement of performance. The emphasis of OT is on performance: specifically, performance of work, play, or activities of daily living. As OTs, the focus has been on reinforcing and enhancing the execution of these occupations and the activities which are part of the occupations. Answers A, B, and C are incorrect because skill acquisition, compensation, and environmental adaptation are methods used to achieve the goal of improving performance, and are, therefore, not the primary emphasis of the profession. See reference: Christiansen and Baum (eds): Baum, C, and Christiansen, C: The occupational therapy context: Philosophy—principles—practice.

197. (D) a small group of patients who are representative of the population, with each individual meeting criteria which validate that they are a representative subset of the population. Answer D is the MOST correct answer because the question asks for a sample (subset) population (defined group of people). Answers A and B are representative of an entire population versus a subset. In research, a sample is a small subset of a group or population. The sample is to be representative of the entire population. Answer C is an example of a system used to identify members of a population to use for a random sampling. See reference: Neistadt and Crepeau (eds): Deitz, JC: Research: Discovering knowledge through systematic investigation.

198. (C) NBCOT The NBCOT grants certification to OT practitioners upon successful completion of the certification exam. Only NBCOT can revoke or suspend certification. An individual may not practice or call himself or herself an OTR or COTA if certification has been suspended or revoked, regardless of location. A state regulatory board (answer B) has jurisdiction only over individuals practicing in that particular state. The AOTA (answer A) has jurisdiction only over its members and can discipline only members. Although it may be important to report the individual to the administration of the facility (answer D), the facility cannot limit the individual's right to practice outside of the specific facility. See reference: Neistadt and Crepeau (eds): Hansen, RA: Ethics in occupational therapy.

199. (A) fail the student. Students should be evaluated at the midpoint of each level-II fieldwork experience as well as at the conclusion. The purpose of the final evaluation is to provide the student with feedback regarding performance during fieldwork as well as to document that entry-level competence has been achieved. A student who does not demonstrate entry-level competence should not be passed. Therefore, answers B, C, and D are incorrect. See reference: Neistadt and Crepeau (eds): Interdisciplinary communication and supervision of personnel.

200. (B) Do not treat the individual based on his refusal and document the interaction in the chart. As stated in principle 1 of the Code of Ethics, "the individual shall inform those people served of the nature and potential outcomes of treatment and shall respect the right of potential recipients of service to refuse treatment." Answers A and C are incorrect in that the therapist proceeded to treat the patient against his wishes. Answer D is incorrect because it does not meet with principle 3 of the Code of Ethics, "the individual shall accurately record and report information." See reference: AOTA: Occupational therapy code of ethics.

SIMULATION EXAMINATION 2

Evaluation

1. **A 4-month-old infant being seen for an OT assessment shows a strong preference for the left hand when reaching for a rattle at midline. Considering the development of dominance in normal children, the OT practitioner should conclude that:**

   A. further observation and evaluation of right-sided dysfunction is indicated.

   B. development of hand dominance is proceeding in a typical manner.

   C. hand dominance will not develop until age 1 year.

   D. unilaterality precedes bilaterality in typical development.

2. **An OT practitioner is evaluating an individual who recently sustained a cerebrovascular accident (CVA). The sensory portion of the test would be invalid for an individual with which one of the following impairments?**

   A. Expressive aphasia

   B. Receptive aphasia

   C. Agnosia

   D. Ataxia

3. **In selecting a standardized test to use with a child, an OT practitioner can assume that the test:**

   A. is valid.

   B. has normative data.

   C. has a standard format.

   D. is reliable.

4. **An OT practitioner is evaluating a client who is unable to name or demonstrate the use of common household objects. The practitioner documents this as:**

   A. apraxia.

   B. stereognosis.

   C. visual agnosia.

   D. alexia.

5. **An OT practitioner is working with a client diagnosed with a mild sprain. The client cradles her hand and appears to be hypersensitive to light touch. The individual also presents with edema, pain, shiny skin, and excessive dryness of the extremity. Based on this, the OT assumes that the client is MOST likely suffering from:**

   A. neuromas

   B. reflex sympathetic dystrophy

   C. carpal tunnel syndrome

   D. desensitization

6. **A preschool child with spastic cerebral palsy uses "bunny-hopping" for functional mobility during an OT evaluation. This indicates that a primitive pattern is being used for mobility. Which of the following reflexes is MOST likely being used by the child:**

   A. symmetrical tonic neck reflex.

   B. asymmetrical tonic neck reflex.

   C. tonic labyrinthine reflex.

   D. neck righting reflex.

7. **An OT practitioner is evaluating a young cabinetmaker who complains of sensory**

changes over the dorsal thumb and proximal phalanx of the index, long, and half of the ring finger. The practitioner will **MOST** likely suspect involvement of the:

A. ulnar nerve.
B. median nerve.
C. radial nerve.
D. brachial plexus.

8. **A child has considerable difficulty with problem solving when playing with Legos™ and becomes frustrated and gives up easily. This MOST likely indicates a problem in which area of play?**

A. Sensorimotor
B. Imaginary
C. Constructional
D. Game

9. **An individual who had a stroke is copying a picture of a clock. The drawing appears as a lopsided circle with a flat side on the left. The numbers 1 through 8 are written in numerical order around the right side of the clock. The hands are correctly drawn on the clock to represent three o'clock. The individual's performance appears to demonstrate:**

A. right hemianopsia.
B. left unilateral neglect.
C. cataracts in the left eye.
D. bitemporal hemianopia.

10. **An individual demonstrates the ability to pick up a penny from a flat surface. This represents which of the following prehension patterns?**

A. Lateral
B. Palmar
C. Tip
D. Three-jaw chuck

11. **An OT practitioner is informing a child's caregiver about when developmental milestones of childhood occupations typically occur. The therapist reports that infants sit without support for a few minutes by:**

A. 3 to 5 months of age.
B. 6 to 7 months of age.
C. 8 to 9 months of age.
D. 13 to 15 months of age.

12. **Of the following, the MOST important aspect of administering a standardized test for an OT practitioner is the use of:**

A. subjective judgment to determine how best to administer the test.
B. previous experience as a way to gauge test results.
C. stated instructions for administration and scoring.
D. practice to learn the best way to administer and score the test.

13. **As part of an initial evaluation of an individual with carpal tunnel syndrome, the OTR evaluates light touch sensation using a cotton ball. After wearing a wrist splint for 2 weeks the patient returns for a reevaluation, which the COTA performs. At this time, the MOST appropriate method for reevaluation of light touch is to use:**

A. a cotton ball.
B. an aesthesiometer.
C. Semmes-Weinstein monofilaments.
D. a pin or straightened paper clip.

14. **An OT practitioner conducting a hand assessment would use which instrument to measure the strength of the three-jaw chuck:**

A. an aesthesiometer.
B. a pinch meter.
C. a dynamometer.
D. a volumeter.

15. **Infants and preschool children with musculoskeletal disorders require ongoing examination of their upper extremity strength, coordination, and functional abilities. The OT practitioner will obtain the majority of assessment information during infancy and preschool through:**

A. assessments related to the specific diagnosis that determine hand function.
B. dynamometer and pinch meter function.
C. observation of play and hand function.
D. functional independence measures.

16. **Which of the following performance components are MOST important to consider when analyzing activities for use with adults with psychosocial problems?**

A. The amount of self-control demands, time management demands, self-expression opportunities, and interest in the activity
B. Age appropriateness, prehension patterns required, and the presence of small pieces that could be mistakenly swallowed
C. Tactile, kinesthetic, visual, and olfactory properties

D. Space requirements, equipment and supply needs, cost, and safety considerations

17. **During the evaluation of a child diagnosed with autism, the child demonstrates a craving for tactile stimulation, rubbing objects on his arms and legs. He also avoids being touched by others. The OTRs FIRST interpretation is that this is a sensory integration problem related to:**

A. poor modulation of tactile input.
B. hypersensitivity to tactile input.
C. hyposensitivity to tactile input.
D. poor modulation of proprioceptive input.

18. **An OT practitioner is treating a client who has a swallowing limitation, partly caused by the inability to receive visual and olfactory stimulation before eating. This limitation typically occurs in which stage of the swallowing process?**

A. Oral preparatory phase
B. Oral phase
C. Pharyngeal phase
D. Esophageal phase

19. **A preschooler with a diagnosis of developmental delay is very withdrawn and passive. While working on toilet skills, the child reaches out for a toothbrush and starts to brush her hair with it. The OT practitioner recognizes the PRIMARY importance of this behavior as:**

A. demonstrating attention-getting behavior.
B. a sign of cognitive limitation.
C. indicating initiative and beginning task-directed behavior.
D. demonstrating misinterpretation of cues because of a visual deficit.

20. **When a new patient is referred for psychiatric services, the COTA and OTR both review the chart. The OTR then completes performance measures, and the COTA performs an interview. The COTA/OTR team relies on the interview part of the assessment to address the individual's:**

A. diagnosis.
B. current medications.
C. ability to concentrate and solve problems.
D. view of the problem and an overall goal.

21. **An OTR observes that an individual on a pureed diet has demonstrated a gurgle or wet voice after swallowing a second**

time. The diet had not been difficult for the individual until this instance. The MOST appropriate recommendation for the OTR to make is for this person to have a:

A. videofluoroscopy.
B. diet change to include thin liquids.
C. tracheostomy.
D. regular diet.

22. **A therapist is evaluating an individual with a peripheral nerve injury for strength, range of motion, and endurance. The MOST appropriate frame of reference on which to base the evaluation is:**

A. rehabilitative frame of reference.
B. neurodevelopmental frame of reference.
C. biomechanical frame of reference.
D. psychoanalytic frame of reference.

23. **An OT practitioner is attempting to decide which type of group to institute within an acute psychiatric setting. The supervising OT suggests the directive group treatment approach because it is MOST appropriate in acute care mental health for individuals with:**

A. substance abuse problems.
B. eating disorders.
C. adjustment disorders.
D. disorganized psychosis.

24. **A toddler diagnosed with developmental delays does not finger-feed when presented with food in the clinic. The BEST way to obtain further information about his feeding skills is to:**

A. interview his parents to determine his favorite foods.
B. observe him in his home during feeding time.
C. review his chart for food allergies.
D. repeat the observation in a quiet area (in order to minimize distractions).

25. **An OT practitioner is assessing the range of motion of an individual who demonstrates internal rotation of the shoulder to 70 degrees. The practitioner would MOST likely document the patient's active range of motion as:**

A. within normal limits.
B. within functional limits (WFL).
C. hypermobility that requires further treatment.

D. limited mobility that requires further treatment.

26. **The OT practitioner is evaluating two-point discrimination in an individual with a median nerve injury. The MOST appropriate procedure is to:**
    A. apply the stimuli beginning at an area distal to the lesion progressing proximally.
    B. test the involved area first, then the uninvolved area.
    C. present test stimuli in an organized pattern to improve reliability during retesting.
    D. allow the individual unlimited time to respond.

27. **While in the hospital, a 48-year-old roofing contractor experienced extrapyramidal syndrome after being placed on neuroleptic medications. The patient is to continue taking the medication after discharge from the hospital. It is MOST important to advise the patient to:**
    A. keep time in the sun as brief as possible.
    B. avoid use of power tools and sharp instruments.
    C. get up slowly from a standing, sitting, or lying position.
    D. be aware of the dehydrating effects of caffeinated drinks and alcohol.

28. **During an initial visit with a 5-year-old child with a suspected learning disability, the OT observes the child run across the room, hop around on one foot, pick up a pencil, and draw a stick figure using a tripod grasp. When asked to complete a four-piece puzzle, the child gives up after several unsuccessful attempts. Which type of assessment would MOST effectively address this child's area of difficulty?**
    A. Fine motor
    B. Gross motor
    C. Developmental
    D. Visual perceptual

29. **In using an assessment that is "norm referenced" for children, the OT practitioner assumes that the test:**
    A. measures normal behavior of children.
    B. compares performance with a normal standard.
    C. is valid and reliable.
    D. should be used with a normal population.

30. **A patient who has had a traumatic brain injury is beginning OT. The OTR practitioner needs to assess whether this person can transfer learning from one activity to another in order to plan treatment appropriately. The MOST appropriate way for an OT to observe this learning ability would be to:**
    A. describe situations that might be unsafe and ask the patient how he would respond.
    B. give the patient a simple jigsaw puzzle to solve.
    C. have the patient get dressed in a certain way, then change the task at the next session.
    D. give the patient simple calculations to perform.

31. **The MOST appropriate assessment instrument for the OT practitioner to use for measuring range of motion of the hand is:**
    A. a goniometer.
    B. a dynamometer.
    C. a pinch meter.
    D. an aesthesiometer.

32. **A client experiences chronic pain while engaged in household chores. Because of this pain, the client avoids actions that require motor performance. OTR observes a MOTOR response to pain, as demonstrated by the patient's:**
    A. inability to concentrate on tasks because of pain.
    B. frequent complaints of aching pain.
    C. repeated protecting of the joints while moving.
    D. refusal to partake in certain ADL to prevent the accompanying pain.

33. **An OT practitioner is working with a client who has been diagnosed with borderline personality disorder. An individual with a personality disorder is MOST likely to demonstrate impaired functioning in:**
    A. activities of daily living (ADL).
    B. instrumental ADL.
    C. relationships with others.
    D. sensorimotor skills.

34. **A client who recently started using a wheelchair will be returning to work and an OTR is evaluating the client's workplace for accessibility, according to ADA guidelines. The doorway to the client's**

office has a clear opening of 28 inches. Which of the following recommendations would be the MOST appropriate to facilitate clear passage of the wheelchair through the doorway?

A. The doorway width needs to be expanded to have a minimum clear opening of 32 inches.

B. The client needs to obtain a wheelchair narrower than 28 inches.

C. The doorway width needs to be expanded to have a minimum clear opening of 45 inches.

D. The doorway width is satisfactory and needs no modification.

35. **An OT practitioner is administering a standardized test to a young client who suddenly becomes uncooperative and complains that the test is "too hard." The MOST appropriate response for the OT practitioner would be to:**

A. switch to easier items to improve the child's self-esteem.

B. terminate the session and schedule another session for the remainder of the test.

C. follow administration instructions and note changes in behavior.

D. adapt the remaining test items to ensure success.

36. **A therapist reviews an individual's chart as part of the screening process. The psychiatrist has written "observe for side effects with current antianxiety medications." The OT practitioner is MOST likely to report about which of the following side effects?**

A. akathisia

B. confusion

C. extrapyramidal syndrome

D. tardive dyskinesia

37. **An OT practitioner is performing a home management evaluation of an ambulatory individual with cerebral palsy (CP) who is cognitively intact but exhibits an ataxic gait pattern. The PRIMARY focus of the evaluation should be on:**

A. safety and stability.

B. the individual's ability to reach and bend.

C. whether the individual has adequate strength to perform homemaking tasks.

D. fatigue and endurance levels.

38. **A child avoids playground equipment that requires her feet to be off the** ground. This behavior MOST likely indicates:

A. tactile defensiveness.

B. developmental dyspraxia.

C. gravitational insecurity.

D. intolerance for motion.

39. **The OT treatment approach that will MOST likely meet the overall needs experienced by individuals with substance abuse problems is to:**

A. assist with skill development in the areas of leisure, cognition and perception, self-expression, and ADL.

B. educate the family members about making safety modifications to the kitchen area.

C. encourage Alcoholics Anonymous (AA) involvement; provide retraining of neglected ADL; explore work-related values.

D. make aftercare arrangements for vocational counseling and AA; provide time management education for self-care activities.

40. **Evaluation results for a person with arthritis will MOST accurately reflect true functional abilities if scheduled:**

A. early morning (8 to 10 A.M.).

B. afternoon.

C. late morning (10 to 11 A.M.).

D. early morning and again in the afternoon.

41. **After many months of therapy, a preschool child with Down syndrome has begun to demonstrate protective reactions when falling forward. Which of the following BEST describes the type of movement that has been demonstrated?**

A. Shoulder flexion, internal rotation, and shoulder adduction

B. Shoulder flexion and abduction and elbow extension

C. Shoulder internal rotation and elbow extension

D. Shoulder hyperextension and external rotation and elbow flexion

42. **An OT practitioner in a work-hardening program needs background information about an individual's work history. The BEST method for obtaining detailed information about the individual's job requirements is:**

A. interviewing the individual.

B. examining an analysis of the individual's job.

C. looking up the individual's job in the Dictionary of Occupational Titles.

D. requesting information from the referring physician.

43. **An OT practitioner is reviewing a patient's chart before evaluating the patient. Based on the physician's history and physical examination, the practitioner is able to identify the patient's deficits and assessments that will best assess the problem areas. This form of clinical reasoning is MOST likely an example of:**
    A. procedural reasoning.
    B. conditional reasoning.
    C. interactive reasoning.
    D. narrative reasoning.

44. **In assessing if a person is a candidate for using a mobile arm support, the OT practitioner would have to determine if the person demonstrates which of the following?**
    A. Incoordination
    B. Lateral trunk stability
    C. Fair plus elbow flexion
    D. Poor head control

Treatment Planning

45. **In planning a therapeutic dressing program for a first grade child who is mentally retarded, the therapist's FIRST consideration should be the need for:**
    A. adaptive equipment.
    B. adaptive clothing.
    C. proper positioning.
    D. adapted teaching techniques.

46. **An OT practitioner is selecting treatment activities to use with a young adult diagnosed with schizophrenia, undifferentiated type, that would help to increase the patient's ability to receive, process, and respond to sensory information. The MOST suitable activities for this patient would include:**
    A. social skills training.
    B. vestibular stimulation and gross motor exercise.
    C. role-playing.
    D. discussion group.

47. **After a radial nerve injury, an individual initially had trace muscle strength in elbow extension. One week later, strength is noted to have increased to poor**

minus. **The individual is ready for which activity?**
    A. Passively self-ranging the injured ar
    B. Extending the elbow in mid range 30 to 40 degrees with the forearm resting on the table
    C. Pushing a cup filled with pennies with the back of the hand, with arm resting on the table
    D. Lifting a book placed on the back of the hand up off the table

48. **A child has poor independent-sitting skills as a result of inadequate postural reactions. The FIRST activity the OTR would use to promote the development of independent sitting is:**
    A. swinging on a playground swing with a bucket seat.
    B. wide-base sitting on the floor while reaching for a suspended balloon.
    C. straddling a bolster swing while batting a ball.
    D. riding a hippity-hop, while using only one hand for support.

49. **An OT practitioner has been asked to develop a program of self-awareness activities for a group of substance abusers. A graded program to develop an individual's self-awareness MUST include activities that:**
    A. encourage self-awareness.
    B. are structured by the OT practitioner to encourage self-reflection and feedback.
    C. provide opportunities for the patient to be self-aware.
    D. allow for increasing social interaction.

50. **An OT practitioner is working with a child who has mild spastic cerebral palsy. The evaluation has shown that the child has poor in-hand manipulation skills. What type of activity would be BEST for practicing this ability?**
    A. Grasping blocks to build a building
    B. Placing pegs from one pegboard to another
    C. Carrying a bag of Lego™ blocks with a handle
    D. Removing a nut from a bolt

51. **An OT practitioner is fabricating a splint for an individual who has carpal tunnel syndrome. Which of the following splint fabrication techniques should be adhered to in order to allow for adequate digit motion?**

A. Trim lines of the splint should extend distal to the MCP crease.

B. Trim lines of the splint should extend proximal to the DIP joint.

C. Trim lines of the splint should extend proximal to the MCP crease.

D. Trim lines of the splint should extend distal to the ulnar 5th MCP crease.

52. **An OT practitioner is beginning training in meal preparation with a homemaker after a traumatic brain injury (TBI). The activity that should be introduced FIRST is:**

A. making a peanut butter and jelly sandwich.

B. preparing a hot cup of tea with sugar.

C. pouring a glass of orange juice.

D. cooking a grilled ham and cheese sandwich.

53. **The occupational therapist is developing a treatment plan for a child with motor planning deficits. The MOST important emphasis of motor planning activities for the child will be on activities that promote:**

A. automatic movement.

B. reflexes.

C. coordination.

D. cognitive planning.

54. **An OT practitioner wants to alter the seating arrangement of a community skills group in order to facilitate communication amongst the members. The BEST arrangement would be to:**

A. provide enough chairs around a rectangle table.

B. provide enough chairs around a round table.

C. provide enough pillows to sit on the floor.

D. use the couches and chairs that are already in the room.

55. **An individual with right unilateral neglect is able to track from the left side to the midline of the body on paper-and-pencil tasks. The BEST treatment activity for this person to work on crossing the midline to improve writing would be to:**

A. have the individual practice wheeling a wheelchair following a taped line on the floor.

B. place commonly used self-care items on the left side.

C. have the individual trace lines across the

page with the right index finger from the left to the right side.

D. place playing cards in a horizontal row from right to left in sequence.

56. **To promote play skills and self-expression in a child who is withdrawn, an OT practitioner should FIRST select activities that:**

A. promote open-ended symbolic play, such as using action figures, puppets, and dolls.

B. provide a defined structure, such as simple craft activities with instructions.

C. promote social interaction, such as a game of tag with peers.

D. provide a means of tension release, such as leather tooling or wedging clay.

57. **An OT practitioner is working with an individual with amyotrophic lateral sclerosis (ALS) who is no longer able to ambulate for kitchen or home management activities. Which of the following interventions BEST addresses the goals of independence in meal preparation for this individual?**

A. Meal preparation techniques using a wheelchair

B. Training in the use of adapted cooking equipment

C. Simple cooking activities while standing at the counter for gradually increasing amounts of time

D. Begin with cold meals and progress to hot meals

58. **An individual with Alzheimer's disease has difficulty following multiple-step instructions. Which method will the OT practitioner instruct the caregiver to use when presenting instructions?**

A. Give one- or two-step instructions frequently repeated.

B. Provide three-step instructions with gestures for demonstration.

C. Write instructions down that are over three steps for the individual.

D. Have individual verbally repeat instructions after the therapist gives them.

59. **An individual with a cognitive disability has recently joined a sheltered workshop setting and has been referred to OT for assignment to the appropriate group. The individual demonstrates the ability to copy demonstrated directions presented one step at a time and can vi-**

sualize an endproduct. However, the individual is unable to recognize errors and may not be able to correct them when they are pointed out. The MOST appropriate group for this individual is the one involved with:

A. sorting plastic utensils into separate containers.

B. assembling packets that include a knife, fork, spoon, and napkin based on a sample.

C. selecting matching shoelaces from a mixed pile and lacing them onto a display card.

D. gluing labels to cans and placing them in the appropriate container according to color.

60. **When providing occupational therapy for children who have been diagnosed with a terminal illness, the PRIMARY focus for OT intervention would be:**

A. educational activities.

B. play and self-care activities.

C. socialization activities.

D. motor activities.

61. **The goal for an adolescent with anorexia is to improve self-concept. Which component of a meal preparation activity BEST addresses this goal?**

A. Participate in a nutrition group and plan a healthy meal

B. Develop a budget and shop for ingredients with three other group members

C. Delegate tasks and prepare the meal with three other group members

D. State strengths and limitations regarding performance in the activity

62. **In establishing long-term goals for an individual with T4 paraplegia in a rehabilitation setting, the OT practitioner would MOST likely predict that the patient will attain what level of independence with bathing, dressing, and transfers?**

A. Complete independence with self-care and transfers

B. Independence with self-care and minimal assistance with transfers

C. Minimal assistance with self-care and moderate assistance with transfers

D. Dependence with both self-care and transfers

63. **A therapist is working with an individual who was admitted to an inpatient psychiatric program for major depression. This individual is also diagnosed with stage 4**

acquired immunodeficiency syndrome (AIDS). The BEST general focus of treatment at this point would be to:

A. restore and maintain functional performance of self-chosen occupations that enhance competent performance of valued occupational roles.

B. increase physical endurance and maintain desired self-care tasks.

C. facilitate resolution of current and anticipated losses through the grieving process.

D. restore and maintain functional performance of the individual's primary work role.

64. **An older adult with diabetes is working on a macramé project as a way of increasing standing tolerance. The MOST relevant safety factor for the OT practitioner to take into consideration is the:**

A. length of the cords she will start with.

B. thickness of the cords she will be using.

C. texture of the cords she will be using.

D. type of surface she will be standing on.

65. **The OT practitioner is selecting activities for an 8-year-old child with Duchenne's muscular dystrophy. Which of the following developmental issues is MOST important to consider when identifying activities for this child?**

A. Establishment of basic trust

B. Freedom to use his initiative

C. Development of self-identity

D. Reinforcement of competence

66. **An OT practitioner working in a partial hospitalization program needs to select a game that allows group members equal opportunities to win and can be played by individuals functioning at various levels. The game type that BEST suits this purpose is:**

A. games of strategy.

B. hobbies.

C. games of chance.

D. competitive games.

67. **An OT practitioner is working with a man diagnosed with schizophrenia. He states that his main goal is to have a girlfriend. Which of the following statements is the MOST appropriate example of a short-term goal?**

A. The client will develop a friendship with a female within 6 months.

B. After each group session, the client will

identify the ways in which his disability has interfered with his thinking processes.

C. The client will initiate appropriate, casual greetings when beginning casual conversations with female staff.

D. During one to two conversations with female group members, the client will make eye contact for 8 to 10 seconds, two times in each half-hour socialization group.

68. An OT practitioner is working with a client in a work program setting. What is the FIRST step to achieving the program objective of preventing reinjury within a work program?

A. Performing a prework screening

B. Learning proper body mechanics

C. Participating in work hardening

D. Engaging in vocational counseling

69. When planning a therapeutic program for a child who has deficits in visual discrimination, the FIRST step is to provide matching activities that require:

A. discrimination among the colors of objects.

B. discrimination among the shapes of objects.

C. discrimination among the positions of objects.

D. the ability to recognize objects.

70. An OT practitioner is fabricating a splint for a client who has rheumatoid arthritis. Which of the following splints is MOST appropriate for the purpose of resting the joints, decreasing pain, and preventing contractures?

A. A protective MP joint splint

B. A wrist stabilization splint

C. An ulnar drift positioning splint

D. A volar resting splint

71. An OT practitioner is using a visual perceptual frame of reference. Which of the following would be the FIRST step in planning a program for a child with visual perceptual problems?

A. Visual memory skills

B. Visual attention skills

C. General visual discrimination skills

D. Specific visual discrimination skills

72. An OT receives a consult for an infant in the neonatal intensive care unit (NICU) with a history of maternal drug abuse during pregnancy. Using a sensory inte-

grative approach, what is the FIRST action the OT should take?

A. Determine the mother's current medical status, parental involvement, and support systems.

B. Recommend a social work referral to address social concerns, provide emotional support and community program information, and make a referral to the department of human services.

C. Modify the environment to protect the infant from excessive and/or inappropriate sensory stimulation prior to direct intervention.

D. Assess motor and behavioral skills to identify areas of developmental delay in order to educate family and medical staff of necessary positional and environmental strategies for skill acquisition.

Treatment Implementation

73. After one session with a new patient in a psychosocial treatment setting, it has become apparent that the patient is highly distractible and cannot complete a magazine collage when in a group. The BEST approach for the OT practitioner to take is to:

A. speak slowly and softly to the patient.

B. coax and praise the patient until she completes the task.

C. ask the rest of the group members to stop talking.

D. position the patient so she is facing a blank wall.

74. An OT practitioner is instructing an individual with left hemiplegia how to remove a t-Shirt. The correct sequence is:

A. (1) remove shirt from unaffected arm; (2) remove shirt from affected arm; (3) gather shirt up at the back of the neck; and (4) pull gathered back fabric off over head.

B. (1) remove shirt from affected arm; (2) remove shirt from unaffected arm; (3) gather shirt up at the back of the neck; and (4) pull gathered back fabric off over head.

C. (1) gather shirt up at the back of the neck; (2) pull gathered back fabric off over head; (3) remove shirt from affected arm; and (4) remove shirt from unaffected arm.

D. (1) gather shirt up at the back of the neck; (2) pull gathered back fabric off over head; (3) remove shirt from unaffected arm; and (4) remove shirt from affected arm.

75. **An OT practitioner is working with a patient who has recently experienced a traumatic amputation of his right upper extremity at the short below-elbow level. Which of the following areas of patient education would the practitioner work on FIRST in the OT intervention program?**

    A. Training to put on and take off the prosthesis
    B. Training in residual limb wrapping
    C. Activities to teach grasp and prehension functions
    D. Training to resume vocational activities

76. **A homemaker who sustained a CVA with subsequent left hemiparesis is returning home to live with her husband and children. To enable the individual to carry out her prior responsibility of meal preparation, which item would MOST likely be recommended for stabilization when cutting a potato?**

    A. A piece of nonskid backing under the cutting board
    B. A plate guard around the edge of the board
    C. A rocker knife
    D. A cutting board with two nails in it

77. **An individual confides to the OT practitioner that he is concerned that lower extremity flaccidity may cause problems during sexual activity. The BEST strategy for the OT practitioner to recommend is:**

    A. use a sidelying position.
    B. use pillows to prop up body parts into the desired position.
    C. incorporate slow rocking into movements.
    D. avoid movements that elicit a quick stretch.

78. **In order for an individual sitting in a wheelchair to achieve maximal pelvic stability, the seat belt should be positioned:**

    A. inferior to the ischial tuberosity.
    B. superior to the iliac crest.
    C. inferior to the anterior superior iliac spine.
    D. superior to the posterior superior iliac spine.

79. **An OT practitioner is treating a patient who has difficulty maintaining attention to a task but is aware of the problem. The BEST example of a strategy that the OT can teach the patient to control effects of attention deficits would be:**

    A. simplifying the instructions given to accomplish the task so only one step is presented at a time.
    B. learning the self-monitoring technique of asking oneself if any part of the task has been missed.
    C. providing practice in shape and number cancellation worksheets.
    D. removing unnecessary objects from around the task area to decrease distractions.

80. **Which of the following pieces of adapted equipment would the OT practitioner MOST likely recommend a client continue to use at home after a total hip arthroplasty?**

    A. A wire basket attached to a walker
    B. A padded foam toilet seat 1 inch in height
    C. A short-handled bath sponge
    D. A long-handled bath sponge

81. **The MOST effective way to adapt a chair to inhibit a child's extensor tone and allow the child to maintain a sitting position is to use:**

    A. lateral trunk supports.
    B. a seat belt placed at a 45-degree angle at the hips.
    C. a wedge-shaped seat that is higher in the front.
    D. a lapboard.

82. **Which of the following sequence of methods is MOST appropriate to achieve sensory desensitization?**

    A. Textured material, rubbing, tapping, and prolonged contact
    B. Massage, facilitory electrical stimulation, and a progressive desensitization program
    C. Pressure, percussion, vibration, icing, and edema massage
    D. Visual compensation and functional use of the extremity

83. **An OTR is implementing cognitive rehabilitation interventions with a client and has given the client the task of finding telephone numbers of specific people in the phone book. The client has also been given a card with a series of questions written on it including, "Do I understand what I am supposed to do?" and "Do I have all the information I need?" and "Is this the best way to do this?" This intervention is MOST accurately described as:**

    A. a self-management task with an environmental cue.

B. a task to improve visual scanning.

C. a memory task with external aid.

D. a problem-solving task with a "self-talk" cueing strategy.

84. An individual with joint changes that limit finger flexion would be MOST comfortable using utensils with:

A. regular handles.

B. weighted handles.

C. a universal cuff attachment.

D. built-up handles.

85. An OT practitioner is working with an elderly woman with a diagnosis of depression and dementia during the clean-up portion of a cooking activity. The patient begins to dry the plates and utensils she has already dried. The OTR should:

A. tell the client that the same dishes and utensils are being redried.

B. put the dried dishes away and begin to hand the client wet dishes.

C. ask the client to stop the activity because it seems too difficult.

D. ask the client to describe what she is doing.

86. An OT practitioner is instructing a client to perform stand-to-sit chair transfers after a total hip replacement. Before sitting down from a standing position, the OTR FIRST instructs the client to:

A. extend the operated leg forward, reach back for the armrests, and slowly sit, while attempting to not lean forward.

B. extend the nonoperated leg forward, while gradually flexing the operated side, reaching back for the arm rests and attempting to not lean forward.

C. flex the operated leg, then flex the nonoperated leg, reach back for the armrests, and slowly sit, while attempting to not lean forward.

D. never perform stand-to-sit transfers with a client with a new total hip replacement until 2 weeks after surgery.

87. An OT practitioner is educating a client with a cumulative trauma disorder about common work-related risk factors. The OTR explains to the client that many of the PRIMARY risk factors are:

A. repetition, high force, and awkward joint postures.

B. progressive resistive exercise, joint mobilization, and weight bearing.

C. inflammation, swelling, and pain.

D. fatigue, muscle cramps, and paresthesias.

88. A client is experiencing acute right upper extremity and hand lymphodema after a recent mastectomy. The client's primary complaint is joint stiffness. The INITIAL techniques the OTR can implement to alleviate joint stiffness would MOST likely be:

A. contrast baths, active and passive range of motion, and retrograde massage.

B. ultrasound, electrical stimulation, and dynamic splinting.

C. resistive exercises, weight bearing, and lifting.

D. joint mobilization, serial casting, and dynamic splinting.

89. Which of the following BEST describes how a OT practitioner would document a normally developing infant's first steps?

A. "The infant uses a narrow base of support and low arm guard position and takes big steps."

B. "The infant uses a wide base of support and is independent in stopping and turning."

C. "The infant uses a narrow base of support and low arm guard position."

D. "The infant uses a wide base of support and high arm guard position and takes short steps."

90. An individual reports that back pain during sexual activity is so severe that it prevents any enjoyment. The BEST strategy for the therapist to recommend is:

A. use a sidelying position.

B. time sexual activity for periods of high energy.

C. do not discuss pain with the sexual partner because it may be a "turn off."

D. identify alternative methods for meeting sexual needs that don't cause pain.

91. The OTR instructs a client with chronic neck pain to use psychosocial pain management techniques. Which of the following BEST represents psychosocial strategies commonly used by OT practitioners?

A. Biofeedback, distraction, and relaxation techniques

B. Specific skill training

C. Strength- and endurance-building techniques

D. Cognitive retraining techniques

92. An OT practitioner is providing instruction to caregivers in a long-term care facility concerning assisting a resident whose severe attention span deficits impair the ability to participate in self-feeding. The OT practitioner is MOST likely to recommend which method?

A. Demonstration of feeding process for the resident

B. Providing verbal feedback to the resident about how he or she is progressing

C. Hand-over-hand assistance

D. Chaining

93. A OTR has been working in a medical setting with a 6-year-old child who has had a traumatic brain injury. At what point should the OTR recommend discharge?

A. When the child refuses to attend OT

B. When the child is ready to make the transition to first grade

C. When the child has achieved a maintenance level of functioning

D. When the child is considered to be completely recovered

94. A child is on a pureed diet because of an inability to chew food. The MOST effective method for the OTR to facilitate the child's ability to chew would be to:

A. encourage the child to remove food from the spoon with his teeth.

B. stimulate the management of texture by using vegetable or beef soup.

C. increase the management of texture by slowly increasing texture of food with a baby food grinder.

D. stimulate biting and chewing by placing a raisin between the child's teeth.

95. When working with clients who experience low back pain, it is important to practice functional techniques such as lifting and carrying. Which of the following BEST represents a correct lifting method?

A. Keep both knees straight, flex the back, and keep object an arm's length away from the body

B. Bend both knees, keep the back straight, and bring object close to the body when lifting

C. Keep both knees and back straight and bring object close to the body when lifting

D. Bend one knee while keeping the other leg

straight and keep the object an arm's length away from the body

96. An individual with Guillain-Barré syndrome complains of pain during passive range of motion (PROM) to the shoulder. Which is the MOST important technique for the OT practitioner to use while performing PROM with this individual?

A. Work proximal to distal.

B. Proceed only to the point of pain.

C. Limit the number of repetitions to 10.

D. Gently encourage the individual to work through pain.

97. A 3-year-old child with a diagnosis of mental retardation is dependent in all areas of dressing. If the OT practitioner uses a developmental approach with this child, which skill should FIRST be addressed?

A. Putting on garments with the front and back of clothing correctly placed

B. Putting on a t-shirt

C. Removing pants

D. Buttoning and tying bows

98. In a long-term care facility, an elderly resident with dementia repeatedly asks for her mother and becomes increasingly upset. The MOST therapeutic strategy for responding to this resident is to:

A. use reality orientation: explain that the person's mother has been dead a long time.

B. set limits: firmly tell the person to stop asking for her mother.

C. therapeutic "fibbing": tell the person that her mother will be coming shortly.

D. respond to the emotional tone expressed by the words: provide extra attention and reassurance.

99. An OT practitioner is planning treatment for individuals with a variety of personality disorders who have inaccurate perceptions of others and unrealistic perceptions of themselves. The treatment method that might BEST address these problem areas is a:

A. small group that provides a wide range of craft activities from which the members are encouraged to select.

B. session focused on understanding and changing the individual's way of relating with the therapist.

C. social skills training program completed in small groups.

D. cooperative group activity that both provides and elicits consistent and accurate feedback about interactions within the group.

100. An auto mechanic is currently in a work hardening program after being in a car accident that left him with numerous upper and lower extremity impairments. The ultimate goal for this individual is to return to full employment as an auto mechanic. Which of the following BEST represents a work hardening activity for this individual?

A. Lifting weights
B. Working on a mock car engine
C. Visiting the work site garage
D. Preparing a light lunch for mealtime

101. An individual with ALS and mild dysphagia becomes extremely fatigued at breakfast, lunch, and dinner. Which is the FIRST intervention the OT practitioner should consider recommending?

A. Speak with the physician about tube feedings
B. Sit in a semireclined position during meals
C. Eat six small meals a day
D. Substitute pureed foods for liquids

102. An individual with MS reports extreme frustration because her house is so dirty. When she does attempt to clean it, she is too exhausted to do anything else afterward. She does not think she can afford to pay someone else to clean. Which of the following strategies is MOST appropriate for this individual?

A. Convince the individual to hire a house cleaner
B. Prescribe activities that will increase strength
C. Use the largest joint available for the task
D. Alternate tasks that require standing with those that can be performed sitting

103. An OT practitioner is fabricating a dynamic splint for a butcher who sustained a low-level radial nerve injury while slicing lunchmeat at the deli where he works. The OTR explains to the client that a dorsal dynamic splint for this type of nerve injury should:

A. provide wrist extension, MCP flexion, and thumb flexion.
B. prevent wrist extension, MCP extension, and thumb extension.

C. prevent wrist extension, MCP flexion, and thumb flexion.
D. provide wrist extension, MCP extension, and thumb extension.

104. While working with a child who has a neuromuscular disorder, the OT practitioner places the child in a sitting position on a therapeutic ball, starts moving the ball and asks the child to reach for a toy while sitting on the moving ball. The primary purpose of this activity is MOST likely:

A. increasing upper extremity strength.
B. facilitating postural reactions.
C. decreasing tactile defensiveness.
D. improving visual perception.

105. A client with hemiplegia and her spouse are working on toilet transfer training activities with the OT practitioner. The BEST way for the OT practitioner to teach the couple to perform transfers will be:

A. only to the unaffected side of the client's body.
B. only to the affected side of the client's body.
C. to both sides of the client's body.
D. only to the side of the body from which the client will be approaching the toilet.

106. An OT practitioner is preparing for the discharge of a preadolescent child with limited strength and endurance. Which of the following home adaptations is MOST important to recommend?

A. Mount lever handles on doors and faucets
B. Remove all throw rugs
C. Install nonskid pads on steps
D. Mount a table-top easel for written home work

107. An OT practitioner is fabricating a static splint to prevent further injury, reduce pain, and encourage proper positioning. Which of the following would BEST address these goals?

A. A resting pan splint for a client after a TBI who has been unresponsive in the intensive care unit for 3 weeks, yet grimaces with passive digit extension
B. A dynamic extension splint for a client with a radial nerve injury sustained after a skiing accident
C. An articular splint after surgical repair of the PIP joint for a burn injury

D. A spring coil splint for a client with a median nerve injury sustained in a boating accident

108. **A child with poor balance is unable to put on and remove lower-extremity clothing. Which of the following approaches would BEST address this functional problem?**

    A. Teach the child to dress in a sidelying position

    B. Add loops to the waistbands of pants and skirts

    C. Use Velcro fasteners in place of zippers

    D. Teach the child to dress in a standing position

109. **An OTR is on the treatment team for patients with lower extremity amputations in a rehabilitation hospital. The PRIMARY role of the OT in the management of lower extremity amputation is:**

    A. fabricating artificial limbs.

    B. providing therapeutic exercise, wound care, pain management and gait training.

    C. providing a program to enhance occupational performance in ADL, work, and leisure.

    D. assessing the client's social environment and making recommendations.

110. **An OT practitioner who is leading a stress management group explains to the members that stressors can be MOST accurately described as the:**

    A. process by which individuals adjust to daily stressful events within their environments.

    B. body's reactions to threat, often described as "fight or flight."

    C. precipitating conditions and events that elicit stress reactions.

    D. process of "fit" between the individual and his or her environment.

111. **An individual demonstrates a left visual field cut as a result of a CVA and demonstrates difficulty crossing the midline during many self-care activities. Which of the following interventions would best represent a REMEDIAL approach to addressing this deficit area?**

    A. Placing self-care supplies to the individual's right side

    B. Patient and family education regarding the effects of visual field loss

    C. Verbal and tactile cueing to look to the right side

    D. Weaving on a wide frame loom

112. **Which of the following is the BEST instruction to impart to a caregiver regarding how to propel a wheelchair down a steep ramp?**

    A. Tip the wheelchair backward and guide it down the ramp backwards

    B. Tip the wheelchair backward and guide it down the ramp forwards

    C. Allow the patient to propel the wheelchair independently

    D. Obtain the assistance of a second individual

113. **A child with athetoid cerebral palsy is learning to use augmentative communication and is frustrated because it takes so long to produce a sentence. Which of the following is the BEST solution for this problem?**

    A. A larger monitor

    B. A voice output tool

    C. Word prediction software

    D. Masking inappropriate keys

114. **A 78-year-old individual who is ambulating with a walker in the home informs the OT practitioner that improving balance is a major concern. Although the patient took showers in the past, now his fear of falling limits him to sponge baths. The OT practitioner tells the individual that it is wise to avoid situations in which the risk of falling is high. Which of the following should the OT practitioner advise the individual to do NEXT?**

    A. Try the bathtub instead of the shower.

    B. Purchase a shower chair.

    C. Describe how using a shower chair improves safety.

    D. Explain that therapy will improve his balance.

115. **The goal for an elderly person with Parkinson's disease is to dress herself independently. The BEST adaptation to compensate for this person's physical deficits would be:**

    A. Velcro closures on front-opening clothing.

    B. large buttons on front-opening clothing.

    C. larger clothing slipped on overhead with no fasteners.

    D. stretchy fabric clothing with tie closures in the back.

116. **The BEST way for an OT practitioner to utilize sensory stimulation for the child with tactile defensiveness is to:**

    A. apply intense light touch stimulation such

as tickling on the abdomen for desensitization.

B. avoid all forms of tactile stimulation to accommodate child's preferences.

C. allow child to self-apply tactile stimuli to maximize child's tolerance.

D. avoid all deep pressure tactile stimuli to decrease defensiveness.

117. An individual consistently confuses white glue with white grout during a tile activity. Which of the following actions would be consistent with an activity adaptation approach?

A. Review with the individual the difference between glue and grout

B. Replace the white glue with blue glue

C. Avoid the use of white tiles

D. Complete the last step of the activity (applying grout) for the individual until the individual has learned how to apply grout

118. A third grade student receives direct OT services provided through the public school system. Which of the following activities should the OT practitioner recommend to the gym teacher to BEST consolidate the child's skills in spatial organization and motor planning?

A. Relay races

B. Obstacle courses

C. The balance beam

D. Freeze tag

119. A patient who is being discharged from a rehabilitation center to home has Parkinson's disease and is at risk for aspiration. When instructing the primary caregiver in proper positioning during feeding, the OT practitioner should recommend:

A. feeding the patient in bed in a supine position.

B. seating the patient upright on a firm surface with the chin slightly tucked.

C. positioning the patient in a semireclined position in a reclining chair.

D. feeding the patient in bed in a sidelying position.

120. An OT practitioner is educating a middle-aged roofer who is recovering from a full-thickness burn about hypertrophic scarring. The OTR should FIRST inform the client that:

A. the depth of the wound and location and the

patient's race and age can all influence scar formation.

B. full-thickness wounds typically heal without significant scar formation.

C. surgical intervention eliminates all risk of hypertrophic scarring.

D. hypertrophic scars involving the joints do not interfere with range of motion.

121. An OT practitioner is instructing a person with arthritis how to maintain range of motion while performing household activities. Which of the following activities MOST effectively accomplishes this?

A. Use short strokes with the vacuum cleaner

B. Keep elbow flexed when ironing

C. Keep lightweight objects on low shelves

D. Use dust mitt to keep fingers fully extended

122. Which of the following is the FIRST step an OT practitioner should take when initiating a safe wheelchair transfer?

A. Have the patient scoot forward to the front of the seat.

B. Position foot plates in the up position.

C. Swing away the leg rests.

D. Lock the brakes.

123. An individual has been referred to OT following open heart surgery and a period of prolonged bedrest. After the individual is able to tolerate sitting unsupported at the edge of the bed, the NEXT activity the OT practitioner should introduce is:

A. peeling potatoes while seated.

B. wheelchair propulsion at 1.2 mph.

C. taking a shower.

D. walking at 1 mph.

124. An OT practitioner is running a discharge planning group in which individuals discuss their personal feelings and concerns about returning to the community. Which of the following would be the BEST method to facilitate this process?

A. Patients write fears and concerns on index cards. The OT practitioner collects and reads the cards to the group for discussion.

B. Patients write fears and concerns on index cards and then take turns reading their cards to the group.

C. Patients each take a turn verbalizing their fears and concerns to the group.

D. The psychologist speaks to the group about discharge fears in general.

125. **A sixth grader with a diagnosis of athe-toid cerebral palsy needs an adapted computer for communication. Her upper-extremity control is poor because of fluc-tuating muscle tone. The BEST way for her to operate her computer is to use a:**

    A. single pressure switch firmly mounted with-in easy reach.
    B. lightweight keyboard placed at midline.
    C. low-resistance mouse and pad.
    D. mercury-switch headband set to respond to minimal movement.

126. **An individual with chronic obstructive pulmonary disease (COPD) with low en-durance is taught to modify his bathing techniques for carryover after dis-charge. The BEST bathing method would be:**

    A. tub bathing with hot water.
    B. standing for a quick shower.
    C. using a bath chair and a hand-held shower with tepid water.
    D. tub bathing using lukewarm water.

127. **Which of the following would be the BEST cup for the OT practitioner to rec-ommend using when working with an in-dividual who tends to drink too quickly?**

    A. A vacuum feeding cup
    B. A "nosey cup" (cut out for the nose)
    C. A mug with two handles
    D. A cup with a large drinking spout

128. **The OTR is organizing a group picnic out-ing to a park. The most important pre-caution for the OTR to implement for those group members taking neuroleptic medications is to:**

    A. encourage the use of PABA-free sunblock and hats.
    B. encourage members to move slowly when changing positions from sitting to standing.
    C. encourage members to use an antiperspi-rant and wear light-colored clothing.
    D. take along such low-calorie snacks as car-rot sticks and celery sticks.

129. **To avoid overstimulation when handling a stable, 12-week premature infant in the NICU setting, an OT practitioner must FIRST:**

    A. provide gentle human touch to enable the infant to slowly respond to intervention.
    B. establish a calm state by utilizing the in-fant's musical mobile.
    C. swaddle the infant in a blanket and cuddle

to provide containment and warmth to as-sist with self-regulation.
    D. establish a bond through visual orientation to the therapist's face.

130. **An individual with complete C7 quadri-plegia demonstrates fair+ strength in the wrist extensors. Which of the follow-ing interventions will MOST effectively increase strength in the wrist extensors?**

    A. A craft activity using increasingly heavy hand tools
    B. Mildly resistive activities that are halted as soon as the individual begins to fatigue
    C. Electric stimulation to the wrist extensors
    D. Moderate resistance during active range of motion to the wrist

131. **Which of the following activities would be BEST to promote prewriting skills with a child in preschool or kindergarten?**

    A. Maneuvering through obstacles and focus-ing on making turns
    B. Having the child create his or her own books on specific topics
    C. Rolling clay into a ball
    D. Drawing lines and shapes using shaving cream, sand, or finger paints

132. **The OTR is teaching a student how to perform range-of-motion exercises with a patient who has quadriplegia. In order to encourage the development of tenode-sis, the OTR must be sure to position the patient's wrist in:**

    A. the neutral position during finger flexion and extension.
    B. flexion during finger flexion and extension.
    C. extension during finger flexion and flexion during finger extension.
    D. flexion during finger flexion and extension during finger extension.

133. **An OT practitioner is performing an as-sistive technology intervention with a client who is has severe limitations of motor function resulting from CP. The FIRST function of the OT in this process is to:**

    A. identify the most appropriate commercially available forms of assistive technology.
    B. identify the abilities, needs, and life goals of the client.
    C. select the appropriate method of accessing the technology.

D. modify the assistive technology device to meet the needs of the client.

134. During an oral motor evaluation, an OT practitioner asks the client to stick out her tongue. Next, the client is asked to move her tongue from side to side. The two functions that the OT practitioner is attempting to facilitate are:

A. protrusion and humping.

B. lateralization and tipping.

C. protrusion and lateralization.

D. lateralization and humping.

135. An OT is running a group for individuals who have difficulty managing anger. Based on a cognitive–behavioral frame of reference, which of the following steps would the OT BEGIN with?

A. Discuss the benefits of alternative beliefs about anger and responses to anger

B. Develop awareness about what produces anger and how the clients respond to anger

C. Role-play a situation that presents minimal difficulty to group participants

D. Role-play a situation that presents significant difficulty to group participants

136. When adapting a toilet for use by a child with poor postural control, the OT practitioner should pay PRIMARY attention to which of the following issues?

A. Can the toilet paper be reached without a major weight shift?

B. Is the flush handle easy to manipulate?

C. Can the child's feet reach the floor?

D. Is a nonskid mat placed on the floor to prevent slipping?

137. A client is having difficulty getting around within her home as a result of low vision. The MOST appropriate strategy to improve accessibility would be to:

A. instruct the client to sit while performing ADL.

B. provide strong color contrast at key areas to identify steps, pathways, etc.

C. recommend the client arrange to get assistance when moving within her home.

D. recommend training in white cane use, for identifying obstacles in the home.

138. A patient with neurological deficits has been unable to carry over skills learned previously in therapy and has exhibited no capacity to learn new information. The MOST appropriate intervention approach to improve ADL functioning for this patient would be:

A. repetitive practice of simple ADL under therapist guidance.

B. recommendation of environmental adaptations and assistance for ADL.

C. ADL training in the familiar home environment.

D. forward or backward chaining techniques.

139. Inpatient OT treatment groups for individuals with schizophrenia are MOST appropriate when they provide the opportunity for group members to:

A. disclose themselves in the groups.

B. develop insight into their feelings.

C. practice social and life skills.

D. deal with expression of anger.

140. A second grade child has a diagnosis of muscular dystrophy. The child operates a manual wheelchair, but his mobility is slow because of muscle weakness. The OT should consider a powered wheelchair when the:

A. child starts junior high school and will be expected to switch classrooms several times daily.

B. child's speed over long distances becomes less than that of a walking person.

C. child's home can be made accessible for a power wheelchair.

D. child becomes unable to propel a manual wheelchair.

141. An elderly man was admitted to the hospital after a car accident. He sustained a right pelvic fracture and verbalizes extreme pain with ambulation. The orthopedic doctor has recommended that the patient perform "toe touch only" weight bearing on his right foot for 6 to 8 weeks. The OT should instruct the patient to use a walker when performing which of the following activities?

A. Transferring on and off a commode seat

B. Working on bed mobility

C. Performing self-feeding

D. Working on distal lower extremity dressing

142. An individual with depression is ready to return to the job held before taking a leave of absence. Which of the following is the FIRST action the OT practitioner should take?

A. Perform a job analysis

B. Request reasonable accommodation

C. Emphasize activities that promote a sense of self-efficacy

D. Encourage the individual to participate in a weekly support group

143. A 1-year-old child is working on increasing neck flexor strength. At this time, the child can maintain head alignment when tilted backward from an upright supported sitting position, to a 45-degree incline, but loses control when tilted further back. The NEXT important step in the intervention is to work on head and neck alignment:

A. in a sidelying position while batting a toy.

B. in a prone position while watching a peek-a-boo game.

C. by tilting backwards up to 60 degrees while rocking.

D. in a supine position, while watching an overhead mobile.

144. An individual with C8 quadriplegia is most likely to require which of the following in order to perform self-feeding?

A. Total assistance

B. Support of the upper extremity against gravity

C. A universal cuff

D. No assistive devices

145. A resident of a long-term care facility has been referred to the OT practitioner because of difficulties with eating. The FIRST step of intervention the OT performs with this resident at mealtime is to:

A. provide skid-proof placemats, plate guard, and utensils with built-up handles.

B. observe for swallowing after each bite of food.

C. instruct the caregivers about a special eating setup for the resident.

D. position the person in an upright posture, make sure head is flexed slightly and in midline.

146. An OT practitioner is working on sequencing skills with a young patient who is s/p TBI. The MOST effective activity to promote development of these skills is:

A. leather stamping using tools in a random design.

B. stringing beads for a necklace, following a pattern.

C. putting together a 20-piece puzzle.

D. playing Concentration.

Effectiveness of Treatment and Discharge Planning

147. The spouse of an individual being treated for bipolar disorder describes the frustration he experiences in regard to the ups and downs of his wife's condition. The support group that the OT practitioner would MOST likely refer this individual to is:

A. Al-Anon.

B. family therapy.

C. National Alliance for the Mentally Ill.

D. Recovery, Inc.

148. By using an interest checklist that includes a report of both interests and actual participation in activities, an OT practitioner will MOST likely collect information on a client's:

A. use of time.

B. developmental level.

C. mood and affect.

D. communication skills.

149. An OT practitioner working in an acute care hospital is writing a progress note in the chart for a treatment session held earlier that day. Medical documentation should include which of the following?

A. Concise objective information

B. Speculative and judgmental information

C. Objective and speculative information

D. Subjective information and personal opinions

150. A young child with a diagnosis of spina bifida has been referred for an assessment. When collecting the initial data by interviewing the child's mother, the OT should focus PRIMARILY on:

A. the mother's concerns and goals for her child.

B. medical management.

C. equipment needs.

D. the physical layout of the home.

151. The treatment environment in which an OTR would be MOST likely to emphasize discharge planning for addressing mental health problems would be a(n):

A. club house.

B. community mental health center.

C. acute care hospitalization.

D. quarterway house.

152. When a therapist reevaluates a client's treatment plan, the therapist would be MOST likely to change activities when the activities:

A. continue to provide some degree of challenge.

B. the activities reflect the client's priorities.

C. the activities help to achieve the client's goals.

D. are easily accomplished by the client.

153. An OT practitioner should discontinue OT services when which of the following has taken place?

A. The goals have been met and the individual can no longer benefit from OT services.

B. The goals have not been met and the individual could benefit from continued services.

C. The goals have been met but the individual could benefit from continued services.

D. The individual feels that he or she has not made gains despite objective measures to the contrary.

154. A school-age child with fine-motor difficulties is ready for discharge from outpatient OT services. Which of the following is the MOST important information to focus on?

A. The child's interests and hobbies

B. The child's writing, dressing, and self-feeding skills

C. The child's academic achievement

D. The availability of the child's parents for follow-up services

155. An OT practitioner in a psychosocial setting is documenting a client's responses to an activity. Which of the following is the most OBJECTIVE statement?

A. "The client did not want to finish her stenciling activity."

B. "The client was hostile to another client in the activity group."

C. "The client independently selected one of six craft designs presented."

D. "The client demonstrated an appropriate level of frustration tolerance during most of the activity."

156. An OT practitioner providing home-based care to an individual with AIDS learns from his caregiver that he has become too weak to turn himself in bed. What is the MOST important modification to the treatment plan for the OT practitioner to recommend?

A. To begin a strengthening program

B. To begin a bed-mobility program

C. To teach the caregiver how to lift and turn the client safely

D. To provide an environmental control unit to the client

157. A preteen with a diagnosis of spastic cerebral palsy is enjoying computer-assisted learning while making significant progress in written communication, but he complains of general fatigue, body aches, and eye strain. Based on this information, which area would be most relevant for the OT practitioner to reassess FIRST?

A. The time he spends at the computer

B. The size of the computer screen

C. The challenge level of the learning program

D. His control of the keyboard

158. During OT treatment, a child has a seizure. The MOST important actions for the OT practitioner during the seizure are to:

A. check breathing and administer mouth-to-mouth resuscitation if necessary.

B. attempt to restrain the child's movements to prevent injury.

C. ease the child to a lying position, remove or pad nearby objects, loosen clothing.

D. take no actions except observation of the child.

159. An individual will be performing sliding board transfers with assistance from family members upon discharge. When ordering the wheelchair, which features will be MOST important to include?

A. One-arm drive and low backrest

B. Reclining backrest and elevating footrests

C. Swing-away footrests and removable armrests

D. Elevating footrests and removable armrests

160. A child's short-term goal is to "demonstrate increased manipulation skills by opening a 3-inch screw-top jar independently." The MOST important tool the OTR will need to reassess the child's progress is:

A. a goniometer.

B. a 3-inch screw-top jar.

C. a dynamometer.

D. a developmental fine-motor assessment.

161. A patient is about to be discharged after completing a rehabilitation program following a total hip replacement. In assessing the home environment, the OT practitioner takes into consideration the patient's poor visual acuity. The MOST appropriate adaptation to ensure that the client can go up and down the stairs safely is:

A. installing a stair glide.

B. installing handrails on both sides of the steps.

C. marking the end of each step with high-contrast tape.

D. instructing the patient to take only one step at a time when going up or down.

162. Which of the following is the MOST important precaution to emphasize to parents when discharging a child with lower extremity paralysis as a result of myelomeningocele?

A. Practice regular skin inspection

B. Avoid feeding the child chewy foods that may cause choking

C. Monitor apnea episodes

D. Avoid situations that can stimulate tactile defensiveness

163. The family of an individual with paraplegia is moving into a new apartment and they need to select a surface for the living area. Finances are limited, but they are looking for the surface that will be easiest for maneuvering a wheelchair. Which of the following is the MOST appropriate surface for this situation?

A. Linoleum floor

B. Short pile carpeting

C. Deep pile carpeting

D. Several area rugs

164. An OT practitioner is writing a daily SOAP note in order to document treatment for a client on the rehabilitation unit. Which of the following documented statements BEST describes an objective basis for judgment?

A. "Patient enjoys reading photography magazines."

B. "Patient likes news magazines."

C. "Patient obviously likes to read a sports magazine."

D. "Patient stated that he likes to read sports magazines."

165. An individual who is being discharged in one week is functioning at Allen's Cognitive Level 4 and needs to take two different psychotropic medications twice daily. Which of the following is the MOST appropriate discharge recommendation?

A. Instruct the client to take medication at 9 A.M. and 9 P.M.

B. Instruct the client to take "one white and one blue pill" with the morning and evening meals

C. Instruct the caregiver to remind the client to take medication twice daily

D. Instruct the caregiver to place pills into client's hands at the designated times

166. An elderly patient has Alzheimer's disease and is about to be discharged to home, where she lives with her husband. She does not always recognize her children, shows a tendency to wander, and has frequent episodes of incontinence. Which of the following is the MOST important item for the OT practitioner to include in the family discharge planning conference?

A. Strategies the patient can use for handling incontinence

B. Strategies the husband can use to prevent the patient from wandering

C. Strategies the patient can use to prevent wandering

D. Reality orientation techniques to increase recognition of her children

167. An OT practitioner is working with an individual who has identified alcohol abuse as a contributing factor to the depression that he has been experiencing. The practitioner is discussing discharge plans with this individual. At discharge, the MOST appropriate type of group to refer this individual to is a(n):

A. advocacy group.

B. self-help group.

C. support group.

D. psychotherapy group.

168. Several clients are about to be discharged from an inpatient psychiatric unit to a variety of community programs. Which of the following areas is

MOST important to address in a discharge planning group?

A. Developing ADL routines
B. Self-awareness
C. Relapse prevention
D. Social skills

Occupational Therapy for Populations

169. An OT manager is preparing the outpatient OT staff for a visit from an accrediting agency. The accrediting agency that surveys inpatient and comprehensive outpatient rehabilitation programs is BEST represented by which of the following:

A. AOTA.
B. JCAHO.
C. CARF.
D. NBCOT.

170. An OT practitioner working in a drug and alcohol rehabilitation center is educating clients about discharge options. The PRIMARY expectation for becoming a member in a self-help group for alcohol problems is:

A. members are encouraged to tell the other members their names and where they live and work.
B. members share their experiences and struggles with alcohol use.
C. members are required to attend a set number of meetings.
D. members are encouraged to give advice to others.

171. Adults with mental retardation can be offered a variety of work alternatives. Which of the following MOST likely involves simple assembly or sorting and packaging tasks with supervision and subcontracted piecework?

A. An adult activity center
B. Supervised employment
C. Job coaching
D. A sheltered workshop

172. An OTR is a team member of a work hardening program. Which of the following would BEST represent the goal that an OT practitioner would document regarding this type of a program?

A. ADL retraining to increase the ability to perform household skills independently

B. Progressive resistive exercise to increase endurance for self-care skills
C. Work simulation to increase strength and endurance for necessary work-related skills
D. Vocational retraining to increase the ability to reenter the job market

173. In establishing a wellness program for older adults, the OT practitioner is MOST likely to incorporate activities that:

A. improve weakness following a CVA.
B. increase physical activity and fitness.
C. improve social skills for depressed elders.
D. increase independent performance of transfers.

174. An OTR is working as a consultant to a health care facility to assist the facility in achieving compliance with the Americans with Disability Act, Title III. The PRIMARY focus of the OT's efforts would be to make recommendations about:

A. improving accessibility in building access, building interiors, and rest rooms.
B. modifying equipment, providing assistive aids, and training in adaptive methods so a disabled person can perform a particular job.
C. providing education to persons who hire personnel concerning nondiscriminatory behaviors and procedures regarding persons with disabilities.
D. assistive technology systems to facilitate job performance of disabled employees.

175. A fall prevention program is being implemented by an OT who works in a life-care retirement community. The BEST way to implement this type of program at the primary level of prevention would be to:

A. develop a protocol for environmental modification to reduce fall risks in the life-care retirement community.
B. observe ADL performance to identify those residents at highest risk for falls.
C. make recommendations for wheelchair positioning for those who have had at least one fall.
D. provide intervention to improve balance with those residents who demonstrate the need.

176. Which of the following activities would be MOST appropriate for vocational skills training for high school students with severe learning disabilities?

A. Stocking the shelves at a local grocery

B. Packaging items in a local sheltered workshop

C. Cleaning the school cafeteria after lunch

D. Reading want ads and role-playing interviews

Service Management

177. **The OT practitioner is leading a grooming group for female clients in a psychosocial treatment setting. Which of the following options BEST complies with universal precautions?**

    A. Use disposable cotton swabs and have clients bring their own cosmetics

    B. Use disposable gloves when combing client's hair

    C. Wash and dry makeup brushes between uses

    D. Avoid bringing cosmetics in glass containers to the group

178. **A COTA and OTR have effectively worked together for the past 5 years. Which of the following BEST describes the supervisory process between a COTA and a supervising OTR at this level?**

    A. A mutual process

    B. A evaluative process

    C. A counseling process

    D. A learning process

179. **An OTR has been working in the area of mental health for 3 years and continues to meet with her supervisor every other week. This therapist has mastered basic role functions, begun specialization, and participates in the education of other personnel. Based on the AOTA document, Occupational Therapy Roles, this OTR is functioning as an:**

    A. entry-level OTR with close supervision.

    B. intermediate-level OTR with minimal supervision.

    C. advanced-level OTR with general supervision.

    D. intermediate-level OTR with routine supervision.

180. **An advanced-level COTA who has worked at an independent living center for the past 7 years has been offered the position of director of the program. There are no funds to pay for OTR supervision.**

According to the AOTA, can the COTA accept the position?

    A. Only if the COTA can find some way to fund OTR supervision.

    B. Yes, as long as state regulations allow autonomous practice and the COTA recognizes situations that require consultation with or referral to an OTR.

    C. No. The COTA cannot work in this practice setting without OTR supervision.

    D. Only if the COTA relinquishes use of the credentials "COTA."

181. **An individual with advanced lung cancer is about to be discharged from an acute care setting to home. She is depressed, and although she remains ambulatory and independent in basic activities of daily living, she tires very quickly and no longer participates in most of her life roles. Which of the following is the BEST action for the OT practitioner to take?**

    A. Provide her with a home program

    B. Recommend home health OT

    C. Recommend discontinuation of OT services

    D. Recommend hospice OT

182. **While practicing wheelchair-to-tub transfers an individual's external catheter is dislodged and urine spills onto the floor. The therapist notes that the urine appears to have blood in it. Which one of the following responses is the MOST appropriate?**

    A. An exposure has not occurred; clean up the area with paper towels and resume treatment as quickly as possible.

    B. An exposure has occurred; close off the area until it can be disinfected and resume treatment as quickly as possible.

    C. An exposure has occurred; clean up the spill with towels, place towels in the dirty laundry bin, and resume treatment as quickly as possible.

    D. An exposure has occurred; put on gloves, clean up the spill with paper towels, put the soiled paper towels in a plastic bag, seal the bag, disinfect the area, and finish the patient's session with whatever time is still left.

183. **An OT manager is attempting to find a way to have financial success in the department while ensuring patient satisfaction. Which of the following is MOST likely to be implemented to assess pa-**

tient flow, develop critical pathways, and cut costs?

A. Quality improvement
B. Peer review teams
C. Cost accounting
D. Interdisciplinary care improvement teams

184. **A client uses a wheelchair and is independent in transfers and basic ADL. With continued OT intervention, he is expected to be able to function independently in the community. The MOST appropriate community living option for him, at this time, would be a(n):**

A. cradle-to-grave home.
B. transitional living center.
C. adult day program.
D. clustered independent living arrangement.

185. **An OT is establishing a department in a rural long-term care facility. When developing the policies and procedures for documentation in the facility, which of the following documents would be MOST useful?**

A. Uniform Terminology for Occupational Therapy
B. Occupational Therapy Code of Ethics
C. Occupational Therapy Standards of Practice
D. Occupational Therapy Roles

186. **An OT practitioner is coordinating a cooking group. As a part of the competency training program for leading the group, the OTR must demonstrate an awareness of the policies and procedures that relate to the storage and maintenance of staple products, as well as food handling. This policy will MOST likely be part of the facility's:**

A. infection control plan.
B. risk management plan.
C. emergency procedures plan.
D. environmental survey plan.

187. **A physician's referral for OT services may be required by which of the following:**

A. AOTA, federal, and state governmental agencies.
B. federal and state governmental agencies and third-party payers.
C. third-party payers, individual facilities, and AOTA.
D. AOTA, third-party payers, and state governmental agencies.

188. **An OT practitioner is graduating from an OT program and is seeking employment. An OT job description would MOST likely contain:**

A. the title of the job, past experience required, and job requirements.
B. a summary of primary job functions, references, and job requirements.
C. the organizational relationships, personality characteristics desired in a job candidate, and accomplishments of the candidate.
D. the title of the job, organizational relationships, essential job functions, and the job requirements.

189. **When working within a school system to assist the mainstreaming of a child with spina bifida into a regular classroom, the OT consults with the classroom teacher. The nature of this "consultation" relationship is BEST characterized by the following statement:**

A. the OT teaches the teacher.
B. the OT provides therapy to the child.
C. the OT directs the teacher.
D. the OT problem solves with the teacher.

190. **The OT department has been asked to provide information to the hospital administration regarding the cost-effectiveness of services provided. Which of the following methods would MOST effectively obtain this information?**

A. Outcomes measurement
B. Utilization review
C. Program evaluation
D. Productivity evaluations

191. **An OT practitioner works with an entry-level COTA on an inpatient psychiatric unit. They each work 4 days a week, overlapping schedules only on Mondays. It would be inappropriate for the OTR to ask the COTA to:**

A. lead the daily craft group.
B. evaluate clients who are admitted on the weekends.
C. assist individuals in carrying out their ADL on Saturday and Sunday mornings.
D. lead a leisure planning group on Saturday afternoon.

192. **A new COTA works in a busy rehabilitation department. Half of the department's OT staff, including the supervisor, is out with the flu. The COTA observes an aide carrying out a session**

of training in **ADL** with a patient who is scheduled for discharge the next day. The **MOST** responsible action for the **COTA** to take is to:

A. allow the aide to finish so the patient will be prepared for discharge.

B. terminate the aide and complete the session herself.

C. bring the issue to the attention of the facility administrator.

D. discuss these concerns with an OTR who is present.

193. **A COTA and OTR jointly decide to discharge an individual after the goal of independence in ADL has been achieved. However, they are instructed by the facility administrator to continue treating, or at least billing, the individual for two sessions per day for the next week, because his insurance will allow it. What is the most appropriate action for the OT practitioners to take?**

A. Continue to work on activities the individual particularly enjoys twice a day whenever possible

B. Discontinue treatment but continue to bill as directed by the administrator

C. Inform the administrator they are unable to provide services to individuals who can no longer benefit from OT

D. Compromise with the administrator and agree to drop in and check on the individual once a day and bill accordingly

194. **A clinical manager of an OT department is reviewing sterilization policies based on universal precautions. The manager revealed that this policy will MOST likely state that:**

A. all equipment is to be sterilized annually.

B. any equipment that has come into contact with body fluids must be sterilized before using the equipment again.

C. all equipment is to be sterilized at the end of each day.

D. all equipment is to be sterilized after each use.

Professional Practice

195. **An OT practitioner in private practice is preparing to act as a consultant to a community agency. The FIRST step would be to:**

A. negotiate the contract.

B. establish trust.

C. assess the environment.

D. identify problems.

196. **A manager of an OT department is attempting to increase the visibility of the OT department within the setting. This type of promotion is commonly done through internal marketing. In order to market internally, the OT manager would MOST likely employ which of the following?**

A. A community newsletter

B. A presentation to physicians

C. A local community workshop

D. A booth at a local health fair

197. **A research question has been identified and a literature review completed by an OT practitioner. The NEXT step for the OT researcher is to:**

A. refine the question and develop the background.

B. decide on methodology.

C. establish boundaries for the study.

D. collect and analyze data.

198. **An OTR/COTA team need to report discharge information and document the information in the patients' chart. At what level does the COTA participate in making discharge recommendations?**

A. An entry-level COTA may perform the task independently.

B. An intermediate-level COTA may perform the task independently.

C. A COTA contributes to the process but does not complete the task independently.

D. A COTA cannot perform the task.

199. **On the way to lunch, an OT practitioner is stopped by a patient's spouse and questioned for 15 minutes about the patient's progress. What is the MOST appropriate action for the OT practitioner to take when determining how the patient will be treated and charged for the scheduled one hour treatment session?**

A. Charge the patient for an additional 15 minutes of treatment for the time spent with family member

B. Reduce the patient's therapy to 45 minutes and charge for 1 hour of treatment to cover the time spent with the family member

C. Reduce the patient's therapy to 45 minutes and charge patient for 45 minutes of treatment

D. Treat the patient as scheduled and charge for the 1 hour of direct time spent with the patient

200. While preparing for his first presentation at a professional conference, an OT realizes he does not have the name of the author of an article containing critical information he planned on photocopying and distributing. Which of the follow-

ing is the MOST appropriate action for the OT to take?

A. Distribute the handout and apologize for not having the author's name.
B. Show the handout with an overhead projector and apologize for not having the author's name.
C. Use the handout only as a resource while developing the presentation.
D. Refrain from using the handout in any way.

ANSWERS FOR SIMULATION EXAMINATION 2

1. (A) further observation and evaluation of right-sided dysfunction is indicated. Answer A is correct because infants usually use a bilateral approach at this age. Although unilaterality occurs several months later, most children alternate hands in many activities until age 6 years. This means that this infant should be observed for possible right-sided dysfunction. Answer B is incorrect because unilaterality at age 4 months is not typical development. Answer C is incorrect because hand dominance begins to develop at age 3 to 6, and answer D is incorrect because bilaterality precedes unilaterality in the course of infant development. See reference: Neistadt and Crepeau (eds): Kohlmeyer, K: Evaluation of sensory and neuromuscular performance components.

2. (B) Receptive aphasia Individuals with receptive aphasia cannot comprehend spoken or written words and symbols; therefore, they cannot understand verbal directions or consistently respond to stimuli. Individuals with receptive aphasia may be able to imitate or follow a demonstration, but these techniques do not work for sensory evaluation. Expressive aphasia (answer A) interferes with an individual's verbal or written expression but not comprehension of verbal or written information. An individual with expressive aphasia would be able to indicate the response by pointing to the stimulus used or a card marked with the correct response. An individual who has agnosia or ataxia (answers C and D) would be able to understand directions but be unable to accurately indicate an area because of impaired recognition of the body part or impaired coordination. The method of response may be adapted by using verbal description of an area or cue cards. See reference: Trombly (ed): Woodson, AM: Stroke.

3. (C) has a standard format. Standardization of a test means that the test is administered in a prescribed manner and that scoring and interpretation of scores are also completed in a prescribed way. The presence of data concerning the test's "norms" and the establishment of reliability and validity (answers A, B, and D) may be, and often are, provided with standardized tests but are not assumed to be

part of the test unless this information is included. The aspects of standardized tests that are always assumed is the specific and standardized method of administration, scoring, and interpretation. See reference: Case-Smith (ed): Richardson, PK: Use of standardized tests in pediatric practice.

4. (C) visual agnosia. Visual agnosia is the inability to recognize common objects and demonstrate their use in an activity. Apraxia (answer A) is the inability to perform purposeful movement on command. A person with alexia (answer D) is unable to understand written language. Stereognosis (answer B) is the ability to identify an object by manipulating it with the fingers without seeing it. See reference: Trombly (ed): Quintana, L: Evaluation of perception and cognition.

5. (B) reflex sympathetic dystrophy This diagnosis is typically "a disabling reaction to pain that is generated by an abnormal sympathetic reflex" (p. 680). Signs include pain, edema, coolness of the hand, and blotchy skin. The level of trauma does not typically correlate to the amount of pain that the client is experiencing. Answer A is more commonly associated with a nerve repair or amputation and presents with symptoms of shooting or sharp pains. Answers C and D do not typically correlate with the symptoms described by patients with reflex sympathetic dystrophy. See reference: Pedretti (ed): Kasch, MC: Hand injuries.

6. (A) symmetrical tonic neck reflex. The correct answer is A because the symmetrical tonic neck reflex, when present, provides the child with bilateral arm extension and hip flexion with the head raised (and bilateral arm flexion and hip extension with the head lowered), which can be used to move forward. Answers B, C, and D are not correct because these primitive patterns do not assist the child into a quadruped position; rather they primarily affect prone and supine positioning. See reference: Neistadt and Crepeau (eds): Kohlmeyer, K: Evaluation of sensory and neuromuscular performance components.

7. (C) radial nerve. Injury to the radial nerve in the

wrist area causes sensory damage only. This damage occurs to the radial two thirds of the dorsum of the hand. Damage to the median nerve at the wrist causes decreased thumb and prehensile strength and complete or partial loss of sensation in the distal portion of the second digit (index finger) and third digits (long finger) with some loss in the fourth digit (ring finger). Damage to the ulnar nerve at the wrist causes decreased grip strength and complete or partial loss of sensation to half of the fourth digit (ring finger) and all of the fifth digit (little finger) as well as the proximal hypothenar region. The ulnar and median nerves are frequently entrapped together. A brachial plexus injury causes peripheral nerve damage to any or all of the fibers from C5 to T1. See reference: Pedretti (ed): Kasch, MC: Hand injuries.

8. (C) Constructional Constructional play involves building and creating things. It is in this area of play that children develop a sense of mastery and problem-solving skills. Sensorimotor play (answer A) generally develops a child's body awareness and sensory experiences. Imaginary play (answer B) involves manipulating people and objects in fantasy as a prelude to dealing with reality. Game play (answer D) requires the ability to learn and apply rules in play. See reference: Kramer and Hinojosa (eds): Luebben, AJ, Hinojosa, J, and Kramer, P: Legitimate tools of pediatric occupational therapy.

9. (B) left unilateral neglect. This is the inability to respond or orient to perceptions from the left side of the body. Evidenced as left unilateral neglect, this deficit is also apparent in the draw-a-man test, flower copying test, house test, and completing a human figure or face puzzle. Unilateral neglect is contralateral to the side of a brain lesion; therefore, left unilateral neglect would result from right-sided brain damage. Left neglect occurs most commonly in right hemisphere lesions. A cataract would cause a visual impairment with detail on both sides of a page. Bitemporal hemianopia (hemianopia is also referred to as hemianopsia) is also known as "tunnel vision," with the individual's peripheral vision lost. The individual would still be able to cross midline with cataracts or bitemporal hemianopsia. A right neglect would not see the right side, and this type of patient would draw all the figures on the left side of the page. Visuospatial deficits are an important factor influencing functional independence outcomes. Visuospatial ability should be taken into account when establishing treatment goals as well as during discharge planning. See reference: Trombly (ed): Quintana, L: Evaluation of perception and cognition.

10. (C) Tip Tip prehension is accomplished by flexing the IP joint of the thumb and the PIP and DIP joints of the finger and bringing the tips of the thumb and finger together. This type of prehension is used to pick up objects such as a pin, nail, or coin. Lateral prehension (answer A) is formed by positioning the pad of the thumb against the radial side of the finger.

This prehension pattern is used for holding a pen, utensil, or key. Palmar prehension (answer B), also known as three-jaw chuck (answer D), is formed by positioning the thumb in opposition to the tips of the index and middle fingers, forming a pad-to-pad opposition. This form of prehension is commonly used to lift objects from a flat surface and tie a shoelace. See reference: Pedretti (ed): Belkin, J, English, CB, Adler, C, and Pedretti, LW: Orthotics.

11. (C) 8 to 9 months of age. "By 8 to 9 months the infant sits erect and unsupported for several minutes" (p. 79). See reference: Case-Smith (ed): Case-Smith, J: Development of childhood occupations.

12. (C) stated instructions for administration and scoring. In standardized assessments, the instructions to the examiner are detailed and fixed so that procedures are followed consistently each time the test is administered. Following these instructions assures the highest level of reliability and validity possible. Subjective judgement (answer A) and previous experience (answer B) may be factors in administration of nonstandardized tests which depend on the skill and judgment of the OT practitioner administering them, but not in the administration and scoring of standardized tests. While practice of a test (answer D) can help to develop competence in the use of the test, it would not influence how to administer and score the test. See reference: Pedretti (ed): Pedretti, LW: Occupational therapy evaluation and assessment of physical dysfunction.

13. (A) a cotton ball. When retesting it is important to use the method used initially in order to make an accurate comparison of status before and after treatment. In addition, evaluation results are more consistent when the individual who performed the initial evaluation performs subsequent reevaluations. An aesthesiometer (answer B) is used to measure two-point discrimination, not light touch. Semmes-Weinstein monofilaments (answer C) are a good tool for assessing light touch thresholds but the results may not be as useful for comparison purposes. A pin or straightened paper clip (answer D) is used for testing superficial pain. See reference: Pedretti (ed): Pedretti, LW: Evaluation of sensation and treatment of sensory dysfunction.

14. (B) a pinch meter. A pinch meter is used to measure the strength of a three-jaw chuck grasp (also known as palmar pinch), in addition to key (lateral) pinch and tip pinch. These tests are performed with three trials that are averaged together and then compared with a standardized norm. The other answers are incorrect. In answer A, the aesthesiometer measures two-point discrimination. In answer C, the dynamometer measures grip strength. In answer D, the volumeter measures edema in the hand. See reference: Pedretti (ed): Kasch, M.: Hand injuries.

15. (C) observation of play and hand function. The observation of play and hand function is the most appropriate way to obtain assessment information during infancy and preschool ages. "Much of the assessment, during infancy and preschool, centers around observation of play and hand function" (p. 609). Answers A, B, and D, are all appropriate choices after the child is old enough for formal assessment. See reference: Neistadt and Crepeau (eds): Atkins, J: Orthopedic and musculoskeletal problems in children.

16. (A) The amount of self-control demands, time management demands, self-expression opportunities, and interest in the activity Components that are primarily within the psychosocial areas and skills of occupational performance are most important to consider with psychosocial populations. Answers B and C are performance components most commonly used with children. Answer D does not address performance components. See reference: Neistadt and Crepeau (eds): Crepeau, EB: Activity analysis: A way of thinking about occupational performance.

17. (A) poor modulation of tactile input. This is the only answer that describes both his hypersensitive and hyposensitive responses to tactile input. The child with autism may be unpredictable in terms of response to sensory stimuli, both avoiding and craving stimulation at various times. Answers B and C are incorrect because they describe only one part of the problem. Answer D is wrong because he appears to be craving deep pressure or proprioceptive input in order to modulate the tactile system. See reference: Case-Smith (ed): Parham, LD, and Maillous, Z: Sensory integration.

18. (A) Oral preparatory phase The oral preparatory phase is typically initiated through the process of looking at and reaching for food. Answer B, the oral phase, typically follows the oral preparatory phase, and the pharyngeal phase (answer C) comes after the oral phase but before the esophageal phase (answer D). See reference: Pedretti (ed): Nelson, KL: Dysphagia: Evaluation and treatment.

19. (C) indicating initiative and beginning task-directed behavior. Because this child is very withdrawn, any spontaneous action should be seen as a very positive sign. It is very important to encourage the child in independent exploratory behavior in order to develop task competence and become less withdrawn. Her use of a toothbrush instead of a hairbrush may indicate cognitive limitations (answer B), possibly caused by a lack of exposure; it could also be caused by a visual deficit (answer D), but the primary importance of the observation lies in C. Attention-getting behavior (answer A) is unlikely in such a withdrawn child. See reference: Case-Smith (ed): Cronin, AS: Psychosocial and emotional domains.

20. (D) view of the problem and an overall goal. The interview is generally the component of the assessment process in which the OT practitioner asks about the individual's goals for treatment and gains an understanding of the problems from the person's perspective. Diagnoses and medications (answers A and B) are most often found in a review of the chart. Abilities (answer C) are determined through performance measures. See reference: Early: Data collection and evaluation.

21. (A) videofluoroscopy. A videofluoroscopy should be performed when it is suspected that the individual is aspirating. An individual who suddenly has a wet voice when there was no prior difficulty may have had a sudden change in medical status causing aspiration. He or she should be reevaluated to determine if there is aspiration into the larynx or trachea. Answers B, a change to thin liquids, and D, a regular diet, would be inappropriate for an individual who does not have a normal swallow or who may be aspirating, because they are too difficult to control. Answer C, a tracheostomy tube, is usually in place prior to the initiation of a feeding program, because the individual was having difficulty with breathing, not swallowing or wet voice qualities. See reference: Pedretti (ed): Nelson, K: Dysphagia: Evaluation and treatment.

22. (C) biomechanical frame of reference. The biomechanical approach is based on enhancing strength, range of motion, and endurance. The biomechanical approach is typically used when impairment does not affect the intact central nervous system. This approach is primarily used for individuals who have had a traumatic injury or illness that has affected the musculoskeletal system. The rehabilitative approach (answer A) emphasizes making an individual as independent as possible and compensating for limitations. The neurodevelopmental approach (answer B) is used for individuals who are born with a central nervous system dysfunction, have experienced an illness, or have had an injury to the neural system. The neurodevelopmental approach is based on using sensory input and developmental sequences to promote function. The psychoanalytic approach (answer D) is based in working with an individual's internal conflicts and past experiences. It is most frequently used in mental health environments. See reference: Trombly (ed): Trombly, CA: Theoretical foundations for practice.

23. (D) disorganized psychosis. Directive group treatment is a highly structured approach that is used in acute care psychiatry for minimally functioning individuals. This approach is useful for disorganized and disturbed functioning with patients with psychoses and other neurological disorders. Task groups are more appropriate for substance abuse disorders (answer A), and psychoeducation groups are most appropriate for eating and adjustment disorders (answers B and C). See reference: Early: Group concepts and techniques.

24. (B) observe him in his home during feeding time. "Considering the context of the child's environments is a critical process in occupational therapy assessments" (p. 167). The reason he does not feed himself may be environmental—for instance, his parents may have taught him not to touch food with his fingers or he may not have learned to feed himself because his grandmother always feeds him. Or the child may not be able to transfer skills learned at home to the clinic—that is, he may believe that "the place to eat is home, not the clinic." Although answers A and C provide useful information for treatment planning, they do not address feeding skills. Answer D does not put the skill to be assessed into an environmental context. See reference: Case-Smith (ed): Stewart, KB: Occupational therapy assessment in pediatrics.

25. (A) within normal limits. The normal range of motion for internal rotation is 70 degrees. Rotation can be assessed with the humerus adducted against the trunk or with the shoulder abducted at 90 degrees. If the humeral movements for internal or external rotation are observed during the performance of activities and found to be adequate for the performance of any functional activities, the range of motion may be noted as WFL. The OT practitioner may choose not to perform a formal joint measurement if the joint is WFL, even though the end of the range may be lacking a few degrees, because the loss of movement may not be significant to the individual. Hypermobility at a joint is motion past the average range of motion, which at the shoulder would be past 70 degrees of internal rotation. If hypermobility is a deformity caused by an unstable joint as might occur after a surgical repair or a disease process, then splinting or another form of stabilization or immobilization can be used to correct the problem. If the practitioner observes hypermobility during range of motion, he or she should compare the range of motion to that on the individual's opposite side in order to assess normal range. A limitation of internal rotation at the shoulder would be less than 70 degrees of motion. If a limitation is apparent, the rehabilitation team may choose not to treat it unless it interferes with the function of the upper extremity. See reference: Trombly (ed): Trombly, CA: Evaluation of biomechanical and physiological aspects of motor performance.

26. (A) apply the stimuli beginning at an area distal to the lesion progressing proximally. The general guidelines for sensation testing are that the person's vision should be occluded, the stimuli should be randomly applied with false stimuli intermingled (opposite of answer C), a practice trial should be performed before the test, and the unaffected side or area should be tested before the affected side or area (opposite of answer B). Also, the tested individual

should be given a specified amount of time in which to respond; therefore, answer D is incorrect. See reference: Trombly (ed): Bentzel, K: Evaluation of sensation.

27. (B) avoid use of power tools and sharp instruments. Individuals experiencing extrapyramidal syndrome, which may cause muscular rigidity, tremors, and/or sudden muscle spasms, should avoid using power tools or sharp instruments. Photosensitivity, an increased sensitivity to the sun, is another side effect often associated with neuroleptic medications that can be addressed by limiting sun exposure (answer A). Answer C is a strategy that can be used to avoid postural hypotension, a sudden drop in blood pressure resulting in feeling faint or loss of consciousness when moving from lying or sitting to standing. Dry mouth is a common side effect of many drugs and can be intensified by the dehydrating effects of caffeinated drinks and alcohol (answer D). All of the above are possible side effects of neuroleptic medications, but answer B is most important because it relates to the only side effect the client has experienced. See reference: Early: Psychotropic medications and somatic treatments.

28. (D) Visual perceptual Running, hopping, using a tripod grasp, drawing a stick figure, and putting together a 10-piece puzzle are all developmentally appropriate skills for a 5-year-old child. Although the child cannot put together the 10-piece puzzle, the gross and fine motor skills that doing a puzzle require have been observed. No fine motor evaluation (answer A) is indicated because the child demonstrates a tripod grasp. No gross motor evaluation (answer B) is necessary because running and hopping skills are evident. Because the child's abilities appear developmentally appropriate, and developmental evaluation (answer C) is not indicated. Because gross, fine, and developmental skills appear to be appropriate, visual perception should be evaluated. See reference: Case-Smith (ed): Case-Smith, J: Development of childhood occupations.

29. (B) compares performance with a normal standard. Norm referencing is a term applied to standardized or formal tests that have been given to a large number of persons in a specific population called the normative sample. When a child is tested with a norm-referenced test, the scores are compared with those of the normative sample; this provides information on how a child performs compared with the average performance of the normative sample. Answers A and D are incorrect. Being "norm referenced" does not guarantee that the test is valid and reliable unless evidence for these characteristics is provided, so answer C is also incorrect. See reference: Case-Smith (ed): Richardson, PK: Use of standardized tests in pediatric practice.

30. (C) have the patient get dressed in a certain way, then change the task at the next session.

Giving the patient a functional task, then changing and observing how he responds will tell the therapist how well the patient can transfer learning to new situations. If the patient can't perform the activity when it is changed slightly, it suggests there may be difficulty with new learning. If the patient can perform the activity with many changes and in a different setting, it suggests that he has more capacity for transfer of learning to new situations. Answers A, B, and D could be ways of assessing different aspects of cognition (judgment, perceptual problem solving and ability to calculate figures), but as described, would not provide evidence of transfer of learning. See reference: Neistadt and Crepeau (eds): Neistadt, ME: Theories derived from learning perspectives.

31. (A) a goniometer. A goniometer measures available joint movement. A pinch meter is used to measure available thumb-to-finger pinch strength in all available positions. A dynamometer measures grip strength in the hand. An aesthesiometer measures two-point discrimination. See reference: Trombly (ed): Trombly, CA: Evaluation of biomechanical and physiological aspects of motor performance.

32. (C) repeated protecting of the joints while moving. An individual's protecting the joints while moving is an example of a motor response associated with chronic pain. Answer A, lack of concentration, is related to a cognitive function secondary to pain. Answer B, aching pain, can be associated with a sensory response to chronic pain, and answer D, the avoidance of certain ADL, is related to self-care responses to chronic pain. See reference: Reed: Chronic pain.

33. (C) relationships with others. The primary problem area for most individuals with a personality disorder is their interactions with others. Specific personality disorder categories indicate that there is some variation among the types of relationships that are impacted. For example, authority relationships seem particularly dysfunctional in those with antisocial personality disorders, and difficulty in establishing relationships is linked to avoidant personality disorders. Answers A and B (ADL) are often problems with mood and thought disorder. Answer D is often a problem in those with schizophrenia. See reference: Early: Understanding psychiatric diagnosis: The DSM-IV.

34. (A) The doorway width needs to be expanded to have a minimum clear opening of 32 inches. According the ADA accessibility guidelines, a doorway needs to have a minimum clear opening of 32 inches with the door open 90 degrees, measured between the face of the door and the opposite stop. In an environmental evaluation process, according to ADA guidelines, the doorway rather than the individual's wheelchair needs to be adapted. See reference: Americans with Disabilities Act: Accessibility Guidelines (ADAAG).

35. (C) follow administration instructions and note changes in behavior. Although the tester may not deviate from the protocol, changes in behavior represent important test data and should be recorded. The responses described in (answers A, B, and D) may make the test results invalid by altering the sequence of test items, the grouping of items, or the actual test item itself. These may not be changed unless it is specified in the test manual. See reference: Case-Smith (ed): Richardson, PK: Use of standardized tests in pediatric practice.

36. (B) confusion Medication side effects are observed and reported by OTs and OT assistants. Anti-anxiety medications often cause confusion. Akathisia, extrapyramidal syndrome, and tardive dyskinesia (answers A, C, and D, respectively) are adverse effects commonly linked to antipsychotic medications. See reference: Early: Psychotropic medications and other biological treatments.

37. (A) safety and stability. Incoordination, tremors, ataxia and athetoid movements may result from conditions that affect the central nervous system, such as Parkinson's disease, CP, multiple sclerosis (MS), and head injuries. "The major problems encountered in ADL performance are safety and adequate stability of gait, body parts and objects to complete the task." Strength (answer C) was not identified as an area of concern for this individual. The ability to reach and bend (answer B) is of primary concern for those with limitations in range of motion. Endurance level (answer D) is a primary concern for individuals with MS, Guillain-Barré syndrome, ALS, and other neurological conditions that cause them to fatigue quickly. See reference: Pedretti (ed): Foti, D, and Pedretti, LW, in Self-care/home management.

38. (C) gravitational insecurity. Gravitational insecurity is described as "excessive fear during ordinary movement activities." The child easily experiences a fear of falling and prefers to keep his or her feet firmly on the ground. Tactile defensiveness (answer A) is a term used to describe discomfort with various textures and with unexpected touch. Developmental dyspraxia (answer B) is a term used to describe a problem with motor planning. Intolerance for motion (answer D) refers to a very similar and often related problem of inhibition of vestibular impulses, but it is usually associated with sensory information received from the semicircular canals. Gravitational insecurity, on the other hand, is associated with the utricle and saccule. See reference: Case-Smith (ed): Parham, LD, and Mailloux, Z: Sensory integration.

39. (A) assist with skill development in the areas of leisure, cognition and perception, self-expression, and ADL. In general, the areas of focus with

OT intervention for individuals identified with substance abuse problems are alternative leisure time use, improved expression of feelings, and the acquiring of social and occupational roles. The approach described in answer B addresses the cognitive disability frame of reference approach. Answers C and D may address specific needs of the patient but not the overall needs of this population See reference: Early: Understanding psychiatric diagnosis: The DSM-IV.

40. (D) early morning and again in the afternoon. Individuals with arthritis should be evaluated at both times to assess the functional abilities of the individual during and after morning stiffness. Evaluating the individual only in the morning (answers A and C) or in the afternoon (answer B) accurately reveals the individual's functional level at only one time of day. Individuals with arthritis have many changes in functional status after morning stiffness has disappeared. See reference: Trombly (ed): Feinberg, JR, and Trombly, CA: Arthritis.

41. (B) Shoulder flexion and abduction and elbow extension Protective arm reactions allow one to return to a support base or to protect the body when there are environmental changes. Answer B is the correct answer because the shoulders flex and abduct while the elbows extend during this protective movement. Facilitation of protective reactions may be a beginning point for the development of arm extension in treatment. Answers A, C, and D are incorrect because these movements are not the major movement components of protective arm reactions. See reference: Neistadt and Crepeau (eds): Kohlmeyer, K: Evaluation of sensory and neuromuscular performance components.

42. (B) examining an analysis of the individual's job. The job analysis is a detailed description of the physical, sensory, and psychological demands of a job. Examples of performance requirements include tasks such as lifting, walking, sitting, standing, and reaching, as well as seeing, hearing, and interpersonal skills. Interviewing the individual (answer A) is useful to obtain information about his or her perception of the injury, motivation for returning to work, and sense of responsibility for rehabilitation. However, the worker may not be able to give an objective, detailed, and concise analysis of the job. The Dictionary of Occupational Titles (answer C) provides generic job descriptions but does not contain as much specific information as a job analysis. A physician (answer D) is unlikely to have the depth of information necessary or the time available to provide the necessary information. See reference: Pedretti (ed): Burt, CM, and Smith, P: Work evaluation and work hardening.

43. (A) procedural reasoning. Reasoning based on corresponding an individual's deficits and physical symptoms with a procedure that may benefit the ar-

ea is referred to as procedural reasoning. Procedural reasoning is the process of identifying a particular treatment or procedure. Conditional reasoning (answer B) is a form of clinical reasoning that takes into account various systems and dynamics involved with the patient and his or her illness or injury. This approach is more holistic in that takes into account the whole patient as he or she functions and interacts within his or her environment. Interactive reasoning (answer C) is a process by which the practitioner and patient collaborate so that the practitioner may better understand the patient's environment and situation. Narrative reasoning (answer D) is a form of story telling in which practitioners share similar experiences, allowing for problem solving to occur. See reference: Mattingly and Fleming: Fleming, MH: The therapist with the three-track mind.

44. (B) Lateral trunk stability An individual who is uncoordinated or has poor head control would not be able to control the mobile arm support to bring the hand safely to the mouth without hitting the face or some other area. Also, poor head control would mean that the individual's head would be out of alignment for the hand to reach, or the person would be unable to see properly to control the mobile arm support. An individual with fair plus (3+) elbow flexion would be able to stabilize the elbow on the table to bring the hand to the mouth and would have enough strength to move the arm without the mobile arm support. For the mobile arm support to perform properly, the individual's trunk needs to be stabilized laterally by his or her own control or with positioning devices to provide a stable base from which the arm may move. See reference: Trombly (ed): Linden, CA, and Trombly, CA: Orthoses: Kinds and purposes.

45. (D) adapted teaching techniques. Answer D is correct because a child with this type of disability characteristically has learning problems that require such teaching methods as "chaining" or behavior modification. Answers A, B, and C are of secondary importance because physical coordination may be impaired or other physical limitations such as abnormal muscle tone or significant problems with balance could also be present. These additional problems may require adaptive equipment, clothing, or techniques. However, all aspects of dressing depend on the child's ability to learn procedures of dressing; therefore, it is necessary to consider task analysis and teaching approach first. See reference: Case-Smith (ed): Shepherd, J: Self-care and adaptations for independent living.

46. (B) vestibular stimulation and gross motor exercise. The sensory integration treatment approach, which aims to improve the reception and processing of sensory information within the central nervous system, uses both vestibular stimulation and gross motor exercises (answer B). Social skills training (answer A), role-playing activities (answer C), and discussion groups (answer D) might be used when an individual needs help in relating appropriately and effectively with others. Although these interventions may be a part of the overall treatment program, this type of individual must be able to receive and process sensory information before embarking on a higher level of social interaction. See reference: Early: Medical and psychological models of mental health and illness.

47. (B) Extending the elbow in mid range 30 to 40 degrees with the forearm arm resting on the table surface Extending the elbow in mid range 30 to 40 degrees while the arm is resting on a table surface would be active assisted range of motion with gravity eliminated. Muscles with poor minus strength would only be able to move a body part through partial range of motion in a gravity eliminated position. The individual would then need assistance to complete the range of motion while using what strength is available in the body part. Answer A is incorrect because PROM would not utilize the increased strength available since the muscle does not contract. Answers C and D are incorrect because both involve resistive activities and a muscle with poor minus strength would be unable to move against gravity or to take any resistance, even with gravity eliminated. See reference: Trombly (ed): Trombly, CA: Evaluation of biomechanical and physiological aspects of motor performance.

48. (B) wide-base sitting on the floor while reaching for a suspended balloon. The child first practices skills in unsupported sitting on a stable surface using a wide base of support. As skills improve, the wide base is reduced to a more narrow one. Reaching activities are used to promote postural reactions, because they involve displacement of the center of gravity and weight shifting. Answers A, C, and D are activities involving unstable support surfaces, typical of more advanced skills. See reference: Case-Smith (ed): Nichols, DS: The development of postural control.

49. (B) are structured by the OT practitioner to encourage self-reflection and feedback. For a graded program designed to develop an individual's self-awareness, the most essential ingredient is the opportunity to verbalize one's ideas and feelings and to receive feedback from others in a safe setting. Therefore, it is not the activities that are graded but the way the OT practitioner structures the activities to encourage self-reflection and feedback. See reference: Early: Analyzing, adapting, and grading activities.

50. (D) Removing a nut from a bolt Answer D describes one type of in-hand manipulation called rotation. Rotation is the movement of an object around one or more of its axes, where objects may be turned horizontally or end over end with the pads of the fingers, as when one would unscrew a nut from a bolt. Answers A, B, and C are incorrect because

they describe hand activities that essentially keep the object in a certain position as it is grasped, released, or carried with no in-hand manipulation required. See reference: Case-Smith (ed): Exner, CE: Development of hand skills.

51. (C) Trim lines of the splint should extend proximal to the MCP crease. Trim lines of a splint that extend proximal to the MCP crease allow for adequate MCP digit extension and flexion. Answers A, B, and D all fall distal to the MCP crease, thus restricting full extension and flexion of the digits at the metacarpal heads. See reference: Pedretti (ed): Belkin, J, and English, CB: Orthotics.

52. (C) pouring a glass of orange juice. Meal preparation is graded from cold to hot foods or beverages and from simple to multiple steps. An individual beginning meal preparation training should start with a cold item involving the least number of steps possible, such as pouring a glass of juice or other cold beverage. Cold sandwich preparation (answer A) adds another step as each topping to the bread is added and as the use of utensils is introduced. After preparation of cold items has been mastered, training in hot food or beverage preparation (answers B and D) may be initiated. See reference: Neistadt and Crepeau (eds): Neistadt, ME: Overview of treatment.

53. (D) cognitive planning Praxis or motor planning refers to the ability to attend to and plan a motor act cognitively, based on adequate sensory input (answer D). Dr. Ayres referred to this function as the highest, most complex of children's motor functions, involving conscious attention that is closely linked to mental and intellectual functions. Automatic and reflex motor activity, as well as coordination of the motor act, do not require attention or volition; it is enough to have a general goal in mind. Therefore, answers A, B, and C are incorrect. See reference: Fisher, Murray, and Bundy (eds): Cermak, SA: Somatodyspraxia.

54. (B) provide enough chairs around a round table. Circular seating arrangements generally facilitate the most communication among members. Rectangular tables can lead to unbalanced communications. Difficulties in maintaining comfort and attention are problems related to floor seating arrangements. Using available chairs and couches frequently provides different seating heights often in rectangular or square arrangements. See reference: Posthuma: Group dimensions.

55. (C) have the individual trace lines across the page with the right index finger from the left to the right side. A person who follows a line when wheeling a wheelchair is focusing on midline positioning, not crossing the midline. Placing objects commonly used on the unaffected side is a compensatory technique that does not involve crossing the midline. The individual with midline problems would need cueing to avoid starting at the midline when attempting to lay cards out from the right to left side. Also, the person would have difficulty accurately completing a sequencing task on the neglected side, making it difficult to complete the midline crossing successfully. However, when tracing a line across the page, the individual receives the same proprioceptive input from the movement, and uses the same amount of space in the visual field, as when writing on paper. This task makes the transfer of skills easier when performing writing. See reference: Zoltan: Body scheme disorders.

56. (A) promote open-ended symbolic play, such as using action figures, puppets, and dolls. Toys that elicit feelings and expression can be used to promote beginning play skills and beginning interaction and communication skills. Inherent in open-ended play is the fact that there is no right or wrong way-that failure is not possible. Structured craft activities (answer B) do not provide sufficient opportunity for self-expression and carry the possibility of failure because since there is a right and wrong way to do them. As an initial activity, a game of tag (answer C), especially one that involves peers, may be perceived as threatening and overwhelming by the child. Activities that promote tension release (answer D) do not directly address play skills; rather, they focus on the powerful motor action only. See reference: Case-Smith (ed): Morrison, CD, and Metzger, P: Play.

57. (A) Meal preparation techniques using a wheelchair As the disease progresses, individuals with ALS lose the strength required for ambulation and begin to use wheelchairs. Therefore, the development of meal preparation skills using a wheelchair, such as transportation of items, addressing work heights, using adaptive equipment (answer A encompasses answer B), and safety issues, is the best answer. Gradually increasing standing tolerance (answer C) is not appropriate for this individual because motoric function will continue to deteriorate. Developing competence in preparing cold meals before advancing to hot meals (answer D) is more appropriate for individuals with cognitive or perceptual deficits. See reference: Dutton: Rehabilitation postulates regarding intervention.

58. (A) Give one- or two-step instructions frequently repeated. The best method to use with an individual with Alzheimer's disease is short instructions of one to two steps keeping them to the point and repeating them frequently. Demonstration with multiple-step instructions (answer B) can be confusing as it provides too much stimulation. Multiple-step written instructions (answer C) are unlikely to be retained in the individual's short-term memory after reading, or remembered in sequence. Also, written instructions could be lost if the individual puts them down. Verbally repeating directions over and over (answer D), or rehearsal, does not enable a person with Alzheimer's disease to retain information in the

memory, and he or she may not repeat the instructions properly. See reference: Neistadt and Crepeau (eds): Holm, M, Rogers, J, and Birge-James, A: Treatment of occupational performance.

59. (B) assembling packets that include a knife, fork, spoon, and napkin based on a sample. This individual is functioning at Allen's Cognitive Level 4. Individuals functioning at this level are able to copy demonstrated directions presented one step at a time. They find it easier to copy a sample than to follow directions or diagrams. Individuals functioning at cognitive level 3 are capable of using their hands for simple, repetitive tasks but are unlikely to produce a consistent endproduct. They are also more successful performing a sorting task (answer A). The shoelace task (answer C) is most appropriate for those functioning at cognitive level 5. These individuals are interested in the relationships between objects and can generally perform a three-step task. Individuals functioning at cognitive level 6 can anticipate errors and plan ways to avoid them, and would be successful with tasks that are more complex and require attention to detail (answer D). See reference: Early: Some practice models for occupational therapy in mental health.

60. (B) play and self-care activities. "When providing OT care for children with terminal illness, the underlying principle is to add quality to their remaining days. There are two performance areas that occupational therapists should address in children with terminal illness: (1) play activities and (2) activities of daily living" (p. 838). Educational activities (answer A) would not address the primary principle of adding quality of life. Play activities help the child to focus interest and express feelings and may incorporate socialization and motor activities (answers C and D), but neither of these types of activities alone would be the primary focus. Self-care activities allow the child to maintain independence and purposefulness. See reference: Case-Smith (ed): Barnstorff, MJ: The dying child.

61. (D) State strengths and limitations regarding performance in the activity Self-concept is defined as the value of one's physical and emotional self. Stating one's strengths and limitations about one's own performance is a reflection of an individual's self-concept. Planning a healthy meal (answer A) addresses the goal of health maintenance. Developing a budget and shopping (answer B) address the goal of money management. Delegating tasks and preparing the meal address the goals of interpersonal skills and meal preparation skills. See reference: AOTA: Uniform Terminology for Occupational Therapy, third edition.

62. (A) Complete independence with self-care and transfers An individual with T4 paraplegia will have sufficient trunk balance and upper extremity strength and coordination to complete self-care and transfers independently. See reference: Pedretti (ed): Adler, C. Spinal cord injury.

63. (A) restore and maintain functional performance of self-chosen occupations that enhance competent performance of valued occupational roles. The depression is likely to be in reaction to the individual's AIDS disease and major loss of functioning at stage 4. Stage 4 of AIDS generally means severe physical and neurological changes. Because the change of function can be broad, answer A is the most comprehensive approach. Answers B, C, and D are too restrictive to be a "major focus." Also, restoration of work is typically unrealistic at stage 4 of AIDS. See reference: Neistadt and Crepeau (eds): Pizzi, M and Burkhardt, A: Occupational therapy for adults with immunological diseases.

64. (C) texture of the cords she will be using. Coarse materials like jute may shred and give splinters or injure the skin on hands and fingers. This is particularly important for individuals with diabetes who frequently have poor sensation and circulation in their extremities. Skin damage must be avoided since healing is compromised. The length of the cord (answer A) would be significant for an individual with limited range of motion. The thickness of the cord (answer B) would be significant for an individual with limited hand function. The type of surface the individual stands on (answer D) would be important to an individual with back pain. See reference: Reed and Sanderson (eds): Diabetes mellitus—type II.

65. (D) Reinforcement of competence According to Erikson, an 8-year-old is usually at the stage of industry versus inferiority, during which he or she develops a sense of competency. For a client who is expected to lose motor function gradually, a treatment plan that will provide him with an ongoing sense of competence (possibly in other areas) is especially relevant. Answers A, B, and C describe other developmental issues identified by Erikson that are typically achieved at other ages: basic trust (answer A) in infancy, initiative (answer B) during the toddler years, and self-identity (answer C) during adolescence. See reference: Case-Smith (ed): Law, M, Missiuna, C, Pollock, N, and Stewart, D: Foundations of occupational therapy practice with children.

66. (C) games of chance. Because winning a game of chance is based essentially on luck, individuals functioning at various functional levels have "equal" opportunities to win. Hobbies (answer B) are not considered a category of games. Competitive and strategy games (answers A and D) both require specific skills to succeed. See reference: Early: Leisure skills.

67. (D) During one to two conversations with female group members, the client will make eye contact for 8 to 10 seconds, two times in each half-hour socialization group. The short-term goal that describes appropriate verbal and nonverbal interactions with female peers is the best answer. A goal set for 6 months (answer A) is a long-term goal. Awareness of thought processes (answer B) is more appropriate to a goal related to self-awareness. Attempting to develop skills with staff (answer C) can pose some confusing boundary and ethical questions in a long-term goal related to developing future personal relationships. See reference: Early: Understanding psychiatric diagnosis: the DSM-IV.

68. (B) Learning proper body mechanics Learning proper body mechanics (along with achieving a good fitness level) is one of the first steps to reducing the risk of reinjury in a work program. Answer C, work hardening, is appropriate to implement after the physical demands of the job specific task are achieved. Answer D, engaging in vocational counseling, is appropriate after it is determined that a client cannot return to the same job or employer. Answer A, a prework screening, is typically completed by the practitioner before the employer offers the new employee a job. See reference: Neistadt and Crepeau (eds): Fenton, S, and Gagnon, P: Treatment of work and productive activities: Functional restoration, an industrial approach.

69. (D) the ability to recognize objects. Answer D is correct because a child must be able to recognize an object before he or she can discriminate among its specific visual attributes. Answers A, B, and C are not correct because the ability to discriminate among colors, shapes, and positions is a skill that develops later. See reference: Kramer and Hinojosa (eds): Todd, VR: Visual information analysis: Frame of reference for visual perception.

70. (D) A volar resting splint A volar resting splint is indicated for acute synovitis of the wrist, fingers, and thumb. Answer B is indicated for wrist pain and to protect the extensor tendons from rupture. Answer C is a splint used to prevent ulnar drift while maintaining joint alignment for grasp and pinch activities. Answer A assists in keeping the MP joints in normal alignment while preventing volar subluxation. See reference: Pedretti (ed): Hittle, JM, Pedretti, LW, and Kasch, MC: Rheumatoid arthritis.

71. (B) Visual attention skills According to Todd, answer B is correct because development of visual attention skills should be worked on first because they prepare and provide foundation skills for other aspects of visual perception. Answer A is incorrect because visual memory skills can only be developed after visual attention skills are established. Answers C and D are incorrect because general and specific visual perceptual skills develop after visual memory. See reference: Kramer and Hinojosa (eds): Todd, VR: Visual information analysis: Frame of reference for visual perception.

72. (C) Modify the environment to protect the

infant from excessive and/or inappropriate sensory stimulation prior to direct intervention. Neonatal Abstinence Score (NAS) infants have multiple sensory needs often resulting in poor self-regulation and behavioral organization. Answers C and D both incorporate sensory integration approaches; however, answer C best demonstrates an initial intervention to promote neurobehavioral organization required to tolerate direct handling. Answers A and B are important in determining appropriate treatment plans for the infant and family. However, a social work referral should be made after initial assessments are completed, to make the most appropriate recommendations for social service involvement if needed. Although identifying maternal medical status and treatment compliance issues are of great importance for an OT to best determine educational and disposition recommendations, it is not the OT's primary sensory intervention focus. See reference: Case-Smith (ed): Hunter, JG: Neonatal Intensive Care Unit.

73. (D) position the patient so she is facing a blank wall. One way to modify the environment for an individual who is easily distracted is to position him or her facing a blank wall (answer D), thereby lessening possible distracters. It may also be necessary to speak loudly in order to get the patient's attention, which is why answer A is not recommended. If the patient is unable to participate in the activity successfully, the OT should direct her to a simpler activity. Coaxing and praising (answer B) will not increase her skill level. Asking the rest of the group members to stop talking (answer C) would probably interfere with the goals of the rest of the group. See reference: Early: Responding to symptoms and behaviors.

74. (D) (1) gather shirt up at the back of the neck; (2) pull gathered back fabric off over head; (3) remove shirt from unaffected arm; and (4) remove shirt from affected arm. Answers A, B, and C are examples of incorrect sequences that would result in failure to remove the shirt successfully. See reference: Pedretti (ed): Foti, D, Pedretti, LW, and Lillie, S: Activities of daily living.

75. (B) Training in residual limb wrapping Residual limb wrapping would help prepare the residual limb by shrinking and shaping it to fit in the prosthesis. Training in how to put on and take off the prosthesis (answer A), and activities to improve grasp and prehension (answer C) come later in the intervention process when the prosthesis has been selected, prescribed, and fitted. Training to resume vocational activities (answer D) would also normally occur later in rehabilitation process, after the patient has mastered the basics of prosthetic use. See reference: Pedretti (ed): Rock, LM: Upper extremity amputations and prosthetics.

76. (D) A cutting board with two nails in it The

potato is placed on the nails to hold it in place while working. The dycem would only hold the cutting board in place, not the potato being cut. A plate guard would not be secured tightly enough to the plate to withstand the force of cutting the potato. A rocker knife would be unable to both stabilize the potato and be used for cutting. See reference: Trombly (ed): Stewart, C: Retraining housekeeping and child care skills.

77. (B) use pillows to prop up body parts into desired position. An individual with low tone may benefit from supportive positioning devices such as pillows, towels, or bolsters that can help to prevent overstretching and fatigue. Slow rocking (answer C) and avoidance of quick stretch (answer D) are both methods for reducing tone and would not be beneficial to an individual having a problem with low tone. A sidelying position (answer A) would be a very difficult position for an individual with lower extremity flaccidity to maintain during sexual activity but may be preferable for someone requiring energy conservation. See reference: Pedretti (ed): Burton, GU: Issues of sexuality with physical dysfunction.

78. (C) inferior to the anterior superior iliac spine. A seat belt placed across the lap inferior to the anterior superior iliac spine prevents the hips from being extended into a posterior pelvic tilt. If the seat belt is placed at an angle inferior to the ischial tuberosity (answer A), it would go across the thighs and allow a posterior pelvic tilt. A seat belt placed superior to the iliac crest or the posterior superior iliac spine (answers B and D, respectively) would be too high, allowing hip extension with posterior pelvic tilt to occur below the seat belt. See reference: Trombly (ed): Deitz, J, and Dudgeon, B: Wheelchair selection process.

79. (B) learning the self-monitoring technique of asking oneself if any part of the task has been missed. Teaching the client to self-monitor is an example of a strategy to control the tendency to miss details involved in the task process. Answer A, simplifying instructions is an example of a method of adapting the amount of information presented during the task. Answer C, practicing shape and number cancellation worksheets is an example of a remedial skill training activity. Answer D, removing unnecessary objects from the task area to decrease distractions is an example of adapting the environment to compensate for attention deficits. See reference: Neistadt and Crepeau (eds): Toglia, JP: Cognitive-perceptual retraining and rehabilitation.

80. (D) A long-handled bath sponge A person with a total hip arthroplasty needs to avoid hip flexion of 80 degrees or more, hip adduction with internal rotation at the knee or ankle, and lifting the knee higher than the hip during self-care or home management activities. A wire basket attached to the walker would not allow the person to come close to a counter without having to step sideways, which causes hip adduction to either move toward or away from the counter. A padded toilet seat of 1 inch height or a short-handled sponge would be inadequate in that it would cause the person to flex the hip past 80 degrees while performing of self-care activities. See reference: Trombly (ed): Bear-Lehman, J: Orthopaedic conditions.

81. (B) a seat belt placed at a 45-degree angle at the hips. A seat belt correctly placed at a 45-degree angle to the child's hips would inhibit extensor tone. Answer A is incorrect because lateral trunk supports support the trunk from sideward movement only. Although a wedge-shaped seat insert (answer C) increases hip flexion more than 90 degrees and inhibits extensor tone, it is not the best choice because it could have the undesirable side effect of tightening hamstrings over time. Answer D is incorrect because, although it may contribute to holding a child in a chair, it does not affect the angle of the hip joint, which is necessary for decreasing extensor tone in sitting. See reference: Case-Smith (ed): Shepherd, J: Self-care and adaptations for independent living.

82. (A) Textured material, rubbing, tapping, and prolonged contact Sensory desensitization helps the individual recalibrate altered sensory perceptions and improve sensibility. This type of program is initiated when light-touch sensation is intact. The above listed modalities are used as graded tactile stimuli. Treatment is most successful when carried out and controlled by the individual. With a severe injury such as a burn, it is also necessary to train the individual in protective precautions. Any techniques that provide an ungraded or nonspecific level of touch, such as massage, pressure, percussion, or electrical stimulation, would be tolerated with difficulty by a person with hypersensitivity, because much of the input is facilitory and would be interpreted as painful. Visual compensation and functional use of the extremity are techniques used with individuals who have impaired sensation. See reference: Trombly (ed): Bentzel, K: Remediating sensory impairment.

83. (D) a problem-solving task with a "self-talk" cueing strategy. Finding phone numbers is a task that requires some problem solving and the cards are a strategy for providing cues for questioning oneself about the process of problem solving. Answer A is incorrect because self-management is a component of psychosocial, rather than cognitive performance. The task requires visual scanning (answer B) of the phone book to accomplish, but that is not the primary focus of the task. Answer C, a memory task, is incorrect because the performance of this task is not primarily dependent on the use of memory skills and the questions posed relate to the problem-solving process. See reference: Neistadt and Crepeau

(eds): Toglia, JP: Cognitive-perceptual retraining and rehabilitation.

84. (D) built-up handles. Built-up handles, without adding extra weight, allow a comfortable grasp that regular utensils do not provide. A weighted handle would cause more rapid fatigue and strain to the joints. An arthritic person most likely has adequate grasp and release with a built-up handle, making it easier to use than a universal cuff. See reference: Trombly (ed): Feinberg, JR, and Trombly, CA: Arthritis.

85. (B) put the dried dishes away and begin to hand her wet dishes. Compensating for mistakes helps to increase the sense of self-worth and integrity of individuals with dementia. This approach is preferable to drawing attention to errors, especially in situations in which safety is not an issue. Answers A, C, and D all draw attention to the individual's errors. See reference: Early: Responding to symptoms and behaviors.

86. (A) extend the operated leg forward, reach back for the armrests, and slowly sit, while attempting to not lean forward. By extending the operated leg forward, reaching back for the armrests, slowly sitting, and attempting to not lean forward, an effective and safe transfer can be accomplished. Answers B and C are incorrect and contraindicated for transfer training with individuals who have total hip replacements. Answer D, prohibiting movement until 2 weeks after surgery, is not considered to be a traditional approach to rehabilitation after a total hip replacement. See reference: Pedretti (ed): Morawski, D, Pitbladdo, K, Bianchi, EM, et al: Hip fractures and total hip replacement.

87. (A) repetition, high force, and awkward joint postures. Repetition, high force, and awkward joint postures are work-related risk factors that are frequently associated with cumulative trauma disorders. Answer B, progressive resistive exercises, joint mobilization, and weight bearing, are not considered to be primary factors that contribute to cumulative trauma disorders. Answers C and D, inflammation, swelling, pain, fatigue, cramps, and paresthesias, are all considered to be potential symptoms of cumulative trauma disorders, not factors that contribute to the condition. See reference: Pedretti (ed): Kasch, MC: Hand injuries.

88. (A) contrast baths, active and passive range of motion, and massage. Contrast baths, active and passive range of motion, and massage are all initial techniques considered for the prevention or relief of joint stiffness. Answers B and D, ultrasound, electrical stimulation, dynamic splinting, and joint mobilization, are all considered treatment techniques for more established joint stiffness. Answer C, resistive exercises, weight bearing, and lifting could all potentially contribute to increasing joint stiffness and pain. See reference: Pedretti (ed): Kasch, MC: Hand injuries.

89. (D) "The infant uses a wide base of support and high arm guard position and takes short steps." Answer D is correct because according to Case-Smith, "The infant's first efforts toward unsupported movement through walking are often seen in short erratic steps, use of a wide based gait, and arms held in a high guard" (p. 80). Answers A, B, and C are not considered typical for a normally developing infant. See reference: Case-Smith (ed): Case-Smith, J: Development of childhood occupations.

90. (D) identify alternative methods for meeting sexual needs that don't cause pain. Because the individual's pain cannot be seen or felt by the sexual partner, communication is particularly important. The couple can discuss alternate positions and methods for achieving sexual fulfillment that are acceptable to them and that do not cause pain, such as alternate positions, masturbation, and fantasy. Good communication will ensure the needs of both partners are met and prevent misunderstandings. Therefore, answer C is inappropriate. A pain-free position is important for successful sexual expression, but there is insufficient information to determine whether answer A, a sidelying position, is a pain-free position for this individual. Timing sex for periods of high energy (answer B) is an appropriate strategy for individuals with low endurance. However, timing sex for periods of lessened pain, such as after taking pain medication, is a useful strategy for individuals with severe pain. See reference: Pedretti (ed): Burton, GU: Issues of sexuality with physical dysfunction.

91. (A) Biofeedback, distraction, and relaxation techniques Biofeedback, distraction, and relaxation techniques are all examples of measures that are implemented to manage pain. Answers B and C, specific skill training and endurance building, are not directly related to pain management techniques and are often associated with cognitive or motor limitations. Answer D, cognitive retraining techniques, is not directly related to pain management techniques, such as psychophysiological imagery that is commonly used with relaxation techniques. See reference: Neistadt and Crepeau (eds): Engel, JM: Treatment for psychosocial components: Pain management.

92. (C) Hand-over-hand assistance In this method, the caregiver places one hand over the resident's hand and provides assistance while guiding the resident's hand through the steps of the task, guiding the hand from the food up and into the resident's mouth. This method provides maximum assistance while still allowing the person to feel involved and connected to the task. Given the resident's attention span deficits, the use of demonstration (answer A), verbal feedback (answer B) and even chaining (answer C) would be insufficient to sustain the

resident's active participation. See reference: Hellen: Daily life care activities.

93. (C) When the child has achieved a maintenance level of functioning Because this child may never be considered completely recovered (answer D) or may refuse OT services because of his head injury (answer A), discharge should be discussed when the child is no longer making significant progress. Transition to the first grade (answer B) is an educational consideration that is not directly relevant to the provision of services under a medical model. See reference: Case-Smith (ed): Case-Smith, J, Rogers, J, and Johnson, JH: School-based occupational therapy.

94. (C) increase the management of texture by slowly increasing texture of food with a baby food grinder. This method offers a gradual increase in texture that encourages chewing. Answer A is not correct because scraping off food from a spoon with the child's teeth does not encourage any voluntary oral motor control. Answer B is incorrect because it combines liquid with pieces of food (soft and chewy), and this combination of textures will be too unpredictable for a child who is having difficulty organizing oral motor skills to manage food. Answer D is incorrect because a raisin is too large of a step in terms of texture from pureed food. See reference: Case-Smith (ed): Case-Smith, J, and Humphry, R: Feeding intervention.

95. (B) Bend both knees, keep the back straight, and bring object close to the body when lifting Bending with both knees while keeping the back straight and the object close to the body will prevent low back bending and strain. Answers A, C, and D are all incorrect methods for lifting and carrying objects. Answers A and C will actually increase an individual's chance of increasing low back strain. See reference: Pedretti (ed): Smithline, J: Low back pain.

96. (B) Proceed only to the point of pain. Care must be taken to avoid fatigue and irritation of inflamed nerves when working with individuals with Guillain-Barré syndrome, so ranging only to the point of pain is the most important concept in this question. While keeping that precaution in mind, the therapist should begin with proximal muscles and move in a distal direction (answer A). The number of repetitions is at the discretion of the therapist (answer C); the quality of the stretch is more important than the quantity. See reference: Pedretti (ed): McCormack, GL, and Pedretti, LW: Motor unit dysfunction.

97. (C) Removing pants Answer C is correct because, according to most developmental scales, children first learn to remove garments, especially socks. Answer A is not correct because the ability to put garments on with the front and back correctly placed is a skill that is developed later. Buttoning and tying bows (answer D) is incorrect for the same reason. Answer B is incorrect because children are able to remove garments before they are able to put them on. See reference: Case-Smith (ed): Shepherd, J: Self care and adaptations for independent living.

98. (D) respond to the emotional tone expressed by the words: provide extra attention and reassurance. Listening for the feelings behind the words will best help to identify and address the needs of the person who has lost ability to use words effectively; the resident's searching for her mother may reflect the resident's sense of loneliness. Explaining the factual truth (answer A) can have the effect of unnecessarily confronting the person with his or her deficits, and the person may respond to the news as if hearing it for the first time. Telling the person to stop the behavior (answer B) will not address the need that is being expressed verbally. Answer C, telling a therapeutic fib, might work for a brief period of time but may backfire if the person continues to question the story given or if it causes sadness or anger. See reference: Hellen: Communication: Understanding and being understood.

99. (D) cooperative group activity that both provides and elicits consistent and accurate feedback about interactions within the group. Because the underlying issues for most personality disorders are related to inaccurate perceptions of the self and others, the selected approach to treatment should directly address these problems. A group format offers a wider variety of feedback about the specific interactions that occur. The group activity should be based on a central goal of reducing misperceptions. Social skills groups (answer C) are often used to address the interaction difficulties experienced with cluster C personality disorders. The question does not specify that cluster C personality disorders are included in the group. Answer B is best used for problems with individuals, not groups. Answer A addresses decision making and not inaccurate perceptions. See reference: Ryan (ed): The Certified Occupational Therapy Assistant: Blechert, TF, and Kari, N: Interpersonal communication skills and applied group dynamics.

100. (B) Working on a mock car engine Working on a mock car engine provides a work simulation that would be required by the client's job. This activity would also assist with increasing his endurance, strength, and productivity. Answer A, lifting weights, is not a work hardening goal when performed in isolation of a simulated work task. Answer C, visiting the work site, would not be a work hardening activity but rather part of the onsite analysis that is typically completed by the practitioner and vocational retraining counselor. Answer D, meal preparation, is not considered to be a demand required by this particular vocation. See reference: Pedretti (ed): Kasch, MC: Hand injuries.

101. (C) Eat six small meals a day An individual with ALS who becomes fatigued eating three full meals a day should attempt eating six smaller meals a day before resorting to tube feedings or pureed diets (answers A and D). Eating regular food is usually more enjoyable than the alternatives and is likely to enhance the quality of life. An upright position is optimal when feeding individuals with dysphagia. A semi-reclined position (answer B) can make swallowing more difficult or dangerous. See reference: Pedretti (ed): Pedretti, LW, and McCormack, GL: Amyotrophic lateral sclerosis.

102. (D) Alternate tasks that require standing with those that can be performed sitting The performance component at issue in this question is fatigue. When fatigue impedes occupational performance, energy conservation techniques should be considered. Alternating sitting and standing activities is one method that can be applied to conserve energy; others include avoiding bending and stooping, avoiding unnecessary trips, using an appropriate work height, and relaxing homemaking standards. Convincing the individual to do something she can't afford (answer A) may not be in her best interests and it is not an example consistent with the OT concept of collaborative decision making. Although increasing strength (answer B) may ultimately be useful, endurance is typically a more pressing issue for individuals with MS. Using the largest joint available for the task is a joint protection technique more appropriate for an individual with arthritis See reference: Pedretti (ed): Hittle, JM, Pedretti, LW, and Kasch, MC, in Rheumatoid arthritis.

103. (D) provide wrist extension, MCP extension, and thumb extension. The purpose of this splint is to prevent the extensor tendons from overstretching as well as provide proper positioning of the hand for functional use. Answers A, B, and C are inappropriate functions for a dynamic radial nerve splint. See reference: Pedretti (ed): Kasch, MC: Hand injuries.

104. (B) facilitating postural reactions. By placing a child in the sitting position on a therapeutic ball, "the therapist can facilitate postural reactions using activities that displace the center of gravity and require corrective or protective responses" (p. 284). The addition of the reaching activity will cause the child to change his or her center of gravity during the reaching phase, which will require a further postural response to compensate for the change of position. See reference: Case-Smith (ed): Nichols, D: Development of postural control.

105. (C) to both sides of the client's body. Answer C is correct because the client must be able to transfer to both sides of the body. It is usually difficult or impossible to arrange the home environment so that the all transfers can be done from one side only. For instance, if the toilet at home is close to the wall, getting on and off the toilet will require transfer first to one side of the body and then to the opposite side. The family also needs to know the different kinds and amounts of support they must use on each side of the client's body. Thus, answers A, B, and D are incorrect because they all involve transfer to only one side. See reference: Trombly (ed): Retraining basic and instrumental activities of daily living.

106. (A) Mount lever handles on doors and faucets For children with reduced strength and endurance, using less complex movements and less force results in energy conservation. Lever handles require less energy than knob handles on doors, faucets, and appliances. Answers B and C are environmental adaptations recommended to minimize the danger of slipping and falling for children with incoordination or postural instability. Answer D is contraindicated because work at a vertical surface against gravity requires more energy than movement in a horizontal plane. See reference: Case-Smith (ed): Dudgeon, BJ: Pediatric rehabilitation.

107. (A) a resting pan splint for a client after a TBI who has been unresponsive in the intensive care unit for 3 weeks, yet grimaces with passive digit extension This type of static splint appropriately positions the wrist and digits in a functional position in order to prevent the development of contractures while providing protection for the hand. Answers B, C, and D are all considered to be dynamic splints. See reference: Pedretti (ed): Belkin, J, and English, CB: Orthotics.

108. (A) Teach the child to dress in a sidelying position The sidelying position eliminates the need for the child to maintain balance in order to dress the lower extremities. Answer B is not correct because the primary purpose of putting loops on waistbands is to help a child with limited grasp strength pull on garments. Answer C is not correct because using Velcro in place of zippers is also an adaptation designed to help children with limited ability to grasp and pull. See reference: Case-Smith (ed): Shepherd, J: Self-care and adaptations for independent living.

109. (C) providing a program to enhance occupational performance in ADL, work, and leisure. The role of the OT on the LE management team is to address occupational performance in areas of function: ADL, such as self-care, functional mobility, community mobility; work or productive activities, such as home management and vocational activities; and leisure activities. The OT may address performance components such as endurance, pain management, and soft tissue integrity to achieve the overall aim of maximizing occupational performance. Answer A is the primary role of the prosthetist; answer B reflects the primary functions of the PT; and answer D is the primary responsibility of the social worker. See reference: Pedretti (ed): Pasquinelli, S: Lower extremity amputations and prosthetics.

110. (C) precipitating conditions and events that elicit stress reactions. The conditions and events that elicit stress reactions are known as stressors (answer C). Stressors can be either short term or long term. Answer A describes coping, answer B describes stress, and answer D describes adaptation. See reference: Christiansen and Baum (eds): Christiansen, C: Performance deficits as sources of stress.

111. (D) Weaving on a wide frame loom Use of and attention to the entire loom area is essential for weaving on a frame loom. The shuttle must slide across the entire width of the loom, which involves crossing the midline. Placing objects within the individual's field of vision and patient education (answers A and B) are both appropriate intervention methods; however, they are adaptive, not remedial, methods. Verbal and tactile cueing (answer C) are remedial methods as well; however, the individual would need to be cued to look to the left, not the right. See reference: Zoltan: Visual processing skills.

112. (B) Tip the wheelchair backward and guide it down the ramp forwards This is the recommended technique for going down a steep ramp. The individual sitting in the wheelchair can also help to control the wheels, if capable of doing so, by grasping the hand rims. It would be difficult for the person guiding a wheelchair backwards down a ramp (answer A) to see where he or she is going. Only very strong individuals can propel themselves independently down a steep ramp (answer C). Using two people to move a wheelchair down a steep ramp could be awkward and dangerous (answer D). See reference: Pedretti (ed): Adler, C, and Tipton-Burton, M: Wheelchair assessment and transfers.

113. (C) Word prediction software Word prediction software anticipates the word desired and increases the speed of input by decreasing the number of keystrokes required. A larger monitor (answer A) or screen may be useful when a child has difficulty seeing the screen or details on the screen. Voice output systems (answer B), which read text and provide cues, can be useful for children with autism, learning disabilities, cognitive delays and visual impairments. Masking inappropriate keys (answer D) reduces the number of options and can help children who have difficulty finding the correct key. See reference: Case-Smith (ed): Swinth, Y: Assistive technology: Computers and augmentative communication.

114. (C) Describe how using a shower chair improves safety. Informing the patient of various options is the first response. By describing the shower chair and how it make showering safer, the OT practitioner is conveying the concept that occupational performance is based on the interaction of performance contexts (physical environment) and performance components (balance) and that there are methods to ensure safety. The OT practitioner would then inquire as to the patient's interest in purchasing a shower chair (answer B). Getting into the bathtub is even more risky than getting into the shower (answer A); therefore, that is not an option for the patient. With a patient who is very focused on deficits and expects therapy to completely remediate these deficits (answer D), answer C refocuses the emphasis on performance of the activity. See reference: Piersol and Ehrlich (eds): Seibert, C: The clinic called home.

115. (A) Velcro closures on front-opening clothing. Velcro closures on front-opening clothing would require the least amount of dexterity, which becomes increasingly difficult with Parkinson's disease. Large buttons on front-opening clothing (answer B) might be easier than smaller buttons, but would still require more manipulation than Velcro closures. Clothing slipped on overhead with no fasteners (answer C) would eliminate the need for dexterity, but having to raise the arms to put on the garment would be problematic because of the rigidity and stiffness of the limbs that typically accompanies Parkinson's disease. Though clothing which stretches freely is easier to put on than tightly constructed clothing, the need to tie the closures in the back of the garment would be difficult for a person with upper extremity rigidity. See reference: Trombly (ed): Newman, EM, Echevarria, ME, and Digman, G: Degenerative diseases.

116. (C) allow child to self-apply tactile stimuli to maximize child's tolerance. Tactile defensiveness is an overreaction or negative reaction to sensations of touch. Answer C is correct. "Generally, tactile stimuli that are actively self-applied by the child are tolerated much better than stimuli that are passively received, as when being touched by another person" (p. 352). Answer A is incorrect because because light touch sensations are particularly disturbing for children with tactile defensiveness and may create overwhelming feelings of anxiety which influence behavior. Answer B is not correct because avoiding all forms of tactile sensation is virtually impossible and such complete avoidance would not help the child to develop coping skills. Answer D is also incorrect because deep touch stimuli is often comfortable for children with tactile defensiveness and can even provide "…relief from irritating stimuli when deep pressure is applied over the involved skin areas" (p. 350). See reference: Case-Smith (ed): Parham, LD, and Mailloux, Z: Sensory integration.

117. (B) Replace the white glue with blue glue Activity adaptations enable the individual to become more functional in his or her task performance. Reviewing the difference between glue and grout (answer A) would be a cognitive approach. Avoiding the use of white tiles (answer C) could be a solution if the problem were figure-ground related. Completing the last step of the activity for the individual (answer D) reflects a forward-chaining approach. See reference: Early: Analyzing, adapting, and grading activities.

118. (B) Obstacle courses This child should be exposed to situations that require problem solving by challenging the child to move his or her body in relation to objects in the environment. Although all of the answers involve motor planning in response to the environment to some degree, running obstacle courses clearly emphasizes the spatial element the most. Obstacles also consist of static items and therefore facilitate success in adjustment (motor planning) more easily than moving objects. See reference: Case-Smith (ed): Parham, LD, and Mailloux, Z: Sensory integration.

119. (B) seating the patient upright on a firm surface with the chin slightly tucked. The best position for feeding an individual with a swallowing disorder is upright and symmetrical, with the chin slightly tucked. "Correct positioning normalizes tone, thereby facilitating quality motor control and function of the facial musculature, jaw and tongue movement, and the swallow process, all of which minimize the potential for aspiration" (p. 180). Supine, semi-reclined, and sidelying positions all place the patient at greater risk for choking and aspiration (entry of food material into the airway). See reference: Pedretti (ed): Nelson, KL: Dysphagia: Evaluation and treatment.

120. (A) the depth of the wound and location and the patient's race and age can all influence scar formation. The depth of the wound and location and the patient's race and age all influence scar formation. Full-thickness wounds typically do heal with significant scar formation (answer B). Also, surgical intervention does not eliminate all risk of hypertrophic scarring (answer C) and hypertrophic scars involving the joints do interfere with range of motion (answer D). See reference: Neistadt and Crepeau (eds): Rivers, EA, and Jordan, CL: Skin system dysfunction: Burns.

121. (D) Use dust mitt to keep fingers fully extended Using dust mitts "keeps fingers straight and prevents the static contraction and potentially deforming forces of holding a dust cloth" (p. 644). Pushing the vacuum (answer A) forward by straightening the elbow completely, then pulling it back close to the body utilizes long strokes and promotes good elbow and shoulder range of motion. When ironing (answer B), trying to get the elbow into full extension helps to maintain elbow range of motion. Keeping lightweight objects (answer C) on high shelves encourages reaching, which helps maintain shoulder range of motion. See reference: Pedretti (ed): Hittle, JM, Pedretti, LW, and Kasch, MC: Rheumatoid arthritis.

122. (D) Lock the brakes. Brakes should be locked first to stabilize the wheelchair. Answers A, B, and C involve movements that could cause loss of balance or wheelchair movement unless the brakes are locked. See reference: Pedretti (ed): Adler, C, and Tipton-Burton, M: Wheelchair assessment and transfers.

123. (D) walking at 1 mph. The MET value for sitting at the edge of the bed is 1.3, and the MET value for walking 1.2 mph is 2. The MET values for peeling potatoes (answer A), propelling a wheelchair at 1.2 mph (answer B), and taking a shower (answer C) are 2.5, 2, and 3.5, respectively. Although it is unrealistic to expect the entry-level practitioner to memorize a MET table, several factors can help the therapist assess the demand of any given task. For example, upper extremity activity work produces a greater cardiovascular response than lower extremity work. Because both peeling potatoes and propelling a wheelchair primarily use the upper extremities, one can deduce that the cardiac demand from those activities would be greater than walking very slowly. Taking a shower not only involves repeated UE use but adds the environmental factor of heat, which also contributes to the demands on the cardiovascular system. See reference: Dutton: Introduction to biomechanical frame of reference.

124. (A) Patients write fears and concerns on index cards. The OT practitioner collects and reads the cards to the group for discussion. This method allows for anonymity by having each patient write down their concerns without including their names, thereby eliminating any fear of embarrassment. Answers B and C require the patients to make public their concerns, which might prevent complete openness when attempting to express their concerns and fears. Although there are certain concerns that might be common to a large number of patients and having a team member address these concerns in general would be helpful (answer D), this approach would not address the specific concerns of the patients in this group. See reference: Early: Group concepts and techniques.

125. (A) single pressure switch firmly mounted within easy reach. A child with fluctuating muscle tone lacks stability and demonstrates extraneous movement; therefore, deliberate motor action is most effectively executed on a securely mounted device using simple movement patterns. Answers B, C, and D involve devices that would respond to slight touch and would therefore not be effective for a person with extraneous movement and difficulty grading motor action. See reference: Case-Smith (ed): Swinth, Y: Assistive technology: Computers and augmentative communication.

126. (C) using a bath chair and a hand-held shower with tepid water. The best bathing method for a person with COPD considers the energy demands of the task as well as the effect of water temperature in light of the person's functional status. A

person with COPD has difficulty breathing when the environment is hot or humid or when there is a high degree of steam. Answer A is incorrect because of the energy demand of transferring into a tub and using hot water may cause difficulty breathing. Answer B, standing for quick shower, is also incorrect because even if brief, standing would be more energy demanding than sitting and an overhead shower can increase humidity because of the method of water dispersion. A lukewarm tub bath (answer D) would provide lower humidity by using the coolest water temperature, but the need to transfer in and out of the tub may make the task very energy demanding. See reference: Trombly (ed): Atchison, B: Cardiopulmonary disease.

127. (A) A vacuum feeding cup Individuals with impulsive behavior or poor judgment often attempt to drink too quickly. The rate of intake can be limited by using a drinking spout with a small opening, pinching a straw, or using a vacuum feeding cup with a control button. A cup with a large drinking spout (answer D) would increase the rate of intake, which could result in choking or spills. A "nosey cup" (answer B) allows individuals with dysphagia to maintain a tucked-chin position while drinking, which is necessary for a good swallow. A mug with two handles (answer C) would benefit an individual with limited grasp or coordination. See reference: Trombly (ed): Konosky, KA: Dysphagia.

128. (A) encourage the use of PABA-free sunblock and hats. Individuals taking neuroleptic medications are prone to photosensitivity and need protection from the sun. A PABA-free sunblock is recommended because this reduces the chance of an allergic reaction to the sunblock. The precautions described in answer B are helpful to the individual experiencing postural hypotension, which can be a side effect of neuroleptic medication but is not an issue for a picnic outing. Answers C and D are not linked to the side effects of neuroleptic medications. See reference: Early: Psychotropic medications and biological treatments.

129. (A) provide gentle human touch to enable the infant to slowly respond to intervention. Although all answers are possible examples of applied calming techniques, the tactile system is the first to develop and the most sophisticated in the young NICU patient. Therefore, answer A is the most suitable for initial interaction contact. Answers B and C involve the auditory and vestibular systems, which are fully operational during the youngest possible gestation viable for life but are still immature, and can be overstimulating for the neonate. The visual system is the last to develop. Answer D is an optimal visual strategy for early infancy after 30 weeks' gestation, when the infant's visual sensory system for visual interaction is maturing. See reference: Case-Smith (ed): Hunter, JG: Neonatal Intensive Care Unit.

130. (A) A craft activity using increasingly heavy hand tools. Progressive resistive exercise is the most effective method for increasing strength in a muscle with fair+ strength. Mildly resistive activities that are stopped as soon as the individual begins to experience fatigue (answer B) are appropriate for maintaining or improving strength in individuals with conditions in which fatigue should be avoided, such as MS, ALS, and Guillain-Barré syndrome. Electric stimulation (answer C) is appropriate for increasing strength in very weak muscles. When performing resisted active range of motion with this individual, the therapist would use maximal resistance. In addition, a craft activity that can be performed against increasing resistance for prolonged periods of time would be more effective than resisted active range of motion (answer D), which is usually only performed one to two times a day. See reference: Dutton: Biomechanical postulates regarding intervention.

131. (D) Drawing lines and shapes using shaving cream, sand, or finger paints The best activity to encourage prewriting would be drawing lines in different sensory media. Answer A, moving through an obstacle course with emphasis on making turns, would be a useful activity to focus on right–left discrimination. Answer B, having the child create his or her own books is useful for increasing orientation to printed language. Answer C, rolling clay into a ball, is recommended for improving the ability to regulate pressure during hand activity. See reference: Case-Smith (ed): Amundson, SJ: Prewriting and handwriting skills. Exner, CE: Development of hand skills.

132. (C) extension during finger flexion and flexion during finger extension. The method used to maintain tenodesis in the hand of a person with quadriplegia is to keep the wrist extended during finger flexion and flexed during finger extension. This allows the finger flexor tendons to shorten so tenodesis action can occur. The other methods would stretch the tendons too much, which would not allow a tenodesis grasp. See reference: Trombly (ed): Holar, L: Spinal cord injury.

133. (B) identify the abilities, needs, and life goals of the client. Identifying the abilities, needs, and life goals of the client occurs before any other steps in the process in order to make a match between the client's abilities, environmental demands, and the appropriate technology to carry out desired daily occupations. Answers A, C, and D are steps which would come later in the process. See reference: Christiansen and Baum (eds): Trefler, E, and Hobson, D: Assistive technology.

134. (C) protrusion and lateralization. Protrusion is the motion of sticking the tongue out of the mouth in a forward manner, and lateralization involves the movement of the tongue from side to side. Answer A, protrusion, is partially correct but is erroneous because the term humping (which is elicited

by having the client say "ng" and "ga"). Answer B, lateralization, is also partially correct, but tipping (the process of touching the tongue to the upper lip) is incorrect. Answer D, lateralization and humping, is also partially incorrect because of the inclusion of humping. See reference: Pedretti (ed): Nelson, KL: Dysphagia: Evaluation and treatment.

135. (B) Develop awareness about what produces anger and how the clients respond to anger All of the answers are steps in the cognitive–behavioral process. Treatment begins, however, with developing awareness of what produces anger and how individuals respond. Next therapy should move to changing behavior to achieve alternate, more healthy ways of responding and examining the benefits of responding in a more healthy fashion (answer A). Graded tasks are used to reinforce the new beliefs, behaviors, and responses, beginning with easier and progressing to more challenging tasks (answers C and D). See reference: Bruce and Borg: Cognitive-behavioral frame of reference.

136. (C) Can the child's feet reach the floor? A relaxed position during toilet use is essential to success in elimination training. The seat should be low enough so the child's feet can be used to help with postural stability. In addition, a seat design featuring a wide base, back support, and placement at a height that enables the child to place the feet firmly on the ground or on foot supports will give the child a sense of comfort and security. Answers A, B, and D describe other useful considerations that should be addressed after the issue of support has been resolved. See reference: Case-Smith (ed): Shepherd, J: Self-care and adaptations for independent living.

137. (B) provide strong color contrast at key areas to identify steps, pathways, etc. Using contrast is a key environmental adaptation strategy for people with visual impairments. The more contrast, the easier it is to locate objects, steps, entrances, and pathways, thereby improving accessibility by maximizing remaining vision. Instructing the client to sit during ADL (answer A) or recommending human assistance (answer C) would not directly address accessibility. Answer D, recommending training in white cane use, is a method of improving mobility for a person who is blind. See reference: Larson, Stevens-Ratchford, Pedretti, and Crabtree (eds): Christenson, MA: Environmental design, modification and adaptation.

138. (B) recommendation of environmental adaptations and assistance for ADL. A patient who exhibits no capacity for new learning will be unable to benefit from therapy interventions that require the ability to transfer learning (answers A, C, and D). A compensatory approach of adapting the environment and recommending assistance for safe performance of daily activities is the MOST appropriate intervention. See reference: Neistadt and Crepeau (eds): Neistadt, ME: Theories derived from learning perspectives.

139. (C) practice social and life skills. Answer C is correct because practicing life skills is essential for learning and has been found to be helpful in improving functional performance. Answers A, B, and D reflect verbally focused, rather than activity-focused group environments that include insight development, self-disclosure, confrontation, and the open expression of anger. Intense treatment milieus that focus on insight development, self-disclosure, confrontation, and the open expression of anger have been found to be contraindicated in the inpatient treatment of individuals with schizophrenia. Structured, supportive milieus with an emphasis on enhancing positive social and life skills have been found to be helpful. See reference: Bonder: Schizophrenia and other psychotic disorders.

140. (B) child's speed over long distances becomes less than that of a walking person. This child should be considered for a power wheelchair when the current means of locomotion proves less efficient and slower than locomotion by walking. Because the child will be experiencing progressive muscle weakness, energy conservation is of primary importance. Answers A and C address valid environmental considerations to be made after determining the general need for a powered chair. Waiting until the child becomes unable to propel the wheelchair (answer D) would make the transition more difficult and prevent the child from getting around independently in the meantime. See reference: Case-Smith (ed): Wright-Ott, C, and Egilson, S: Mobility.

141. (A) Transferring on and off a commode seat The patient will most likely utilize a walker to transfer on and off a commode seat. In this case, the assistive device (the walker) will permit the patient to adhere to the mandated toe touch precautions, while providing balance, decreasing pain and encouraging safe transfers. Answer B, bed mobility, does not indicate the need for a walker. In this case, the patient may benefit from the use of a trapeze attached to the bed to increase the use of both upper extremities while performing bed mobility. Answer C, self-feeding, can be performed in bed, or at the patient's bedside prior to performing a kitchen/meal preparation task which would include the use of an assistive device. While answer D, distal lower extremity dressing , can be performed in bed with devices such as a long handled shoehorn, sock aid, dressing stick, elastic shoelaces and reacher, most of these activities can be initiated at the bedside in a chair without the use of a walker. See reference: Bernstein (ed): Bernstein Lewis, C and Daleiden, S: Clinical implications of neurologic changes in the aging process.

142. (A) Perform a job analysis Job analysis identifies essential functions of a particular job. Based on the results, the OT practitioner can then work with the individual to maximize performance or request reasonable accommodation (answer B). Activities that promote self-efficacy (answer C) are beneficial for individuals with depression but should not be used at this stage of the individual's program. A weekly support group may be an effective way for the individual to obtain support and can be recommended by the OT practitioner, but it is not the FIRST action the OT practitioner would take. See reference: Early: Work, homemaking and childcare.

143. (C) by tilting backwards up to 60 degrees while rocking. By lowering the child backwards from the sitting position, the child is required to activate increasing degrees of antigravity control in the neck musculature. As the child's strength increases, the degree of incline can be increased. Answers A, B and D do not address antigravity control using neck flexor musculature. See reference: Case-Smith (ed): Nichols, DS: Development of postural control.

144. (D) No assistive devices A person with a spinal cord injury at the C8 level would have full upper extremity function and would be able to perform self-feeding independently without using equipment. A person with an injury at C1, C2, or C3 would have no upper extremity movement and would not be able to perform self-feeding at all (answer A). An injury at C4 or C5 would allow scapular elevation and would allow the individual to self-feed using a mobile arm support, which supports the upper extremity against gravity (answer B). At the C6 and C7 levels, an injury would allow enough upper extremity function to use a universal cuff independently (answer C). See reference: Pedretti (ed): Adler, C: Spinal cord injury.

145. (D) position the person in an upright posture, make sure head is flexed slightly and in midline. Making sure that the resident is correctly positioned is the first step in addressing eating problems. Improper posture can result in difficulties with swallowing. Depending on the particular problems of the person, providing adaptive devices (answer A) may or may not be helpful but would not be the first step or given without assessment of need. Observing for swallow after each bite (answer B) and instructing caregivers (answer C) as to proper setup would also be important steps but these would occur later in the intervention process. See reference: Larson, Stevens-Ratchford, Pedretti, and Crabtree (eds): Foti, D: Evaluation and interventions for the performance area of self-maintenance.

146. (B) stringing beads for a necklace, following a pattern. This is the only activity of those listed that requires the individual to follow a sequence in order to achieve the desired outcome. Leather stamping in a random design (answer A) does not require sequencing skills but does require coordination, visual-motor integration, and strength. Putting together a puzzle (answer C) requires perception of spatial relations. Playing Concentration (answer D) requires memory and attention span. See reference: AOTA: Uniform Terminology for Occupational Therapy, third edition.

147. (C) National Alliance for the Mentally Ill. This is a support group that is open to clients and families and focuses on education and support related to all mental illnesses. Al-Anon (answer A) is a support group for family members of alcoholics. Family therapy (answer B) is not a support group. Recovery, Inc. (answer D) is a self-help support group for individuals with mental disorders. See reference: Neistadt and Crepeau (eds): Perinchief, JM: Management of occupational therapy services.

148. (A) use of time. By comparing interests and actual participation reported, the OT practitioner may identify discrepancies between interests and actual play and leisure behavior. This information can help address the client's use of time and facilitate temporal organization. The issues in answers B, C, and D are not directly addressed using this method. See reference: Case-Smith (ed): Cronin, AF: Psychosocial and emotional domains.

149. (A) Concise objective information All medical documentation should be accurate, concise, and objective. Personal opinions and statements that are speculative, judgmental, or subjective are not appropriate to be included into the patient's chart. Therefore, answers B, C, and D are incorrect. See reference: AOTA: The Occupational Therapy Manager: Acquaviva, JD: Documentation of occupational therapy services.

150. (A) the mother's concerns and goals for her child. The caregiver's concerns are essential in planning effective intervention within the context of the family. Medical management (answer B), equipment needs (answer C), and the physical layout of the home (answer D) are important issues as well but can be addressed at a later time. See reference: Case-Smith (ed): Stewart, KB: Occupational therapy evaluation in pediatrics.

151. (C) acute care hospitalization. The emphases of acute care hospitalization are symptom reduction, medications, and discharge planning. The club house treatment format emphasizes belonging and security. Community mental health centers focus on medication management, crisis intervention, and outpatient therapy. Quarterway houses emphasize increasing autonomy and decreasing supervision. See reference: Neistadt and Crepeau (eds): Freda, M: Facility-based practice settings.

152. (D) are easily accomplished by the client. Answer D is correct because activities which are easily accomplished offer no challenge and, there-

fore, will not enhance learning of skills and development of competence. During the process of reassessment, such activities require changing through the process of grading to make them somewhat more difficult. Activities which continue to provide some level of challenge (answer A), or which reflect the client's priorities (answer B), or which directly relate to the client's goals (answer C) will all continue to motivate the client to continue with therapy. See reference: Neistadt and Crepeau (eds): Neistadt, ME: Overview of treatment.

153. (A) The goals have been met and the individual can no longer benefit from OT services. Discontinuation of OT should occur when an individual has met the goals and further progress is not anticipated within the therapeutic environment. Answer C is incorrect in that individuals may often achieve their goals and new goals are established because it is anticipated that further progress may be made. Answer B is incorrect in that if the practitioner does not anticipate progress and the goals have not been met, it is necessary for the practitioner to discharge the individual. Depending on an individual's status at discharge, recommendations may be made for community services, outpatient care, day care, or home health services. A vital role of OT practitioners is to provide appropriate linkages to the community for those individuals served. The preparation for discharge planning should include the patient's support system, discharge environment, and possible need for continued health care services. Answer D is incorrect in that discharge of an individual should be made on objective information. If an individual does not "feel" that he or she is making progress, the therapist should be able to clarify with the individual his or her status based on objective measurements and observations. See reference: Neistadt and Crepeau (eds): Perinchief, JM: Management of occupational therapy services.

154. (B) The child's writing, dressing, and self-feeding skills Because the child was being treated for difficulties with fine motor skills, discharge criteria should focus on fine motor function. Answers A, C, and D describe information that is relevant in overall discharge planning but is not relevant in determining readiness for discharge. See reference: Case-Smith (ed): Case-Smith, J, Rogers, J, and Johnson, JH: School-based occupational therapy.

155. (C) "The client independently selected one of six craft designs presented." The notation of the client's response to treatment that contains the MOST objective information is answer C. The notations that address the client's wants and hostility are interpretations of behavior versus directly observable responses. The use of the word "appropriate" reflects the OT practitioner's judgement. See reference: Early: Medical records and documentation.

156. (C) To teach the caregiver how to lift and

turn the client safely Individuals unable to move themselves and those with sensory loss are susceptible to the development of decubiti. Skin damage results from pressure on the skin over a prolonged period of time. The skin over bony prominences is particularly prone to the development of decubitus ulcers. Frequent position changes are essential for these individuals to prevent skin breakdown and the risk of serious infection. If the patient were already involved in a strengthening program (answer A), it may be appropriate to change it to a maintenance program at this point. A bed-mobility program (answer B) and an environmental control unit (answer D) would be appropriate if the individual has potential in these areas, but instructing the caregiver in how to reposition the patient is the highest-priority modification. See reference: Trombly (ed): Bentzel, K: Remediating sensory impairment.

157. (A) The time he spends at the computer Since computer work requires very little active movement, and lower extremities, trunk, and neck are generally held in a static position, it is essential to assess how much time the child spends in this position. The OT practitioner needs to instruct the child to take regular breaks and maintain proper positioning while at the computer to avoid further strain. Answers B, C, and D address other relevant factors in computer use but none that would directly produce the symptoms described. See reference: Ryan (ed): The Certified Occupational Therapy Assistant: Ryan SE, Ryan BJ, and Walker, JE: Computers.

158. (C) ease the child to a lying position, remove or pad nearby objects, loosen clothing. The most important action to take is to protect the child during the seizure by preventing injuries which can occur from falling or hitting objects during movements. Other protective measures include loosening clothing that is restrictive and placing a blanket or cushion underneath the child if possible. Answer A is incorrect because checking breathing would not be done until the seizure has stopped. Answer B is incorrect because any attempt to restrain the child could result in injury. While it is important to let the seizure end without any interference, Answer D, taking no actions and only observing, would not help to protect the child from environmental hazards. See reference: Case-Smith (ed): Rogers, SL, Gordon, CY, Schanzenbacher, KE, and Case-Smith, J: Common diagnosis in pediatric occupational therapy practice.

159. (C) Swing-away footrests and removable armrests After swinging away the footrests and removing the armrests, the individual can perform a sliding board transfer without being blocked by the wheelchair. Answers A and B include nothing that would facilitate a sliding board transfer. One-arm drive is useful for individuals with the use of only one upper extremity. A low backrest is useful for those who require minimal trunk support because it allows greater freedom of movement for the arms and shoulders. A reclining backrest benefits individuals who are unable to sit upright for prolonged periods of time or who need to recline for weight shifts. Elevating footrests may be desirable for individuals with lower extremity edema. Answer D is incorrect because although removable armrests may make transfers easier, elevating footrests would not. A footrest would need to be detachable or a swing-away type for it to be moved out of the way. See reference: Pedretti (ed): Adler, C, and Tipton-Burton, M: Wheelchair assessment and transfers.

160. (B) a 3-inch screw-top jar. Since the goal was written as a functional behavioral objective, the OTR should reassess the child for functional progress made in performance areas. Assessing progress by measuring range of motion with a goniometer (answer A), the strength of grip using a dynamometer (answer C), or degree of coordination using a fine-motor scale assessment may provide useful information of individual performance components addressed; however, none of these will provide sufficient information to measure progress on a functionally written goal. See reference: Case-Smith (ed): Richardson, PK, and Schultz-Krohn: Planning and implementing services.

161. (C) marking the end of each step with high-contrast tape. Difficulty in seeing contrast and color are two forms of decreased visual acuity that cannot be addressed by corrective lenses. Two effective environmental adaptations to these deficits are increasing background contrast and increasing illumination. Using tape or paint to make the edge of each step contrast sharply with the rest of the step is an inexpensive way to adapt the environment for the patient. Installing a stair glide or installing handrails (answer A and B) are more costly adaptations that do not address the problems of decreased visual acuity. Instructing the patient to take only one step at a time when going up or down may cause the individual to be unnecessarily slow and does not address the problems of decreased visual acuity. See reference: Pedretti (ed): Warren, M: Evaluation and treatment of visual deficits.

162. (A) Practice regular skin inspection Children with lower extremity paralysis resulting from myelomeningocele usually experience impaired lower extremity sensation, placing them at risk for developing decubitus ulcers or burns due to contact with hot water or objects. Generally, children with myelomeningocele do not have oral motor or eating problems (answer B) or apnea episodes (answer C) unless Arnold-Chiari deformity is present. Tactile defensive behaviors and other sensory integrative disorders (answer D) can be present in children with spina bifida and myelomeningocele, but the issue of skin breakdown is more essential at this time. See reference: Neistadt and Crepeau (eds): Erhardt, RP, and Merrill, SC: Neurological dysfunction in children.

163. (A) Linoleum floor Linoleum floors are the easiest and least expensive surface over which to maneuver a wheelchair. Although it is possible to find inexpensive short pile carpeting (answer B), a smooth, uncarpeted surface is still the easiest to negotiate. The friction provided by deep pile carpets (answer C) makes them difficult to push a wheelchair across, and wheeling over the edge of an area rug (answer D) also increases the level of difficulty for wheelchair users. See reference: Christiansen (ed): Bates, PS: The self-care environment: issues of space and furnishing.

164. (D) "Patient stated that he likes to read sports magazines." This statement provides a basis for an objective judgment on what the patient likes because it has been made by the patient. Answers A, B, and C are examples of assumptions by the practitioner. See reference: Early: Medical records and documentation.

165. (B) Instruct the client to take "one white and one blue pill" with the morning and evening meals Cognitive disabilities' levels of function distinguish the types of assistance an individual needs to safely complete everyday tasks. Cognitive level 4 functioning involves having a routine goal in mind. Linking medications with meals helps the goal become routine. Answer A is consistent with cognitive level 5, answer C is consistent with level 3, and answer D is consistent with level 2. See reference: Early: Some practice models for occupational therapy in mental health.

166. (B) Strategies the husband can use to prevent the patient from wandering Although wandering, incontinence, and failure to recognize family members (answers A, C, and D) are all issues, wandering is the only potentially dangerous one. Because the patient's dementia is advanced, most of the discharge planning is directed toward the husband. Discussion with the patient will have no effect on her ability to manage her incontinence. At this point, environmental adaptation will be more effective than attempting to change the patient's behavior. See reference: Early: Understanding psychiatric diagnosis: The DSM-IV.

167. (B) self-help group. Self-help groups are supportive and educational and focus on personal growth around a single major life disrupting problem. Support groups (answer C) focus on assisting members who are in crisis until the crisis is past. Advocacy groups (answer A) focus on changing others or changing the system versus changing one's self. Psychotherapy groups (answer D) focus on understanding the influence of past experiences on present conflicts. See reference: Posthuma: Self-help groups.

168. (C) Relapse prevention Relapse prevention, symptom identification and reduction, and medica-

tion management are the areas that are emphasized in discharge planning groups. Developing ADL routines, self-awareness, and social skills (answers A, B, and D) are all areas that would be addressed throughout hospitalization, and perhaps after discharge as well. See reference: Early: Treatment settings.

169. (C) CARF. The Commission on Accreditation of Rehabilitation Facilities (CARF) is the regulatory agency for the provision of rehabilitation services. AOTA (answer A) was formed in March of 1917 as the National Society for the Promotion of Occupational Therapy. JCAHO (answer B) is the Joint Commission on Accreditation of Hospital Organizations. The JCAHO reviews the medical care provided by hospital organizations. The NBCOT (answer D) is the agency that develops and administers the examination for registration as an OT; therefore, answers A, B, and D are incorrect. See reference: Neistadt and Crepeau (eds): Bailey, DM: Legislative and reimbursement influences on occupational therapy: Changing opportunities.

170. (B) members share their experiences and struggles with alcohol use. Shared experiences can build feelings of understanding, hope, and acceptance among the members of a self-help group. Answers A, C, and D are all examples of member roles that are NOT typically encouraged in self-help groups. See reference: Posthuma: Self-help groups.

171. (D) A sheltered workshop Sheltered workshops are designed to help individuals master basic work skills. Answers B and C are similar in that they incorporate actual job sites for developing work skills. Answer A focuses on work-related and leisure activities. See reference: Neistadt and Crepeau (eds): Baloueff, O: Developmental delay and mental retardation.

172. (C) Work simulation to increase strength and endurance for necessary work-related skills Work simulation is considered to be a primary goal of work hardening, in addition to increasing productivity and feasibility through work-simulated activities. Answers A and B, ADL retraining and progressive resistive exercises, are not typical goals associated with the description of a work hardening program. Answer D, vocational retraining, is incorrect. It is vital that a work hardening program be viewed as an adjunct to vocational retraining, not as a vocational training program in and of itself. OTs typically measure and assess a client's overall physical ability to perform the requirements of a particular job. See reference: Pedretti (ed): Kasch, MC: Hand injuries.

173. (B) increase physical activity and fitness. Wellness programs focus on developing personal control of behaviors through educational approaches and active participation in activities that promote health, such as increasing level of physical activity to improve physical fitness. Answers A, C, and D reflect traditional occupational therapy therapeutic interventions to improve performance in specific deficit areas rather than promoting general good health. See reference: Cottrell (ed): Swarbrick, P: A wellness model for an acute psychiatric setting.

174. (A) improving accessibility in building access, building interiors, and rest rooms. Title III of the ADA addresses accessibility of facilities used by the public and focuses on removal of structural barriers to allow access to the premises and use of the facilities, including, parking areas, walks, ramps, entrances, etc. Answers B, C, and D may be relevant areas for OT consultation; however, these relate to Title I of the ADA which addresses employment of persons with disabilities. See reference: Pedretti (ed): Smith, P: Americans with Disabilities Act: Accommodating persons with disabilities.

175. (A) develop a protocol for environmental modification to reduce fall risks in the life-care retirement community. Developing a protocol for environmental modification of general hazards to reduce falls throughout the community is an example of a primary prevention strategy. Activities which focus on eliminating fall risk factors specific to individuals represents secondary prevention (answers B, C, and D). See reference: Larson, Stevens-Ratchford, Pedretti, and Crabtree (eds): Cook, M, and Miller, PA: Prevention of falls in the elderly.

176. (A) Stocking the shelves at a local grocery OT interventions for the transition from school to adult life should focus on real-life functional activities in actual work settings. Working in the natural setting affords students opportunities to develop skills necessary for success in community jobs. Working in a sheltered workshop in their own school environment does not provide real-life settings for job training. Reading want ads and role-playing interviews (or answer D) are not considered vocational training. See reference: Case-Smith (ed): Spencer, K: Transition services: From school to adult life.

177. (A) Use disposable cotton swabs and have clients bring their own cosmetics Universal precautions are related to the prevention of the spread of infection. Using disposable cotton swabs and having clients use their own cosmetics would be effective in reducing the risk of infection. Combing someone's hair (answer B) does not usually involve risks related to blood or bodily fluids. Washing equipment (answer C) that is used near eyes and mouths by several individuals is inadequate. Avoiding glass containers (answer D) is a safety precaution that is related to self-harm and not universal precautions. See reference: Early: Safety techniques.

178. (A) A mutual process The supervisory process is one that requires the attention of both parties involved. The COTA needs to develop his or her own role and identity within the institution and profession. In addition, the OTR supervisor needs to provide the COTA with opportunities for growth and development. As part of this relationship, ongoing evaluation and counseling may take place to enhance learning and role development. Although answers B, C, and D are necessary to the supervisory process, the best answer is A. See reference: Early: Supervision.

179. (D) intermediate-level OTR with routine supervision. Supervision is the oversight required of an OT and may be at any one of four levels based on the expertise of the professional. This therapist sees the supervisor every other week, indicating a routine or general level of supervision which is appropriate for an intermediate-level practitioner. An intermediate therapist will have gained skill mastery, begun to specialize, and have the ability to participate in education of others. However, he or she has not yet gained the refinement of special skills to be considered advanced. Answers A, B, and C are incorrect in that they match the skill level of the therapist with inappropriate levels of supervision. See reference: AOTA: Occupational therapy roles.

180. (B) Yes, as long as state regulations allow autonomous practice and the COTA recognizes situations that require consultation with or referral to an OTR. OT plays a significant role working with consumers in the independent living movement by working both with individuals and their environments. According to the AOTA position statement The Role of Occupational Therapy in the Independent Living Movement, AOTA "supports the autonomous practice of the advanced COTA practitioner in the independent living setting." In this situation, it would be the responsibility of the COTA to recognize and seek out OTR consultation when appropriate. However, this does not supersede state regulations when they prohibit autonomous practice by the COTA. Other options for this COTA would be to find some way to fund the necessary OTR supervision (answer A) or to work as a program director and not use the COTA credentials (answer D). See reference: AOTA: Occupational therapy roles.

181. (D) Recommend hospice OT OT in hospice care focuses on role performance, the components of which are quality of life, locus of control, and adaptation. This type of intervention may bring quality and meaning to the individual's remaining days. It is unlikely that this individual, who is depressed about a terminal illness, will actually carry out a home program (answer A). Not all home health OT practitioners (answer B) have the expertise to work with terminally ill patients using a hospice approach. Discontinuing OT services altogether (answer C) would not facilitate continuation role performance. See reference: Neistadt and Crepeau (eds): Griswold, LS: Community-based practice arenas.

182. (D) An exposure has occurred; put on gloves, clean up the spill with paper towels, put the soiled paper towels in a plastic bag, seal the bag, disinfect the area, and finish the patient's session with whatever time is still left. The Occupational Safety and Health Administration (OSHA) has identified materials that require universal precautions to include blood, semen, vaginal secretions, cerebrospinal fluid, synovial fluid, pleural fluid, any body fluid with visible blood, any unidentifiable body fluid, and saliva from dental procedures. Items OSHA has identified as not needing universal precautions include feces, nasal secretions, sputum, sweat, tears, urine, and vomitus. Because the urine had blood in it, in this case it WOULD be considered an exposure (answer A). Hospitals have policies regarding response to exposures such as this. Answer A is incorrect because it indicates that an exposure has not occurred. Leaving the area unavailable for other therapists and their patients who might need to use it (answer B) would be inconsiderate. Contaminated linens and towels (answer B) need to be placed in a specially designated laundry area. See reference: Early: Safety techniques.

183. (D) Interdisciplinary care improvement teams Healthcare professionals who are part of an interdisciplinary care improvement team work together to "address such issues as patient flow, the discharge process, patient outreach, and promotion and cost-efficiencies" (p. 47). Quality improvement (answer A) is a systematic approach to monitoring patient care. Peer review (answer B) is a component of quality improvement. Cost accounting (answer C) is a method of tracking the costs of specific services or costs incurred by diagnosis-specific groups. See reference: Jacobs and Logigian (eds): Logigian, MK: Cost management.

184. (B) transitional living center. Transitional living centers "provide temporary living arrangements for individuals who are in a transitional phase between hospital or institution and independent community living. Professional staff, including occupational therapists, assist the residents in gradually assuming responsibility in self-maintenance" (p. 362). Cradle-to-grave homes (answer A) are houses designed with accessibility in mind at the time of construction. Should an individual begin to use a wheelchair later in life, his home would already be wheelchair accessible. Adult day programs (answer C) are rehabilitation-oriented day programs for clients who live in the community. They are not residential. Clustered independent living arrangements are usually comprised of "apartment clusters or other types of housing in close proximity to each other, in which groups of residents with disabilities share services such as attendants and transportation" (p. 362). See reference: Trombly (ed): Law, M, Stewart, D, and Strong, S: Achieving access to home, community, and workplace.

185. (A) Uniform Terminology for Occupational Therapy Uniform Terminology is a document that defines OT in relationship to performance areas and performance components. This document provides a common language for OTs to use to describe individuals and their performance abilities. The Code of Ethics (answer B) is a document that outlines the standard for the conduct expected of OT professionals. The Standards of Practice for Occupational Therapy (answer C) defines the minimal standards for provision of OT services as well as the different roles of the OT and OTA in OT service delivery. The Occupational Therapy Roles document (answer D) defines the various educational levels and skills of OT professionals. See reference: AOTA: Uniform Terminology for Occupational Therapy, third edition.

186. (A) infection control plan An infection control plan most likely includes appropriate techniques and procedures for storing and handling foods within the OT department. Such plans specify the shelf lives of certain foods, standards for storage of food, use of hair nets, and cooking temperatures and times. A risk management plan (answer B) addresses the issue of liability in reference to negligence and malpractice issues. Emergency procedures (answer C) specify the procedures and techniques to be used in a critical situation (i.e., fire, code blue, severe weather alert). An environmental survey plan (answer D) inspects a service area for potential hazards and dangers and corrects the situation. See reference: Ryan (ed): Practice Issues in Occupational Therapy: Jones, RA: Service operations.

187. (B) federal and state governmental agencies and third-party payers. AOTA (included in answers A, C, and D) does not require physician referral for the provision of OT services. Federal, state, and local government agencies; third-party payers; regulatory and state agencies; and individual facilities may require physician referral. See reference: AOTA: Statement of occupational therapy referral.

188. (D) the title of the job, organizational relationships, essential job functions, and the job requirements. Job descriptions usually contain the title of the job, organizational relationships, essential job functions, work performed, job requirements, and environmental risks. Items that are not required but may complement an individualized job description are personality characteristics, past experience requirements, and accomplishments. Answers A, B, and C include items that are not typically found in a job description but are more appropriately located on a resume. See reference: AOTA: The Occupational Therapy Manager: Boyt Schell, BA, and Schell, JW: Personnel management.

189. (D) the OT problem solves with the teacher. Answer D is correct because the consultation relationship in the school is based on a shared relationship with the school staff for whom the OT is hired to consult. Answer A is incorrect as the teaching role is usually associated with monitoring type of service. Answer B is incorrect as a provision of therapy is direct service. Answer C is incorrect because it describes an authoritarian approach, which would take away the teacher's commitment to solving the problems of mainstreaming a child with a disability. Answer D reflects one of the essential tenets of consultation—that the consultee, by sharing in problem solution, will become committed to a child's program. See reference: Case-Smith (ed): Case-Smith, J, Rogers, J, and Johnson, JH: School-based occupational therapy.

190. (D) Productivity evaluations "Productivity is the ratio between the output and the resources expended to obtain the desired output" (p. 780). High productivity is often associated with cost-effectiveness. Analysis of productivity data can contribute to program development, improving staff effectiveness and containing costs. Outcomes measurements (answer A) are taken at the completion of service intervention and are used to evaluate the effectiveness of the intervention. Utilization reviews (answer B) assess the care that is provided to ensure that services were appropriate and not overutilized or underutilized. Program evaluation (answer C) is a method used to determine how well the program's goals have been achieved. See reference: Neistadt and Crepeau (eds): Perinchief, JM: Management of occupational therapy services.

191. (B) evaluate clients who are admitted on the weekends. The primary role of the COTA is to implement treatment such as that described in answers A, C, and D. AOTA guidelines about OT roles (AOTA, 1993) indicate that a COTA may not independently evaluate patients. Depending on the site and its policies, the COTA may be able to begin the process of assessment by making contact with the client and collecting data that the OTR would use in performing the evaluation. See reference: Neistadt and Crepeau (eds): Sands, M: Practitioners' perspectives on the occupational therapist and occupational therapy assistant partnership.

192. (D) discuss her concerns with an OTR who is present. Although the COTA's own supervisor is absent, an OTR present would become the acting supervisor for the COTA for the day. The COTA should always discuss concerns with the supervisor first. Going to the administrator (answer C) would not only disregard the chain of command but could escalate a problem that should be handled internally. Training in ADL is a skilled service beyond the scope of service of an aide. The COTA should not allow the aide to finish the treatment session (answer A). It may not be feasible for the COTA to complete the session herself (answer B), but it would also be inappropriate to terminate the aide when simple review of procedures and role delineations would be indicated in this case. See reference: Early: Supervision.

193. (C) Inform the administrator they are unable to provide services to individuals who can no longer benefit from OT Answers A, B, and D involve falsifying documentation, financial exploitation of insurance carriers, and inaccurate recording of professional activities, and are violations of the Code of Ethics. It is unethical to bill for services not rendered or to provide services to individuals who can no longer benefit. In this case, the individual reached his full potential for independence in self-care and no longer requires OT services. See reference: AOTA: Occupational therapy code of ethics.

194. (B) any equipment that has come into contact with body fluids must be sterilized before using the equipment again. OSHA has set out strategies to protect individuals from potential exposure to HIV and hepatitis B virus. This situation would be an example of an engineering control. These controls are to modify the work environment to reduce risk of exposure. Other examples are using sharps containers, eyewash stations, and biohazard waste containers. Answers A, C, and D would not meet guidelines set forth by OSHA. See reference: Early: Safety techniques.

195. (A) negotiate the contract. Many OT practitioners have moved into consultation roles. The first step in the consultation process should include negotiation of a contract. This immediately establishes the general terms of agreement and a focus of the activities that are to be completed by the therapist. Answers B (establish trust), C (assess the environment), and D (identify problems) should follow after the contract has been negotiated. See reference: AOTA: The Occupational Therapy Manager: Jaffe, EG, and Epstein, CF, Consultation: A collaborative approach to change.

196. (B) A presentation to physicians Answer B, a presentation to physicians, is correct because this is an example of internal marketing. Other internal marketing strategies are site-based open houses, progress notes, service reports, and in-services for nursing staff. Answers A, C, and D are all examples of external marketing strategies. See reference: Jacobs and Logigian (eds): Jacobs, K: Marketing occupational therapy services.

197. (A) refine the question and develop the background. Once the question has been identified, a review of the literature should occur. The next step in research is to refine the question and develop the background. Answer B is the next step of the process, which is deciding on the methodology. Answers C and D come later in the research, as the researcher establishes the boundaries and then collects and analyzes data. See reference: Royeen: Quality in research.

198. (C) A COTA contributes to the process but does not complete the task independently. The

COTA participates in this process by providing factual information to the OTR and collaboratively identifying discharge needs (answer C). However, because of the analytical nature of provision of discharge recommendations, the COTA does not complete this activity independently. Answers A and B are incorrect because they do not take into account the analytical nature of the task. Answer D is incorrect because it does not allow for the input of data from the COTA. See reference: AOTA: Occupational therapy roles.

199. (D) Treat the patient as scheduled and charge for the 1 hour of direct time spent with the patient This answer is correct in that this meeting was not part of the planned intervention and had occurred spontaneously and without measurable goals. Based on the Standards of Practice, if collaboration with the individual or family was included as a part of the intervention plan, the patient could be billed for the time. See reference: Kornblau and Starling: Legal issues in ethical decision making.

200. (C) Use the handout only as a resource while developing the presentation. The Code of Ethics states that "Occupational therapy personnel shall accurately represent the qualifications, views, contributions, and findings of colleagues" (p. 1038). The options presented in answers A and B do not give the necessary credit to the author for his or her contribution. It is not necessary to discard the article altogether (answer D). See reference: AOTA: Occupational therapy code of ethics.

SIMULATION EXAMINATION 3

Directions: Circle the correct answer to the following questions. When you have completed this examination, check your answers against the answer key that follows. As you will see, an explanation is given for each answer along with a reference for further study. The book author is listed as well as the chapter author. See the bibliography for complete references. Study the areas in which your comprehension was low, then test yourself again by taking Simulation Examination 4.

Evaluation

1. **To assess an individual who is suspected of having carpal tunnel syndrome, the OTR tests for Tinel's sign by gently tapping the median nerve at the level of the carpal tunnel with the person's wrist positioned in:**
   A. 10 degrees of ulnar deviation.
   B. 10 degrees of radial deviation.
   C. 20 degrees of flexion or 20 degrees of dorsiflexion.
   D. neutral.

2. **In the assistive technology evaluation process, the OT on an assistive technology team is MOST likely to:**
   A. make recommendations for ways of accessing the technology.
   B. recommend communication strategies.
   C. seek funding sources for the technology.
   D. solve mechanical or software problems.

3. **An OTR has asked a COTA to identify how a patient spends his leisure time, which leisure activities he especially enjoys, and which others he has participated in that he would be interested in renewing. The MOST appropriate tool for the COTA to use is:**
   A. an evaluation of living skills
   B. an interest checklist.
   C. an activity configuration.
   D. a self-care evaluation.

4. **The OT practitioner is making recommendations to a community living site for a 13-year-old child who has mental retardation. Which of the following statements most accurately describes the functional ability of this child who is in the moderate (trainable) range of intellectual ability?**
   A. The client requires nursing care for basic survival skills.
   B. The client can usually handle routine daily functions.
   C. The client requires supervision to accomplish most tasks.
   D. The client is able to learn academic skills at the third to seventh grade level.

5. **Before treating a client referred to the hand center for a nerve injury, the OTR must understand the nerve pathways that innervate the hand. The nerves of the hand are MOST commonly referred to as:**
   A. lateral, medial, and central.
   B. femoral, obdurator, and sciatic.
   C. radial, median, and ulnar.
   D. dorsal, lateral, and volar.

6. **An OT practitioner observes the following: A patient who is asked to show the path she would take to get from her room to the therapy clinic at the other end of the corridor becomes easily confused and makes several wrong turns. This behavior MOST likely indicates:**
   A. spatial relations disorders.
   B. figure-ground discrimination deficits.
   C. topographical disorientation.
   D. form discrimination deficits.

7. **A person with functional limitations in shoulder abduction and external rotation is performing self-care activities. The OTR is MOST likely to observe the client having difficulty during which self-care activity?**
   A. Buttoning a shirt
   B. Combing the hair
   C. Tucking in a shirt in the back
   D. Tying a shoe

8. **A teenage patient is hospitalized with anorexia nervosa. An OT practitioner has been assigned to collect data on the child's family background, education, and habits through a chart review. Where will the practitioner MOST likely find this information?**
   A. In the nurse's notes
   B. In the doctor's notes
   C. In the social worker's notes
   D. In the admitting note

9. **While observing a newly referred child in the playground, the OT practitioner suspects that the child has dyspraxia. The MOST relevant assessment to determine the child's level of performance will be one which determines the child's ability to:**
   A. print or write.
   B. read.
   C. calculate mathematics.
   D. plan new motor tasks.

10. **An OTR is performing an UE functional assessment on an elderly client with rheumatoid arthritis. The OTR is MOST likely to determine that the client has limited internal rotation if the client is unable to touch the:**
    A. back of the neck.
    B. top of the head.
    C. lower back.
    D. opposite shoulder.

11. **An adolescent patient is attending a craft group for the first time. The OT practitioner is observing the patient closely for signs of aggressive and violent behavior. This individual has MOST likely been diagnosed with:**
    A. hyperactivity.
    B. attention deficit disorder.
    C. conduct disorder.
    D. oppositional defiant disorder.

12. **A child with a learning disability has difficulty integrating visual, auditory, vestibular, and somatosensory stimuli, and responds to stimuli primarily with defensiveness. The area of the central nervous system that serves as a center for these functions is the:**
    A. reticular formation.
    B. superior and inferior colliculi.
    C. cerebral cortex.
    D. cerebellum.

13. **An OT practitioner is working with a client who sustained a traumatic injury to the right upper extremity during a motorcycle accident. The client states that he does not understand why he has paralysis to the deltoid, brachialis, biceps, and brachioradialis muscles. In addition to this, the client's arm hangs limply with minimal functional movement noted in the hand. The OTR suggests that this injury MOST accurately describes:**
    A. a brachial plexus injury.
    B. a long thoracic nerve injury.
    C. an axillary injury.
    D. a Volkmann's contracture.

14. **Which of the following instructions should the OT practitioner follow when administering standardized tests to young children?**
    A. Test in a stimulating environment
    B. Follow test manual directions
    C. Always administer tests in a single session
    D. Carry on a conversation with the child

15. **An individual that an OT practitioner is treating is suddenly diagnosed with a disabling condition. Which would be the FIRST adaptive response that would MOST likely pass in time without intervention?**
    A. A dependency reaction
    B. A stress reaction
    C. A grief response
    D. A desire to set unrealistic goals

16. **In an OT clinic, a patient with severe hand weakness as a result of arthritis is preparing for discharge. The OT is performing an evaluation to determine the person's ability to function at home. In terms of home safety, the skill that would be MOST important for this person to demonstrate would be the ability to:**

A. work locks and latches on doors or windows.
B. manipulate built-up utensils while eating.
C. demonstrate energy conservation techniques.
D. manipulate fasteners on clothing for easy dressing and undressing.

17. An OT practitioner is performing an environmental assessment to determine accessibility for a client who will be returning home. The FIRST step in this process is to:

A. identify the barriers to movement and function in the home environment.
B. identify and analyze the tasks and occupations that the client will be performing in the home.
C. identify the aspects of the environment which support movement and function in the home.
D. determine the social environment of the client.

18. An OT practitioner asks a client who recently sustained a head injury to repeat a random list of numbers 1 minute after hearing the list. The OTR is MOST likely evaluating:

A. short-term recall.
B. attention.
C. hearing.
D. abstraction.

19. An OT practitioner observes a child with a learning disability use an unusually tight grip when writing with a pencil. The child also frequently breaks his pencil from applying too much pressure on the paper. This type of problem is MOST likely caused by inadequate sensory information from the:

A. vestibular system.
B. auditory system.
C. somatosensory system.
D. visual system.

20. On an assessment report, the OT practitioner documents that a person exhibits elbow flexion strength of grade 1. According to the manual muscle test system of letters and numbers, the word that would be the equivalent of grade 1 would be:

A. absent.
B. trace.
C. good.

D. normal.

21. A child with motor delays is being evaluated to determine how he performs self-care activities. Which evaluation procedure is MOST likely to provide relevant information about self-care function?

A. Standardized tests of motor development
B. Review of the medical record
C. Developmental screening test
D. Home observation and parent interview

22. Which of the following activities would MOST effectively evaluate group interaction skills?

A. The clients make individual collages, sharing a set of magazines to complete the activity.
B. All group members construct one tower that incorporates all of the pieces provided in a set of constructional materials (e.g., Legos™, Tinkertoys™, or Erector™ set).
C. All group members work together to make pizza and salad for their lunch that day.
D. Each client selects a short-term craft activity from four available samples.

23. A client who was fitted for an upper extremity prosthesis complains of pain at the stump site. The client comments that the absent limb still feels intact and that the pain is severe. This is MOST likely an example of:

A. paresthesias.
B. phantom link sensation.
C. neuromas.
D. phantom limb pain.

24. An OT practitioner is working with the caregiver of a newly diagnosed client with Alzheimer's disease. The caregiver insists on keeping the client out of a skilled nursing facility. In this case, caregiver education is vital. It is important to make the caregiver aware that the early stages of dementia, Alzheimer's type, may be detected in behaviors such as:

A. difficulty swallowing food.
B. forgetting to turn off the stove burner.
C. angry outbursts at close family members.
D. restless pacing around the house.

25. A 3-year-old child is able to use the toilet independently except for wiping and readjusting clothing afterward. This behavior indicates the child is performing at which of the following levels?

A. significantly below age level.
B. slightly below age level.
C. at age level.
D. above age level.

26. **During a tub transfer training session, an individual requires cueing to lock his wheelchair brakes and requires assistance to lift his legs from the wheelchair into and out of the tub. He is able to scoot himself from the wheelchair to the tub bench with occasional loss of balance. How should the individual's performance be documented?**
A. Dependent
B. Minimal assistance
C. Moderate assistance
D. Maximal assistance

27. **An OTR observes a child with autism waving his hand in front of his eyes repeatedly in an apparently purposeless manner. The MOST relevant observation is the:**
A. child's ability to focus his eyes at close range.
B. degree of wrist mobility.
C. hand preference.
D. presence of self-stimulatory behavior.

28. **During an initial evaluation, an OT practitioner documents that the client's chart reveals a history of both depression and substance abuse. The term that indicates a diagnosis from two mental diagnostic categories is:**
A. dual diagnosis.
B. multiply handicapped.
C. axis I and II duplicity.
D. primary and secondary diagnoses.

29. **The OT practitioner is evaluating a client who has position-in-space difficulties. When assessing the sense of proprioception at an individual's joint, movement within the range would BEST be performed:**
A. until pain is elicited.
B. until the stretch reflex is elicited.
C. at the end ranges of the joint.
D. at the midrange of the joint.

30. **An OT practitioner is assessing a client's ability to perform work and productive activities. Examples of these occupational performance areas include:**

A. health maintenance, socialization, and community mobility.
B. feeding, eating, and sexual expression.
C. clothing care, cleaning, and volunteering.
D. reading, watching television, and doing small handicrafts.

31. **An 11-month-old child who was born 3 months prematurely is being evaluated at an OT outpatient clinic. The MOST accurate assessment profile can be obtained if the OTR compares this child's abilities with those of a normal child aged:**
A. 11 months.
B. 14 months.
C. 8 months.
D. 10 months.

32. **The OT practitioner is assessing an individual who demonstrates normal range of motion when flexing the elbow but hyperextends by 15 degrees when the elbow is extended. The practitioner will MOST LIKELY record the measurement as:**
A. -15 to 140 degrees.
B. 0 to 140 degrees.
C. 15 to 140 degrees.
D. -15 to 120 degrees.

33. **During the evaluation of a 6-month-old baby the OT practitioner gently pulls the infant from a supine position into a sitting position by the hands. The child demonstrates the ability to hold her head and trunk in alignment against gravity. This observable movement can MOST accurately be described by the OT as a:**
A. protective reaction.
B. flexion righting reaction.
C. body righting on body reaction.
D. optical righting reaction.

34. **An OT practitioner is working with a motivated and alert adult who recently had a cerebrovascular accident (CVA) affecting the parietal lobe. The client appears to be unaware of his limitations and is unable to learn compensation techniques for neglect despite many training sessions regarding ADL. This condition can MOST be described as:**
A. a visual field cut.
B. apraxia.
C. aphasia.
D. anosognosia.

35. **An OT practitioner is assessing a client's mental status, oral structures, and motor control abilities of the head, extremities, and trunk. The practitioner has MOST likely received a referral for a:**

    A. TMJ evaluation.
    B. cranial nerve evaluation.
    C. dysphagia evaluation.
    D. dysmetria evaluation.

36. **When deciding if a standardized test is valid, the MOST important aspect for the OT practitioner to determine is whether the test:**

    A. measures the skill or function it claims to measure.
    B. provides similar scores on serial test administrations.
    C. provides similar scores when administered by two different examiners.
    D. is based on a normative population.

37. **A parent observes her infant "cruise," while holding onto furniture, and asks the OT practitioner at what age a normal child begins to cruise, while holding onto furniture. The OT practitioner tells the parent that this behavior typically occurs between the ages of:**

    A. 3 and 5 months.
    B. 6 and 8 months.
    C. 9 and 12 months.
    D. 13 and 15 months.

38. **During a functional assessment of a person's strength, the therapist observes that the individual can move the arm through the full range of motion to reach a high bathroom shelf, but can lift and place nothing heavier than a can of spray deodorant on the shelf, suggesting that the person can tolerate only minimal resistance against gravity during arm motion. The strength according to the manual muscle test (MMT) is:**

    A. fair minus (3–).
    B. fair (3–).
    C. fair plus (3+).
    D. good minus (4–).

39. **When working with a child who exhibits tactile defensiveness, which of the following areas should be evaluated FIRST?**

    A. Reading skills
    B. Dressing habits
    C. Social skills
    D. Leisure interests

40. **The OT is assessing sensory awareness in an individual whose diagnosis is CVA. The MOST appropriate technique to use is to:**

    A. test the individual's affected extremity before the unaffected extremity.
    B. demonstrate the procedure on the unaffected extremity, then occlude the individual's vision.
    C. demonstrate the procedure on the affected extremity, then establish rapport with the individual.
    D. interview the individual and assess only the areas that he or she reports are impaired.

41. **What should the OT practitioner do FIRST to obtain accurate information about a patient's family situation and occupational, cultural, and educational backgrounds?**

    A. Read the medical record
    B. Interview the patient's family
    C. Interview the patient
    D. Read the social worker's report

42. **Which of the following children with neuromotor impairment would benefit MOST from using a prone scooter for exploratory play?**

    A. A child with cerebral palsy (CP) with predominant extensor tone
    B. A child with low tone who is easily fatigued
    C. A child with cognitive limitations and poor sensory awareness
    D. A child with spina bifida with lower extremity paralysis

43. **An infant has begun to sit and is leaning forward onto its arms. The OT practitioner notes during assessment that the infant is able to coactivate muscle groups around the shoulder and arm in order to bear weight on arms in sitting. This demonstrates that the infant has MOST likely developed which type of reactions?**

    A. Protective
    B. Equilibrium
    C. Rotational righting
    D. Support

44. **An OT instructor is teaching a group of OT students about various hand grips and their relationship to specific muscles and nerves. A hook grasp, for example, would MOST likely be used to hold:**

    A. a sewing needle while it is being threaded.

B. a tall glass half filled with water.

C. a heavy handbag held by the handles.

D. a key while it is being placed in a lock.

Treatment Planning

45. **A therapist who is planning treatment for a child with athetoid CP is concerned about the child's inability to control flexion and extension of the arm when reaching for a toy. The child flexes too much or extends too much, which makes placement of the hand very difficult. The MOST appropriate goal for this type of problem in hand function would be to improve the:**

    A. ability to isolate movement.

    B. ability to grade movement.

    C. ability to control how fast movement occurs.

    D. bilateral integration of arm movements.

46. **An OT practitioner has been assigned to develop an expressive activity group for women who have experienced emotional and physical abuse. The BEST choice would be:**

    A. mediation and yoga exercises.

    B. writing a soap opera.

    C. personal hygiene and grooming classes.

    D. aerobics and fitness program.

47. **An individual with poor writing skills needs to produce large amounts of legible material upon returning to work. The MOST appropriate method of compensation the OT could recommend would involve having the person:**

    A. learn to type.

    B. practice fine motor coordination exercises.

    C. practice letter or shape formations.

    D. strengthen the finger flexors and extensors.

48. **Which individual would benefit the MOST from using a wrist-driven flexor hinge splint during a prehension activity?**

    A. A client with a C1 injury

    B. A client with a C3 injury

    C. A client with a C6 injury

    D. A client with a T1 injury

49. **When developing play activities for a child with acute juvenile rheumatoid arthritis, which of the following precautions should the OT practitioner follow?**

A. Avoid light touch

B. Avoid rapid vestibular stimulation

C. Avoid resistive materials

D. Avoid elevated temperatures

50. **The OT is developing a treatment plan to promote developmental acquisition for an infant in the neonatal intensive care unit. Which of the following actions will have the most PERMANENT impact?**

    A. Modify the environment to protect the infant from additional stressful stimuli

    B. Recommend early intervention referral to assess infant upon discharge home

    C. Complete the neurobehavioral assessment and identify interventions emphasizing developmental skill acquisition

    D. Create a comfortable foundation for fostering parent skills through parent-therapist collaboration

51. **An OT practitioner is working with a group of individuals with substance abuse disorders. The practitioner wants to use an activity that will allow the clients to experience success after making a mess and one that will delay gratification. The activity process that BEST provides this experience is:**

    A. working in a group with three other individuals.

    B. selecting the design pattern for a tile trivet.

    C. applying grout to a tile trivet and waiting for it to dry.

    D. encouraging the individual to clean off the table at the end of the group.

52. **A treatment plan for a child with a visual discrimination problem would MOST likely include which of the following adaptations of visual materials?**

    A. Low contrast and defined borders

    B. High contrast and defined borders

    C. High contrast and unclear borders

    D. Low contrast and unclear borders

53. **An OT practitioner is working with a group of individuals with Parkinson's disease in an aquatic exercise program. The three performance components MOST important for successfully walking across the pool are:**

    A. strength, fine motor coordination, and kinesthesia.

    B. visual motor integration, postural control, and gross motor coordination.

C. vestibular processing, postural control, and muscle tone.

D. range of motion, praxis, and crossing the midline.

54. An OT practitioner is planning to use remedial strategies to prepare individuals treated in a psychosocial setting for job hunting. The activity MOST consistent with this approach is:

A. reviewing an interest checklist

B. holding a class about job-seeking strategies.

C. modifying the work environment to reduce stress.

D. using an expressive group magazine collage using pictures of different types of jobs.

55. An OT practitioner is leading a group session on the topic of "handling anger" with a group of clients who have deficits in psychosocial functioning. The MOST effective way for an OT practitioner to structure this group would be to:

A. begin with "Today we are going to discuss how we handle anger" and wait for discussion to start.

B. start by having the members make a collage or drawing which symbolizes how they handle anger.

C. ask each member what activities they would like to do during this session.

D. begin with a personal anecdote related to handling anger, and ask each member to do the same.

56. A school-age child with multiple handicaps is beginning to develop some controlled movement in the upper extremities. It would be MOST appropriate to introduce switch-operated assistive technology when the child:

A. develops tolerance of an upright sitting posture.

B. can reach and point with accuracy.

C. demonstrates any reliable, controlled movement.

D. develops isolated finger control.

57. An OT practitioner is using a sensory integration approach with a group of regressed individuals with limited attention spans. Most group members can tolerate a group situation for no more than a half-hour. Which of the following

activities would be BEST for beginning the session?

A. Go around the circle and ask each patient to introduce himself or herself

B. Pass around a scent box and ask each patient to smell the contents

C. Ask each patient to select a favorite poem and read it

D. Discuss the lunch menu and healthy eating habits

58. An OT practitioner is treating a client who developed a severe PIP joint contractures in the third digit, 2 months after a burn injury. Which of the following static splinting techniques would BEST address the needs of this individual?

A. Plaster cylindrical splint

B. Dynamic outrigger splint

C. Blocking splint

D. PIP-DIP splint

59. After completing the initial evaluation of a home care patient, the home care OTR expects the patient to achieve independence in self-care activities at different times—that is, grooming first, then upper and lower extremity dressing, then toileting. When writing the treatment goals, which of the following choices MOST appropriately reflects incremental improvements?

A. Patient will be independent in self-care in 3 weeks.

B. Patient will be independent in grooming, dressing, and toileting in 3 weeks.

C. Patient will be independent in grooming in 1 week, in upper and lower extremity dressing in 2 weeks, and in toileting in 3 weeks.

D. Patient will be independent in upper extremity dressing in 2 weeks and independent in lower extremity dressing in 3 weeks.

60. An OT practitioner is working with a homemaker who sustained a mild head injury. The client frequently forgets appointments and wakes up late for work. The practitioner suggests the use of external memory devices. Examples of external memory devices that might assist this individual would be:

A. visual imagery and a diary.

B. labeling and calendars.

C. mnemonics and verbal cues.

D. log and repetition.

61. **A child with behavioral problems has difficulty with peer interactions. Which of the following aspects of the treatment plan is MOST important?**

    A. Provide activities in an authoritarian environment
    B. Allow the child the opportunity to develop basic social skills on his own
    C. Provide enjoyable activities in a safe and accepting environment
    D. Strictly enforce rules for group play

62. **A child with poor anticipatory postural control demonstrates inadequate playground skills, losing her balance when trying to anticipate movement. Which of the following activities will BEST promote the development of these skills?**

    A. Ballet
    B. Soccer
    C. Basketball
    D. Ping-pong

63. **An OT practitioner is simulating cylindrical grasping activities with a client who desires to work on the skills necessary to be a carpenter. Which of the following activities would MOST likely address these needs?**

    A. Positioning a nail on a piece of wood
    B. Hammering a nail into a piece of wood
    C. Carrying a pail of bolts
    D. Unscrewing a lunchbox thermos

64. **When planning treatment for individuals diagnosed with eating disorders the OT practitioner's initial OT treatment goals would MOST likely address:**

    A. increasing self-awareness through expressive activities.
    B. increasing awareness of nutritional issues.
    C. improving school performance skills.
    D. making recommendations or referrals for family therapy.

65. **A fifth grade child with significantly low muscle tone caused by Duchenne's muscular dystrophy is losing trunk control in sitting. Which of the following frames of reference should the OT practitioner consider when reevaluating the treatment program?**

    A. Neurodevelopmental treatment
    B. Sensory integration
    C. Biomechanical
    D. Visual perceptual

66. **A child's long-term goal is to increase fine motor skills. The assessment has revealed a deficit in tactile discrimination, specifically stereognosis. The MOST relevant short-term goal would be:**

    A. "The child will correctly identify five out of five fingers touched when given tactile stimulus."
    B. "The child will correctly identify five out of five shapes drawn on the dorsum of her hand."
    C. "The child will correctly identify five out of five matching textures."
    D. "The child will correctly identify, by feel only, five out of five common objects."

67. **Staff members in a group home report to the OT practitioner that several of the men repeatedly try to touch female clients and staff and often make sexual gestures and comments. Which of the following environmental modifications would be MOST likely to reduce this behavior?**

    A. Provide a relatively active and stimulating environment with opportunities for these individuals to engage in real-life activities
    B. Stand to the side of these individuals instead of face to face during interactions with them
    C. Avoid having these individuals in close proximity to others to reduce opportunities for physical contact
    D. Advise these individuals in a calm, nonjudgmental manner about the behavior you expect

68. **An individual who previously worked as a cashier in a clothing store has been referred to a work-hardening program following knee surgery. Limitations are present in standing tolerance and balance. The activity that will BEST prepare this individual to return to work is:**

    A. moving piles of clothing from one end of the clinic to the other.
    B. folding laundry and putting it in a basket while standing.
    C. washing dishes while standing.
    D. putting price tags on clothing while sitting.

69. **When providing adaptive equipment to an individual with arthritis, the OT practitioner would explain that the PRIMARY purpose of using this equipment is to:**

    A. decrease joint stress and pain.
    B. correct deformity.

C. simplify work.

D. decrease independence.

70. **After administering an interest check-list, the therapist documents that the individual has identified a few solitary leisure interests and no interests involving social interaction. Based on this information, what is the BEST activity to use in the next session of a leisure counseling group?**

A. A leisure inventory assessment

B. An activity exploring leisure opportunities and problems

C. A magazine picture collage

D. A calendar of community leisure activities for the first week after discharge

71. **An adolescent with mental retardation is planning to enter a supported employment program in the community after leaving school. Which area of intervention would the OT practitioner be MOST likely to focus on?**

A. Developing the student's leisure interests and play skills

B. Developing the student's vocational interests, social skills, and community mobility skills

C. Facilitating development of the student's gross motor skills

D. Facilitating development of the student's fine motor skills

72. **The MOST effective method of compensation for both unilateral neglect and absence of sensation in an upper extremity with good motor control is to:**

A. avoid the use of sharp tools or scissors and to avoid extreme water temperatures.

B. wear noisy bracelets on the wrist or ankle as a reminder to visually scan toward the affected side.

C. use an electric shaver.

D. wear elbow pads on the affected side.

Treatment Implementation

73. **A client who is s/p traumatic brain injury (TBI) exhibits good strength with ataxia in both upper extremities. The writing adaptation that would be MOST appropriate in compensating for the patient's deficit areas would be:**

A. using a keyboard.

B. a universal cuff with pencil-holder attachment.

C. using a balanced forearm orthosis with built-up felt-tip pen.

D. a weighted pen and weighted wrists.

74. **An OT practitioner is working with an older adult who has diabetes, poor vision, and peripheral neuropathies. The client also has difficulty discriminating between medications. The BEST adaptation for the OTR to provide is:**

A. Braille labels.

B. labels with white print on a black background.

C. a pill organizer box.

D. brightly colored pills with each type of medication a different color.

75. **While participating in the first session of a relapse prevention group, a client reports that he often misses a dose of his medication because he forgets when to take it. Which of the following actions should the OT take FIRST?**

A. Ask group members to discuss how they feel about taking their medications.

B. Suggest using a diary to record each dose of medication.

C. Instruct him in the use of a timer to assist in medication management.

D. Make sure he knows what his medication schedule is.

76. **The goal for a patient who has had a CVA is to be able to put on a shirt independently. The MOST effective way to structure dressing training for maximum learning retention and generalization of this skill is:**

A. teaching and practicing each segment of the dressing procedure during consecutive treatment sessions.

B. practicing the whole task of putting on a shirt in a setting similar to the real environment.

C. providing dressing simulation activities (button boards, etc).

D. allowing the client to view a videotape on how to put on a shirt and written directions for completing steps for dressing.

77. **The benefits that a correct sitting position has in relation to hand function is explained to the parents of a child with CP. The child currently uses compensatory movements because of the inability to sit**

independently. Which aspect of therapeutic positioning should the OTR stress?

A. Stabilizing the trunk
B. Placing weight on the arms
C. Stabilizing the pelvis, hips, and legs
D. Stabilizing the head and neck

78. **An individual with a fast-growing brain tumor has begun ignoring food on the left side of the meal tray. Which of the following approaches would be MOST appropriate for this individual?**

A. Focus on remediation
B. Educate the patient to increase left-side awareness
C. Implement compensatory strategies
D. Select appropriate adaptive equipment

79. **A first grade child with a diagnosis of attention deficit disorder, hyperactivity type, is receiving OT to increase his attention span. Keeping this in mind, the OT practitioner introduces a construction activity. When blocks were placed in front of the child, the child swept many of them onto the floor and started throwing the remaining ones around the room. How can the OT practitioner most effectively restructure the activity to facilitate a successful experience for this child?**

A. Use soft foam blocks
B. Provide blocks of one color only
C. Use interlocking blocks
D. Present only a few blocks at a time

80. **A patient with an indwelling catheter asks his therapist for advice concerning sexual activity. Which of the following responses is MOST appropriate?**

A. Refer the patient to his physician
B. Discuss precautions necessary for sex when an indwelling catheter is present
C. Teach the individual how to remove and replace the indwelling catheter
D. Explain that it is dangerous and difficult to have sex when an indwelling catheter is present

81. **A client is participating in an assertiveness training group within a work setting. The expected outcome of this intervention is that the client will MOST likely improve the ability to:**

A. engage in relevant conversations with coworkers.

B. use appropriate facial expressions when disagreeing with coworkers.
C. express disagreement with coworkers in a productive manner.
D. use courteous behavior when disagreeing with coworkers.

82. **An individual is unable to bring her hand to her mouth for feeding because of weakness in supination. The MOST helpful adapted utensil for this person would be a:**

A. spoon with an elongated handle.
B. spork.
C. spoon with a built-up handle.
D. swivel spoon.

83. **A client with CP has severe motor impairment resulting in insufficient arm and hand motion, and insufficient grasp or prehension to access a computer keyboard. The BEST low-technology solution for improving his ability to access keys would be a(n):**

A. head pointer and slanted keyboard.
B. typing splint.
C. adapted mouse.
D. built-up pencil to press the keys.

84. **An OTR is preparing to do a parachute activity as part of a sensory integration program and several of the patients in the group are taking antipsychotic medications. The OTR should be alert for which possible side effect that could occur as a result of this activity?**

A. Postural hypotension
B. Photosensitivity
C. Excessive thirst
D. Blurred vision

85. **A child with a diagnosis of athetoid CP would like to be able to dress herself independently. Which of the following clothing features could the OT practitioner recommend that would be MOST useful in facilitating self-dressing?**

A. Mini tees made of elasticized fabric
B. Dresses with side zippers and zipper pulls
C. Oversized t-shirts and elastic-top pants
D. Shirts with front closures, such as snaps or large buttons

86. **An individual who sustained a C7-8 spinal cord injury 5 years ago has been admitted to an inpatient psychiatric unit. The OT practitioner should inform the**

staff that this individual will **MOST** likely be able to perform wheelchair-to-commode transfers at which of the following levels?

A. Independent with a sliding board
B. Assisted, using a stand-pivot transfer
C. Dependent in all transfers
D. Independent without adaptive equipment

87. **During an interview, the OT practitioner decides to respond to an individual by paraphrasing. The PRIMARY reason for this type of response is to:**

A. refocus or redirect the individual's comments.
B. show acceptance and understanding to the individual.
C. force the individual to make a choice.
D. encourage an individual to give additional information.

88. **An individual who is being discharged home after participating in an inpatient pulmonary rehabilitation program for chronic obstructive pulmonary disease (COPD) is given a list of tips to use in the home to promote function. Which one of the following items is MOST likely to be on the list?**

A. Perform pursed lip breathing when doing activities
B. Use a long-handled sponge while in the shower
C. Take hot showers to reduce congestion
D. Avoid air conditioned rooms during warm months

89. **An individual attending an adult day program has expressed interest in obtaining employment. In groups, however, the individual grabs tools from others, frequently acts out of turn, and has difficulty accepting feedback. Participation in which one of the following interventions is MOST appropriate for addressing this individual's limitations and helping to prepare the individual for a work environment?**

A. Operating the photocopy machine in a clerical group
B. Handing out trays and utensils in a food service group
C. Placing books back on the shelves in a library group
D. Balancing the books at the end of the day in a thrift store group

90. **An individual who is several days s/p myocardial infarction experiences nausea during a bathing evaluation. Which of the following is the FIRST action the OT practitioner should take?**

A. Stop the activity
B. Document the symptoms
C. Instruct the individual to sit and then continue the activity
D. Ask the individual if he feels like he can continue the activity

91. **An OT practitioner who needs to transfer an obese man is not confident she can manage the transfer alone. The BEST action for the OT practitioner to take is to:**

A. use proper body mechanics.
B. ask someone from PT to do the transfer.
C. ask another OT practitioner for help.
D. refrain from transferring the patient.

92. **An individual in an adult day program demonstrates poor social skills and frequent sexual acting-out. The activity that would MOST effectively provide release for this individual's sexual tension is:**

A. jogging.
B. macramé.
C. reading *Playboy* magazine.
D. ballroom dancing.

93. **A patient is beginning to demonstrate return in the right upper extremity following a CVA, but has mildly impaired proprioception in the right hand, which results in uneven letter formation during writing activities. Which would be the BEST method to help improve letter formation?**

A. The OT practitioner verbally describes how to make a letter as the individual writes.
B. The individual watches her grip on a felt-tip pen while writing.
C. The individual works with thera-putty to strengthen her hand.
D. The individual traces letters through a pan of rice with her fingers.

94. **An OT is explaining to a teacher the kind of high-technology aid that can be used to help a multiply handicapped student with speech and writing deficits function in the classroom. The OT is MOST likely to describe a(n):**

A. environmental control unit.

B. Wanchik writer.

C. head pointer.

D. electronic augmentative communication device.

95. An individual with paraplegia wishes to become independent in driving an automobile. The most appropriate piece of adaptive equipment for this individual is:

A. a palmar cuff for the steering wheel.

B. a spinner knob on the steering wheel.

C. pedal extensions for acceleration and braking.

D. hand controls for acceleration and braking.

96. An OT practitioner is working with a client who is has had a TBI and demonstrates deficits in sequencing and problem solving. The client has successfully prepared a cold meal in today's treatment session. The next meal preparation activity the OTR should have the client prepare is a:

A. fruit salad.

B. cup of instant soup.

C. casserole.

D. spaghetti dinner with salad and garlic bread.

97. A child diagnosed with mental retardation has been participating in a craft group structured as a parallel group. The child is now developing skills such as sharing materials and interacting with other group members. The NEXT level of structured activity which the OT practitioner would recommend for the child is in a(n):

A. egocentric cooperative group.

B. project group.

C. cooperative group.

D. mature group.

98. An individual with a history of substance abuse lives in a group home. The residential manager has asked the OT practitioner to work with the individual to develop house cleaning skills. Which of the following interventions is most appropriate when a COGNITIVE approach is desired?

A. Reward the individual with a snack bar token when chores have been successfully completed

B. Praise the individual when chores have been successfully completed

C. Post a schedule of each individual's chore responsibilities in a highly visible location

D. Conduct a group discussion about responsibilities people have when living in a group home

99. An OT practitioner has been working with a cognitively intact patient to train him in the safe use of a tub bench for transferring for several sessions. According to motor-learning principles, the BEST way to give feedback about the person's performance to ensure that this person learns the skill is to provide:

A. summary feedback, given at the end of the patient's attempts.

B. continuous feedback to let the person know how he is progressing.

C. feedback about the performance whenever the patient makes a mistake.

D. give no feedback during or after the practice session.

100. During a home visit, a client with rheumatoid arthritis informs the OT practitioner that her joints have recently become very painful and inflamed. She reports she has been performing her activity program despite the pain and demonstrates a series of briskly executed active range of motion movements. The BEST response of the OT practitioner is to instruct the client to:

A. continue performing her program as she has been.

B. instruct her to perform gentle active range of motion with weight as tolerated.

C. eliminate all range of motion exercises for a week.

D. perform only gentle active range of motion.

101. The OT is working with an individual in a psychosocial partial hospitalization program who is having difficulty making decisions. The therapist has suggested a baking activity but the client as unsure if she wants to do this activity. The therapist's response that would BEST facilitate decision making is:

A. "I think baking would be a helpful activity to try. Baking something you like offers you several choices and decisions. You wanted to bake cookies today, didn't you?"

B. I think baking would be a helpful activity to try. Baking something you like offers you several choices and decisions. Why do you want to bake?

C. I think baking would be a helpful activity to try. Baking something you like offers you several choices and decisions. These choices and decisions can help you feel more positive about making other decisions. You can choose a cake mix or a cookie mix. Which would you like?

D. I think baking would be a helpful activity to try. Baking something you like offers you several choices and decisions. These choices and decisions can help you feel more positive about making other decisions. Do you want to bake cookies?

102. A client's family wants to build a ramp to the primary entrance of the home. The OT practitioner advises the family that the ramp should be graded with a maximum slope of:

A. 1 inch of ramp for every foot of rise in height.

B. 1 foot of ramp for every inch of rise in height.

C. 10 inches of ramp for every 2 inches in height.

D. 1 foot of ramp for every foot of rise in height.

103. An OT practitioner positions an infant in the supine position and places attractive toys overhead to provide an opportunity to work against gravity. This position is MOST effective for developing which ability?

A. Shoulder flexion and protraction

B. Shoulder extension and retraction

C. Development of head control

D. Development of trunk control

104. A person with a long history of Parkinson's disease is experiencing considerable fatigue during the day. The OT practitioner's MOST appropriate response to help the person maintain his or her level of function is to teach the person how to:

A. "work through" the fatigue.

B. perform desired activities in a simplified manner, to conserve energy.

C. perform additional exercises to increase energy level.

D. eliminate activities and reduce activity level as much as possible.

105. An OT practitioner is performing a kitchen evaluation with an individual with limited shoulder range of motion the day before discharge. The individual demonstrates difficulty retrieving items from the higher shelves. Which of the following recommendations will BEST facilitate home management for this individual?

A. Store the most frequently used items on the shelves just above or below the counter

B. Use the largest joint available to move or lift items from high shelves

C. Perform shoulder range of motion exercises 10 times each, twice a day

D. Continue reaching for items on high shelves because it will help improve range of motion

106. A young client who is diagnosed with depression tells an OT practitioner about feelings associated with being alone and afraid. A chart review reveals that the individual leads a very isolated lifestyle. The BEST way for the practitioner to respond is to:

A. reassure the client that they can be friends.

B. tell the client, "I know how you feel."

C. encourage the client to socialize more often.

D. use active listening techniques.

107. An individual uses a mouthstick when working with a computer. Which of the following devices will prevent the mouthstick from accidentally striking other keys?

A. A moisture guard

B. A keyguard

C. An auto-repeat defeat

D. One-finger-access software

108. A child with CP demonstrates poor head control, high lower extremity extensor tone, and high upper extremity flexor tone. The BEST device for positioning this child for feeding is a:

A. prone stander with lateral trunk supports.

B. corner chair with head support and padded abductor post.

C. wedge that positions the hips in 15 degrees of flexion when the child is supine.

D. bolster chair without back support.

109. An individual with an IV drug use problem has developed acquired immunodeficiency syndrome (AIDS). The OT evaluation revealed that the individual's major problems are with daily tasks, self-esteem, physical deconditioning, and anxiety.

Which of the following approaches would be MOST beneficial to the client?

A. Have the patient use stress reduction using meditation, yoga, and energy conservation techniques

B. Have the patient participate in aerobic activities to combat deconditioning

C. Provide video lectures on AIDS to educate the client about the disease process

D. Incorporate energy conservation techniques and daily aerobic activities into the client's ADL

110. A patient with a short below-elbow amputation is lacking sensation in the residual limb. The MOST appropriate intervention would be for the OT to teach the patient:

A. techniques of tapping, rubbing, and application of textures to the residual limb.

B. to routinely inspect the skin closely for signs of skin breakdown.

C. to perform deep massage on the residual limb.

D. the necessary procedures of proper skin hygiene.

111. A client with paranoia prefers to stay away from the group, working alone at another table. The BEST action for the OT practitioner to take is to:

A. encourage the client to join the group.

B. tell the client he is required to sit with the group.

C. tell the client it is okay to work where he is until he feels comfortable in joining the group.

D. stay with the client until he is ready to join the group.

112. A 16-year-old boy with juvenile rheumatoid arthritis is ready to begin shaving but has difficulty as a result of limited range of motion in his shoulders and elbows. Which of the following is the BEST adaptation for him to use?

A. Electric razor attached to universal cuff

B. Safety razor with built-up handle

C. Safety razor with extended handle

D. Safety razor attached to universal cuff

113. After wearing a new splint for 20 minutes, an individual develops a reddened area along the ulnar styloid process. The MOST important first modification the OT practitioner should make to correct the splint is to:

A. line the splint with moleskin.

B. line the splint with adhesive-backed foam.

C. flange the area around the ulnar styloid.

D. reheat and refabricate the entire splint.

114. An individual with Guillain-Barré syndrome demonstrates poor to fair strength throughout the upper extremities. Which is the most appropriate approach for the OT practitioner to use in the EARLY stages?

A. Gentle, nonresistive activities

B. Progressive resistive exercise

C. Fine motor activities

D. Active range of motion against moderate resistance

115. An OT practitioner realizes that an adult worker with a developmental disability is having difficulty learning an assembly sequence. The practitioner decides to use backward chaining. Backward chaining can BEST be implemented by:

A. encouraging the individual to reverse the packaging sequence.

B. having the worker put only the last piece into the game package.

C. putting only the pencil or the pad into the game box.

D. having the therapist demonstrate and repeat the correct sequence before each of the worker's attempts.

116. An early intervention OT practitioner is working with a toddler whose significant physical disabilities have limited the child's ability to explore the environment. The BEST "low-tech" assistive technology play aid to allow the child to experience cause and effect and some control over an aspect of his or her environment would be:

A. a tape recorder for the child to listen to music.

B. a switch-adapted battery-operated toy car that knocks down a block tower.

C. storybook software for use on a computer

D. powered wheelchair

117. An individual in the early stages of amyotrophic lateral sclerosis (ALS) has been referred for OT in an outpatient setting. Which of the following interventions is MOST appropriate for this individual?

A. Work simplification and energy conservation

B. Progressive resistive exercises

C. Splinting

D. Active and passive range of motion exercises

118. A child has mastered brushing her teeth with the OT practitioner giving verbal and physical cues. What would be the NEXT step in the process of reducing the intrusiveness of cues?

A. Verbal cues

B. Verbal and gestural cues

C. Physical cues

D. Verbal and physical cues

119. In a work-hardening program, an OT practitioner is teaching a man with an excessive anterior pelvic tilt how to use proper body mechanics during lifting tasks. The MOST appropriate emphasis of the instruction should be correction of:

A. stenosis.

B. scoliosis.

C. kyphosis.

D. lordosis.

120. A patient who sustained head trauma is receiving an OT program of repetitive pegboard, paper-and-pencil tasks, and computer activities to remediate attention and memory deficits. The type of client MOST likely to benefit from this type of cognitive remediation is one who has:

A. cognitive deficits which must be treated within a short treatment time frame.

B. awareness, minimal deficits, and learning potential.

C. difficulty transferring learned skills to new situations.

D. a history of cognitive deficits resulting from a head trauma years ago.

121. A first grader has difficulty with poor finger isolation. The MOST appropriate activity for the OT practitioner to recommend to the teacher is:

A. crayon drawing on sandpaper.

B. copying shapes from the blackboard.

C. rolling out Play Doh with a rolling pin.

D. picking up raisins with pair of tweezers.

122. An OT practitioner is interviewing a client who believes she is suffering from chronic low back pain. As part of the educational process, the OTR explains the differences between acute versus chronic pain to the client. Chronic pain is:

A. pain that is associated with an inflammation or irritation that lasts for a brief period of time.

B. pain as a result of disease or injury that persists for long segments of time and has not resolved itself in the anticipated time.

C. pain as a result of surgery that lasts for hours, days, or weeks.

D. pain that presents itself through motor behaviors such as limping.

123. An individual with Parkinson's disease exhibits a lack of facial expression, resulting in decreased communication. The BEST strategy to promote improved social interaction through facial expression is to:

A. teach caregivers to give patient time to reply and to ask questions so that short responses are required.

B. give a word chart or communication board to prevent frustration.

C. teach use of mirror feedback to make the person aware of his or her facial expression.

D. instruct in deep breathing, articulation, speech volume, breaking up sentences into segments.

124. A client with cognitive deficits exhibits little transfer of skills from one activity to the next. Which intervention would be BEST to assist this client in performing the steps of doing his laundry?

A. Performing memory drills of the steps involved in doing in a laundry activity

B. Placing serial pictures of a laundry activity in sequence

C. Making a checklist of steps in the process, then consulting the list while doing laundry in the actual setting

D. Reading a story about a person doing laundry with the client, then discussing the story

125. The adaptation that provides the MOST benefit for an individual with paraplegia in the area of dressing is:

A. a buttonhook zipper pull device.

B. a clip-on tie.

C. adapted shoes.

D. loose-fitting clothing.

126. A child with a physical disability and poor postural stability is developmentally

ready for toileting. Which of the following elements of the treatment plan should be considered FIRST?

A. Training in management of fasteners
B. Provision of foot support
C. Provision of a seatbelt
D. Training in climbing onto the toilet

127. An individual with a low back injury lives alone and must be able to do laundry independently. Which of the following recommendations will BEST protect the back from reinjury?

A. Place the clean laundry basket on the floor next to a chair and sit for folding
B. Stop the activity when pain becomes severe
C. Divide the laundry into several small loads for carrying
D. Carry the laundry in one or two large loads

128. The MOST appropriate treatment sequence for an OT practitioner to follow when providing a cold pack to an individual with edema of the hand is:

A. precede the cold packs with purposeful activity.
B. provide the cold packs followed by purposeful activity.
C. provide the cold packs as the main focus of intervention.
D. OT practitioners should never provide this type of intervention.

129. A resident of a long-term care facility is being seen by the OT practitioner in the mornings to help the resident reestablish dressing routines after a period of illness. The client is in a weakened condition and has mild cognitive deficits. The BEST way to structure the task is to:

A. have the resident select the clothing they prefer, then dress the client.
B. have the resident dress in bed with garments which are stretchy and one size larger than usual; preview each step of the process with the resident.
C. have the resident walk to retrieve clothing garments and encourage independent performance.
D. place clothing within close reach of the resident, encourage the resident to proceed as you provide distant supervision.

130. A child with athetoid CP demonstrates a jaw and tongue thrust when a food-filled spoon is placed in his mouth. To decrease this problem, the therapist is

MOST likely to recommend a positioning strategy that includes increased:

A. neck flexion.
B. shoulder retraction.
C. hip extension.
D. neck extension.

131. The OT practitioner is treating a person with mild carpal tunnel syndrome. The MOST important instruction for the therapist to give the patient is to avoid:

A. extension.
B. flexion.
C. ulnar deviation.
D. radial deviation.

132. Which of the following is the MOST important adaptation to recommend to an individual returning home following a total hip replacement?

A. Move items from high cabinets to lower locations
B. Obtain a raised toilet seat
C. Place high-contrast tape at the edge of each step
D. Install a handheld shower head

133. An OT practitioner is running a living skills group. Before the active involvement of the participants, the practitioner needs to review lecture materials for 30 minutes. The group composition that is MOST LIKELY to result in an increased focus on the group leader and decreased interaction among the group members is a:

A. group size of fewer than five members.
B. group made up of members of differing ages.
C. group size between 7 and 10 members.
D. group with members who have similar goals and abilities.

134. When a fifth grader with hypertonicity is seated for schoolwork, she tends to adduct her legs and extend her hips and spine. The BEST way for the OTR to position the child in order to give her better postural control in sitting would be:

A. tilted forward 20 to 30 degrees.
B. upright.
C. reclining 45 degrees.
D. in a lateral tilt of 45 degrees.

135. What wheelchair feature would be MOST appropriate to recommend for an individual who will be traveling by car with the family to community outings and bringing his or her wheelchair?

A. A lightweight folding frame
B. A one-arm drive
C. An amputee frame
D. A reclining backrest

136. **An individual with C4 quadriplegia is able to independently use a mouth stick to strike keys on a computer keyboard for 15 minutes. To upgrade this activity, the therapist should:**

A. provide a heavier mouth stick.
B. have the individual work at the keyboard for 30 minutes.
C. progress the individual to a typing device that inserts into a wrist support.
D. teach the individual how to correctly instruct a caregiver in use of the keyboard.

137. **An OT practitioner has been asked to design a series of stress management sessions for individuals with multiple sclerosis (MS). The FIRST session should include:**

A. time management techniques.
B. self-assessment.
C. aerobic exercise.
D. progressive resistive exercise.

138. **A young child with hypertonicity is unable to bring his hands to midline to reach for a toy while in the supine and sitting positions. The BEST position to use in order to reduce the effects of abnormal patterns and facilitate midline grasp is:**

A. the standing position.
B. the prone position.
C. the sidelying position.
D. the quadruped position.

139. **An OT practitioner enters the room of a patient who recently had a RCVA with flaccidity to the left upper extremity. The therapist begins to perform upper extremity passive range of motion (PROM) treatment when marked pitting edema of the left hand is noted. What is the FIRST thing the OTR should do?**

A. Perform PROM and then position and elevate the affected extremity.
B. Fabricate a resting splint for the affected extremity.
C. Take no action at this time and wait for the edema to subside.

D. Have the individual attempt to squeeze a ball.

140. **The OT practitioner is instructing a patient who has had a myocardial infarction in energy conservation techniques. The BEST example of limiting the amount of work needed for a task is:**

A. using a side-loading washer.
B. wearing permanent-press clothing.
C. using an extended-handle dustpan.
D. using good body mechanics.

141. **A child diagnosed with ataxic CP exhibits tremors in the upper extremities. When she feeds herself, the tremors cause most of the food to fall off her spoon before it can reach her mouth. Which of the following adaptations should the OT practitioner recommend?**

A. Replace the spoon with a blunt-ended fork
B. Build up the handle of the spoon
C. Give the child a swivel spoon
D. Bend the spoon handle 45 degrees

142. **When ordering a wheelchair for an individual with MS, the MOST important consideration is the adaptability of the wheelchair in anticipation of:**

A. gradual gains in strength.
B. growth of the individual
C. further decline.
D. improved wheelchair mobility.

143. **A 60-year-old automobile mechanic with diabetes has been referred to OT following an above-knee amputation. The patient has impaired sensation in the remaining lower extremity and will be using a wheelchair for the foreseeable future. The FIRST patient education subject the OT practitioner should cover is:**

A. skin inspection.
B. grooming techniques (shaving, trimming toenails, etc).
C. retirement planning.
D. returning to work.

144. **An OT practitioner is working with an individual who is unable to complete the multiple steps that are necessary to brush his teeth. In response to this, the practitioner modifies the activity by having the client perform the task one step at a time while gradually adding on more steps with each success. The OT is at-**

tempting to employ which of the following?

A. Repetition
B. Cueing
C. Rehearsal
D. Chaining

145. An individual in the late stages of AIDS is bedridden, and flexion contractures have begun to develop in his right hand. Which of the following types of splints would be MOST appropriate for this individual?

A. Dorsal wrist splint
B. Functional-position resting splint
C. Volar wrist-cock-up splint
D. Dynamic finger-extension splint

146. A woman who had a CVA exhibits random movements in all four extremities. What is the MOST appropriate switch to use on the controls for her wheelchair?

A. Infrared switch
B. Sip and puff switch
C. P switch
D. Rocking lever switch

Effectiveness of Treatment and Discharge Planning

147. An elderly client was hospitalized for an episode of acute depression after the death of his spouse. The client is preparing for discharge and would like to return to his home but is fearful of spending his days alone. The BEST environment for the client to continue socialization and participation in meaningful occupation would be:

A. partial hospitalization.
B. adult day care.
C. home health care.
D. psychosocial rehabilitation center.

148. An OT practitioner is preparing an individual with burns to perform a home program of positioning and splinting. To prevent deformity, the OT practitioner would be MOST likely to recommend that the individual:

A. discontinue the positioning and splinting program upon returning home.
B. continue the same positioning and splinting program that was indicated before discharge.

C. continue with the positioning and splinting program only during the day.
D. continuing with positioning and splinting program only during the night.

149. An OT practitioner is working on lower extremity dressing with a young adult with a spinal cord injury. As the client attempts to put on his underwear, he notices an erection and asks the practitioner how it is possible for him to have an erection and if he will be able to have sexual intercourse. The OT practitioner is slightly embarrassed and uncomfortable with the question. The BEST action for her to take is to:

A. tell him she will find out the answers to his questions and get back to him with an answer by the next morning.
B. answer his questions to the best of her ability and quickly return to the lower extremity dressing program.
C. refer him to his psychiatrist.
D. refer him to her OTR supervisor, who has attended a workshop on sexuality and spinal cord injury.

150. A 9-year-old with a diagnosis of mental retardation has been receiving OT in order to become independent in dressing and feeding and is now being discharged. The BEST advice for the OT practitioner to give his parents in order to maintain the child's independence in dressing at home is:

A. give assistance when the child asks for it to provide a successful experience.
B. give praise for completed dressing; do not help the child get dressed.
C. give him oversize clothing with Velcro closures and large snaps.
D. give him verbal prompts when needed and help with closures only.

151. An individual about to be discharged from an inpatient psychiatric unit asks, "When I apply for jobs, what should I put down when it asks if you have been hospitalized in the past 6 months?" The therapist's response should include strategies that address:

A. developing assertiveness.
B. improving self-esteem.
C. anger management.
D. managing stigma.

152. When preparing to discharge a child with juvenile rheumatoid arthritis, what is the MOST important information to share with the child's teacher?

A. A summary of the child's cognitive and visual perceptual skills

B. Methods of accommodation in the classroom

C. Information on the child's range of motion status

D. A summary of the child's progress in OT

153. A patient is being discharged after hospitalization for a cerebrovascular accident and a 2-week inpatient rehabilitation program. He requires minimal assistance in advanced ADL but is independent in most basic ADL, and his RUE function is improving. He plans on eventually returning to work as a cashier. What would be the MOST appropriate recommendation concerning OT services?

A. Home health OT

B. Outpatient OT

C. A work-hardening program

D. Discontinuation of OT services

154. A client diagnosed with schizophrenia is taking a neuroleptic medication to control hallucinations. While in the hospital, the client experienced postural hypotension as a side effect of the medication. Before discharge, the MOST important advice to give this client concerning medication management is:

A. to keep time in the sun as brief as possible.

B. to avoid using power tools and sharp instruments.

C. to get up slowly from a standing, sitting, or lying position.

D. about the dehydrating effects of caffeinated drinks and alcohol.

155. A preteen with a history of TBI is relearning to prepare simple foods but has been having difficulties with sequencing so the OT practitioner has provided the patient with a chart of steps to follow. The child has just learned to prepare his favorite sandwich without "losing his place" in the process but continues to need occasional verbal reminders to look at the chart and to ensure safety. At this point, the child's MOST recent level of independence would be documented as:

A. independent.

B. independent with setup.

C. supervision.

D. minimal assist.

156. A young individual with MS is about to be discharged to home. The client is independent in bathtub transfers using a grab bar. The MOST important self-care recommendation the OT practitioner can make regarding bathing is to:

A. use cool water.

B. use moderately heated water.

C. take showers and avoid bathing.

D. bathe at the sink with a basin.

157. An OT practitioner is considering possible topics for a discharge planning group for individuals on an inpatient psychiatric unit. Which of the following topics would be MOST important to cover because it is significantly related to the possibility of rehospitalization?

A. Managing family conflicts

B. Living skills needed for keeping aftercare appointments

C. Coping strategies for continuing medication compliance

D. Education about problems with alcohol and substance use

158. An 8-year-old boy is being treated in OT for social withdrawal and depression. At the time of discharge, the BEST recreational activity for the OT practitioner to recommend for the child is:

A. swimming lessons.

B. Boy Scouts.

C. computer games.

D. piano lessons.

159. The OT practitioner has completed patient education with an individual who has just received a splint for carpal tunnel syndrome. When documenting this session, the OT practitioner will indicate that the patient was instructed in precautions, wearing schedule, and care of a:

A. wrist cock-up splint.

B. thermoplastic splint.

C. resting hand splint.

D. dynamic MP flexion splint.

160. A client that the OT practitioner is working with uses a wheelchair and requires minimal assistance with all transfers

and basic **ADL. The client is expected to remain at this functional level. Which of the following would be the MOST appropriate community living option for this client at discharge?**

A. A cradle-to-grave home

B. A transitional living center

C. An adult day program

D. A clustered independent living arrangement

161. **The OT practitioner has fitted a 6-year-old child for an adapted seat for use in the home for mealtime and other table-top activities. Which of the following instructions is MOST appropriate to convey to the parents?**

A. Adapt the seat as needed

B. Bring the seat in for each weekly therapy session in order to adjust it according to the child's growth

C. Bring the seat in for reevaluation within 6 months

D. Keep the seat until the end of the IEP

162. **An OT practitioner is helping a family plan a wheelchair ramp to the front door of their home. What is the minimum amount of space needed in front of the door to allow easy access by wheelchair?**

A. 3 feet by 5 feet

B. 4 feet by 4 feet

C. 4.5 feet by 3 feet

D. 5 feet by 5 feet

163. **The discharge disposition of an individual is: "The patient will return home upon discharge and receive services from the Bureau of Vocational Rehabilitation for vocational placement." This type of discharge plan is BEST described as:**

A. a follow-up plan.

B. aftercare.

C. a home program.

D. home health services.

164. **The OT observes that a child moves from a completely prone position to a prone-on-elbow position. In reporting the child's progress, the OTR documents that the child is gaining control in the midline position through the development of:**

A. primitive reflexes.

B. prehensile reactions.

C. righting reactions.

D. equilibrium reactions.

165. **In preparing a patient with a unilateral below-knee amputation for discharge from a rehabilitation facility, the MOST important adaptive equipment for the OT to recommend is:**

A. lightweight cooking utensils.

B. a tub bench and toilet rails.

C. long-handled dressing devices.

D. a reacher.

166. **"The patient arrived without her walker 3 out of 3 days this week." The MOST appropriate section of a SOAP note for the OT practitioner to place this statement is the:**

A. subjective.

B. objective.

C. assessment.

D. plan.

167. **Each day, an OT practitioner spends a portion of the day on documentation procedures. One of the MOST important purposes of documentation is to:**

A. occupy the therapist's time between treatments.

B. satisfy accrediting agencies.

C. be used as a research tool.

D. facilitate effective treatment.

168. **An individual was unable to achieve the goal "the client will initiate two requests to other group members for sharing materials within a 1-week period." The BEST revised goal is:**

A. "The client will initiate two requests to other group members for sharing group materials within a 2-week period."

B. "The client will initiate one request to one other group member for sharing or using group materials within a 1-week period."

C. "The client will initiate two requests to each of the five group members for sharing one group tool within 2 weeks."

D. "The client will say hello to the group leader at the start of each group session."

Occupational Therapy for Populations

169. **An OT practitioner in a long-term care facility would like to provide an activity to engage a number of residents with dementia who wander and pace the halls throughout the day. The BEST type of ac-**

tivity to plan for these residents would be:

A. reminiscing about previous jobs.
B. walking as part of a walking club.
C. singing oldies in a group.
D. a craft activity requiring concentration.

170. An OT practitioner who makes recommendations to improve accessibility in the community and advocates the rights of individuals with disabilities for employment, housing, public accommodations, public service, public transportation, and telecommunications is working to implement:

A. the Architectural Barriers Act of 1969.
B. the Federal Rehabilitation Act of 1973.
C. the Fair Housing Amendment Act of 1988.
D. the Americans with Disabilities Act of 1990.

171. In a long-term care facility, a number of residents have Parkinson's disease and would benefit from regular group activity which would help decrease the effects of muscular rigidity. The BEST activity the OT could recommend for this purpose would be:

A. weight training.
B. walking.
C. Tai Chi.
D. gardening.

172. The OT is using the Five-Stage group process for adults diagnosed with moderate levels of mental retardation. As a closure activity, which one of the following is the MOST appropriate?

A. Reviewing the rules for appropriate behavior in the group
B. Discussing emotional reactions to the crafts activity done earlier in the group
C. Walking through an obstacle course to music
D. Sitting in a circle and reciting a short poem

173. An OT has been hired to develop social skills training programs for persons with long-term mental illness in a community mental health facility. The OT needs to select a behavior to assess as an outcome measure. Which would BEST indicate that the program was successful in achieving goals for this population?

A. Improved ability to balance rest, work, and play and leisure

B. Improved verbal and nonverbal communication skills
C. Improved ability to identify areas for vocational exploration
D. Improved ability to perform daily self-care and home management activities

174. Which of the following is the most appropriate emphasis for a cooking group for young women with eating disorders?

A. Increasing knowledge of a variety of weight-loss techniques
B. Information on the caloric content of different foods
C. Preparing and consuming nutritional and normal-sized portions of food
D. Preparing healthy and appealing looking meals

175. An OT practitioner is requested to evaluate and make recommendations to a job site that is in search of ergonomic adaptations. An example of this type of adaptation might be:

A. introducing relaxation seminars for employees to decrease stress while on the job.
B. treating corporate clients for cumulative trauma disorders.
C. initiating a smoking cessation program.
D. suggesting furniture and accessories that promote better positioning at work.

176. Following initial evaluation of children needing early intervention services, the OT should:

A. independently develop an IEP.
B. collaboratively develop an IEP.
C. independently develop an IFSP.
D. collaboratively develop an IFSP.

Service Management

177. Which of the following is the BEST method for demonstrating service competency in a standardized evaluation?

A. Observe performance of the standardized test by a competent OT practitioner
B. Observe a competent OT practitioner, then practice, then teach another individual how to administer the test
C. Follow procedures exactly as outlined in the test manuals
D. Obtain the same results as another OT practitioner who has demonstrated service competency

178. A clinical manager of OT supervises an employee who has demonstrated specialized skills in treatment and serves as an expert for her peers. This practitioner has completed research, leadership training, and assisted in continuing education activities. The manager of the department is MOST likely to supervise this individual at what level?

A. Close supervision

B. Intermediate supervision

C. Advanced supervision

D. Educator supervision

179. OT services in a long-term care facility are provided by two OTRs and one COTA through a contract agency. When the absence of one of the OTRs creates a staffing shortage, the administration instructs the present OTR to perform evaluations only and instructs the COTA, a new graduate, to perform all treatment planning and implementation until they are full staffed again. No time is designated for supervision. What is the MOST appropriate way for the OT staff to respond?

A. Follow the administrator's instructions.

B. Express concern to the administrator about inadequate supervision and then follow administrator's instructions.

C. Express concern in writing to contract agency and then carry out the administrator's instructions.

D. Explain to the administrator this is not an appropriate solution and then develop an alternate solution.

180. The precaution MOST frequently used by OT practitioners and others in the health care field to prevent infection is:

A. the wearing of goggles.

B. the wearing of a mask.

C. frequent handwashing.

D. the wearing of a gown over work clothes.

181. An OT practitioner is working to reduce the application of restraints for the population of a long-term care facility. The MOST appropriate form of intervention for the OT to provide is:

A. identifying legal issues related to restraint reduction.

B. providing staff education, recommendations, and support for restraint alternatives.

C. investigating incidents of resident abuse related to restraint reduction.

D. assessing the level of risk and liability involved with restraint use.

182. During a group community reentry outing, one of the individuals complains of chest pain. The OT practitioner monitors the client's heart rate and blood pressure. The therapist interprets the client's resting heart rate at 120 bpm, and blood pressure at 220/180 mm Hg. The MOST appropriate action for the OT practitioner to take is to:

A. continue the community reentry outing.

B. immediately return the patients to the hospital.

C. help the patient lie down and wait until his vital signs return to normal.

D. call 911.

183. An elderly patient was hospitalized for a total hip replacement and is preparing to be discharged to a caregiver's home. The OT practitioner has recommended a program to address the patient's decreased mental abilities, specifically poor memory and difficulty with orientation to place and time. The BEST way for this individual to receive OT services is:

A. partial hospitalization.

B. adult day care.

C. home health care.

D. a psychosocial rehabilitation center.

184. An OTR has requested that a COTA document an initial note in the chart of a new patient. The COTA should document which of the following in the initial note?

A. The treatment and changes in the patient's condition

B. The source of the referral, the reason for the referral, and the date the referral was received

C. A summary and analysis of the patient's assets and deficits

D. The projected outcome of treatment

185. When an experienced OT practitioner completes a range of motion evaluation of an individual and asks the supervisor to retest the person to check the results, the OT practitioner is MOST likely seeking:

A. supervisory feedback.

B. evidence of competence.

C. evidence of interrater reliability.

D. evidence of incompetence.

186. **An OT practitioner is working in a psychiatric OT department that uses a variety of craft paints, stains, and sharp tools. In order to ensure patient safety, the practitioner MUST complete which of the following activities on a daily basis?**

    A. Label chemicals used within the department.
    B. Complete a tool count of departmental sharps.
    C. Obtain a locked storage cabinet for sharps.
    D. Decline suicidal clients the opportunity to participate in craft groups.

187. **An OT practitioner is collecting data for a quality assurance project. The advantage of asking a closed question is that the format:**

    A. allows the therapist to obtain facts.
    B. avoids emphasizing feelings being expressed by the patient.
    C. can help the therapist who is in a hurry.
    D. forces the person to give the answer that the therapist needs.

188. **When there is not a referral for OT services, it is MOST important for the COTA involved in the provision of services to know that:**

    A. the OTR is operating outside the scope of practice and regulating agencies should be notified.
    B. the OTR must assume responsibility for all OT services delivered.
    C. a written letter of consent must be received from the patient or a significant other.
    D. the COTA should seek a referral from the patient's family physician.

189. **An OT practitioner in a busy rehabilitation department consistently exemplifies the abilities and performance skills of an outstanding clinician. The manager of the department may financially reward this particular employee through:**

    A. disciplinary actions.
    B. performance reviews.
    C. clinical education.
    D. merit increases.

190. **The manager of an OT department is planning for reallocation of space that the department occupies. The manager studies and identifies the flow of staff** and patients through the clinic, offices, and ADL apartment. In so doing, the manager has MOST likely:

    A. identified elements critical for selecting a new location for the department.
    B. determined equipment needs.
    C. analyzed the work flow.
    D. determined functional areas.

191. **An OT practitioner is treating a middle-aged client who has carpal tunnel syndrome. The industrial nurse indicated that the condition was a result of repetitious fine motor skill execution required as an essential job function. The OT suggests to the client that the payment program MOST likely to reimburse for OT services is:**

    A. Medicare.
    B. Medicaid.
    C. workers' compensation.
    D. the Education for All Handicapped Children Act.

192. **A COTA frequently administers the Allen Cognitive Level Test and then discusses it with the supervising OTR. Which of the following MOST accurately describes the OTR's role during these discussions?**

    A. Determine the COTA's service competency
    B. Collect data on the patient's performance
    C. Interpret the results based on data collected by the COTA
    D. Develop the treatment plan

193. **A supervising OT asks an experienced COTA to complete a portion of an assessment. The portion that is MOST appropriate for the COTA to complete independently would be:**

    A. collecting chart review information.
    B. analyzing and interpreting assessment information.
    C. establishing the treatment goals.
    D. establishing the treatment plan.

194. **An OTR is working with an individual who tests positive for human immunodeficiency virus. The individual is working on a copper tooling project when he cuts his finger on the edge of the copper. Which of the following are the MOST APPROPRIATE precautions to follow?**

    A. Suicidal precautions
    B. Universal precautions
    C. Escape from unit precautions
    D. Medical precautions

Professional Practice

195. A hospital's public relations department plans to take some pictures of the OT staff working with patients. Before proceeding, which of the following MUST be obtained?

A. The correct spelling of the patients' names for the photograph caption

B. The patients' written consents to take the photographs and use them for publicity

C. The department head's written consent to take the photographs and use them for hospital purposes

D. The correct spelling of the patients' diagnoses and names for the photographs' captions

196. The OT practitioner is attempting to better understand a particular phenomenon by conducting a small research study. Initially, the OTR identifies a potential research question. The NEXT step in the process would be to:

A. state the purpose.

B. design the research.

C. complete a review of the literature.

D. establish boundaries for the study.

197. An OTR who has demonstrated service competency in the use of paraffin baths moves from one state to another to take a position in a hand rehabilitation center. The licensure act in the new state prohibits OT practitioners from using PAMs. The MOST appropriate action for the therapist to take is:

A. to use PAMs only under the supervision of a licensed PT.

B. to use PAMs only under the supervision of a doctor.

C. to use only paraffin.

D. not to use PAMs in the new state.

198. The FIRST step a COTA should take upon receiving a written referral for OT services for an acute care patient being discharged in 2 days is to:

A. initiate the ADL component of the evaluation.

B. begin a chart review.

C. notify the OTR.

D. screen the patient.

199. An OTR arrives for a home health visit on a Thursday morning (1/14/01), but the client is not feeling well, so they reschedule for the following day. The practitioner's charges for the week are due on alternating Thursday afternoons. Anticipating a follow-up visit with the client the next day (1/15/01) and reluctant to wait another 2 weeks to submit for payment, the practitioner bills for treatment using the 1/14/01 date. The OT practitioner's action is:

A. acceptable because treatment has been scheduled for the next day.

B. acceptable if the agency she works for allows it.

C. unacceptable because it violates the Code of Ethics.

D. unacceptable because if the patient is still ill and unable to participate in therapy on 1/15/01, a delay of more than 1 day is unacceptable for billing purposes.

200. An OT public relations campaign is being instituted in your state. It was suggested by the OT state representative that a committee be formed in order to externally educate potential consumers of OT. Which of the following BEST represents an appropriate form of external marketing?

A. Community newsletter

B. Departmental open house

C. In-service to all rehabilitation nurses

D. Participation in conference

ANSWERS FOR SIMULATION EXAMINATION 3

1. (D) neutral. Answer D describes the test position for the Tinel's sign, which is with the wrists in neutral. "Tinel's sign is positive if there is tingling along the course of the nerve distally when purcussed" (p. 665). The positions indicated in answer A, wrists ulnarly deviated, and answer B, wrists radially deviated, would not provide compression to the median nerve to elicit such a sensory change. Answer C is incorrect in that flexion/dorsiflexion is representative of the Phalen's test. However, in the Phalen's test, the wrists are positioned at the end point of range for flexion and dorsiflexion to elicit the greatest amount of compression on the median nerve. See reference: Pedretti (ed): Kasch, MC: Hand injuries.

2. (A) make recommendations for ways of accessing the technology. The OT on the assistive technology team usually determines which part of the body has sufficient motor control for accessing technology and then recommends the type of input access device (switch, keyword, software, etc.) that will best meet the client's needs. Answer B, recommending communication strategies, is most often the job of the speech and language pathologist. A social worker or other specialist in funding is usually responsible for answer C, seeking funding sources. Answer D, solving mechanical and software problems, is usually the role of the rehabilitation engineer. See reference: Angelo and Lane (eds): Angelo, J: A guide for assistive technology therapists.

3. (B) an interest checklist. An interest checklist is frequently used to initiate discussion of how a patient usually spends his leisure time and to identify areas of specific interest. Although the evaluation of living skills and the self-care evaluations (answers A and D) address the use of leisure time, they are used primarily to assess skills in personal care, safety and health, money management, transportation, use of the telephone, and work. An activity configuration (answer C) is used to assess the patient's use of time and his feelings about all of the activities he performs in a typical day or week. See reference: Early: Data gathering and evaluation.

4. (B) The client can usually handle routine daily functions. Answer B is correct because it describes the skills of an individual with moderate or trainable mental retardation. This child would most likely be able to complete ADL, live in a group home setting, and do unskilled work in a sheltered workshop. Answer A describes a child with profound mental retardation, answer C describes a child with severe mental retardation, and answer D describes a child who is mildly mentally retarded and educable. See reference: Case-Smith (ed): Rogers, SL, Gordon, CY, Schanzenbacher, KE, and Case-Smith, J: Common diagnosis in pediatric occupational therapy.

5. (C) radial, median, and ulnar. Radial, median, and ulnar are the terms used to describe the nerves that supply the hand. Answer B, femoral, obdurator, and sciatic nerves, supply the lower extremities. Answers A and D are not associated with the terminology used to describe the nerves that innervate the hand but typically describe the anatomical positioning of the body. See reference: Pedretti (ed): Belkin, J, and English, CB: Orthotics.

6. (C) topographic disorientation. Topographical disorientation is difficulty in finding one's way in familiar surroundings or in learning new routes and would be exhibited as the patient's inability to find the therapy clinic. Spatial relations disorders (answer A) would be exhibited as difficulties in relating objects to each other. Figure-ground discrimination deficits (answer B) would be exhibited as difficulty in differen-

tiating objects in the foreground from the background. Form discrimination deficits (answer D) would be exhibited as the inability to distinguish between different types of forms. See reference: Unsworth (ed): Arnadottir, G: Evaluation and intervention with complex perceptual impairment.

7. (B) Combing the hair An individual normally abducts and externally rotates the shoulder to comb his or her hair. Shoulder abduction is not required for buttoning a shirt (answer A) or tying a shoe (answer D). Tucking in a shirt in the back (answer C) requires shoulder abduction and internal rotation. Tying shoelaces (answer D) is less dependent on shoulder motion than on hip and spine flexibility. See reference: Pedretti (ed): Foti, D, Pedretti, LW, and Lillie, S: Activities of daily living.

8. (C) In the social worker's notes The social worker's notes include "details about the patient's family and occupation, education, cultural background, financial situation, and habits" (p. 341). The nurse's notes (answer A) provide information about the patient's adjustment to hospitalization and ongoing functioning in the hospital. The doctor's notes (answer B) document changes in diagnosis or medication. The admitting note (answer D) includes data on circumstances of the hospital admission, the tentative diagnosis, and any known history. See reference: Early: Data collection and evaluation.

9. (D) plan new motor tasks. Dyspraxia refers to difficulty planning new motor tasks (answer D). Inability to print or write (answer A) is termed "dysgraphia." The term "dyslexia" (answer B) literally means dysfunction in reading. Inability to perform mathematics (answer C) is known as dyscalcula. See reference: Case-Smith (ed): Rogers, SL, Gordon, CY, Schanzenbacher, KE, and Case-Smith, J: Common diagnosis in pediatric occupational therapy practice.

10. (C) lower back. Touching the lower back requires shoulder abduction and internal rotation. Answer A, back of the neck, and answer B, top of the head, are incorrect because they would require external shoulder rotation. Answer D, opposite shoulder, is also incorrect because horizontal adduction is required for this motion. See reference: Trombly (ed): Trombly, CA: Evaluation of biomechanical and physiological aspects of motor performance.

11. (C) conduct disorder. Conduct disorders often involve aggression toward people or animals and property destruction. Individuals with hyperactivity (answer A) demonstrate extremely high energy and activity levels. Attention deficit disorders (answer B), involve impulsive but not typically violent behaviors. Oppositional defiant disorders (answer B) involve similar but less severe behaviors than conduct disorders. See reference: Early: Understanding psychiatric diagnosis: The DSM-IV.

12. (B) superior and inferior colliculi. The correct answer is B because the inferior and superior colliculi are the areas that integrate stimuli from the visual, auditory, vestibular, and somatosensory systems. They also respond to stimuli of a protopathic nature and play an important role in spatiotemporal orientation. Answer A is not correct because the brainstem reticular formation is responsible for regulation of reflex centers for eye movements, sleep-wake cycles, heart rate, respiration, perspiration, salivation, and vomiting. Answer C is not correct because the pathways of the dorsal medulla are an extension of the dorsal column (carrying kinesthetic information). Answer D is not correct because the ventral aspect of the brainstem contains descending pathways responsible for voluntary control and coordination of skilled functions, relaying signals from cortical to subcortical structures, and modifying incoming sensory stimuli. See reference: Christiansen and Baum (eds): Dunn, W: Implementing neuroscience principles to support habilitation and recovery.

13. (A) a brachial plexus injury. A brachial plexus injury is a lesion that is typically a result of a traumatic injury. The nerve roots innervating the upper extremity originate between C4 and T1. Answer B, a long thoracic nerve injury, innervates C5-C7, affecting the serratus anterior muscle. Answer C, an axillary nerve injury, includes the C5-C6 spinal nerves and typically affects the deltoid and teres minor muscles. "The axillary nerve is rarely damaged by itself, it is often damaged along with traumatic lesions to the brachial plexus" (p. 753). Answer D, a Volkmann's contracture, is a fracture of the distal end of the humerus that interferes with the blood supply of the forearm. See reference: Pedretti (ed): McCormack, GL, and Pedretti, LW.: Motor unit dysfunction.

14. (B) Follow test manual directions When administering a standardized test, directions from the test manual should be followed closely to ensure reliability of test results. The test environment should be free of visual or auditory distractions or the child may have difficulty concentrating; therefore, answer A, "test in a stimulating environment" is incorrect. Answer C is incorrect because there are times when "...a child's fatigue, behavior, or time constraints" make it impossible to give the complete test in one session, and "most tests provide guidelines about how the test can be administered in two sessions" (p. 239). Answer D is wrong because, although the overall success of an evaluation can depend on the OT practitioner's ability to establish a rapport with the child and the family, too much conversation with the child may be distracting and prevent optimal performance. See reference: Case-Smith (ed): Richardson, PK: Use of standardized tests in pediatric practice.

15. (C) A grief response Grief is an adaptive mechanism used for dealing with a disabling condition because a loss of function has occurred. Dependency, stress reactions, and unrealistic goals are responses that would not normally pass with time. They also interfere with the recovery process when they are present in the extreme, as with grief. See reference: Trombly (ed): Versluys, HP: Evaluation of emotional adjustment to disabilities.

16. (A) work locks and latches on doors or windows. Checking the individual's ability to work the locks and latches on the doors and windows at home needs to be assessed because the style and stiffness may vary from those available in the clinic. The locks and latches may not be maintained in the same way and may be stiffer or smoother to work. The ability to work the locks and latches is also a safety concern because the individual may not be able to open them to let family into their home or close them to keep intruders from entering. Answers B, built up handles; C, energy conservation techniques; and D, adaptations to clothing fasteners, are all adaptations or activities that could be easily performed in the clinic because clothing and utensils are able to be transported to the clinic and energy conservation may be incorporated into treatment activities. See reference: Trombly (ed): Feinberg, JR, and Trombly, CA: Arthritis.

17. (B) identify and analyze the tasks and occupations that the client will be performing in the home. The first step in the process is to analyze the tasks and occupations that the client will be performing at home because this forms the basis of the entire assessment and recommendations that will be offered. This will also provide a framework for determining how well the client can perform the tasks within the particular environment being surveyed. Answers A, C, and D are also important aspects of the process but occur after the initial step. See reference: Pedretti (ed): Smith, P: Americans with Disabilities Act: Accommodating persons with disabilities.

18. (A) short-term recall. Short-term recall is the ability to recall all information that has just been received and to hold it in temporary use from 1 to 5 minutes or more. Short-term recall is not just a selected part of the information. Attention (answer B) allows the person to retrieve information from a long series and to single out a specific part of the information for use. A person who is being evaluated for hearing (answer C) would be checked for the accuracy of sound at different pitches, not a specific sound. Abstraction (answer D) is the ability to extrapolate information from an idea to generalize to another situation. See reference: Zoltan: Orientation, attention and memory.

19. (C) somatosensory system. Many children who use an excessively tight grip on the writing tool and press too hard with the pencil on their paper have poor proprioceptive awareness (somatosensory). Answer A, vestibular system, is not the most correct answer because, although it is difficult to completely separate one sensory system from another, the vestibular system primarily affects balance and general motor coordination. Answer B, the auditory system, is not the most correct answer because the auditory system interprets sound for use in language. Answer D, the visual system, is not correct because although the visual system can monitor motor control such as pencil grip and pressure, use of a pencil requires unconscious awareness of body position and pressure at times when the task is not monitored visually. See reference: Case-Smith (ed): Amundson, SJ, and Weil, M: Prewriting and handwriting skills.

20. (B) trace. Trace muscle strength equals a 1 on the numerical scale of muscle testing. The other answers would be incorrect, since answer A, absent strength would equal 0, answer C, good strength would equal a 4, and answer D, normal strength would equal a 5. See reference: Pedretti (ed): Pedretti, L: Evaluation of muscle strength.

21. (D) Home observation and parent interview "Observation of children in familiar settings and routines allows more characteristic views of their abilities and may be actually more reflective of how children can be expected to perform....." (p. 207). Parent interviews provide information about the child's abilities from the parent's point of view and can identify the priorities of the child's caregiver. Answers A, B, and C provide necessary information about performance components, development, and other parameters but are not as effective in helping the evaluator learn about the child's self-care functioning. See reference: Case-Smith (ed): Stewart, KB: Purposes, processes, and methods of evaluation.

22. (B) All group members construct one tower that incorporates all the pieces provided in a set of constructional materials (e.g., Legos™, Tinkertoys™, or Erector™ set). Activities used in evaluation groups should require group collaboration that can be done in approximately 45 minutes and emphasize process rather than endproduct. The collage and crafts are individual and do not demand group interaction. Making pizza for lunch is an endproduct that serves the group as a whole and usually takes longer than 45 minutes. The pizza activity and format is typically not an evaluation group but is better suited as a task-oriented group activity in which self-awareness and self-understanding are primary goals. See reference: Mosey: Evaluation.

23. (D) phantom limb pain. Phantom limb pain is present when the amputated limb is perceived to be present with accompanying pain. Answer A, paresthesias, are not related to an absent limb's being intact, but to feelings of numbness and tingling. Answer B, phantom limb sensation, is associated with the feeling of the limb's being intact after surgery but

without the associated pain. Answer C, a neuroma, can cause pain because of nerve tissue, but it is not associated with feelings that the limb is intact. See reference: Pedretti (ed): Pasquinelli, S: Lower extremity amputations and prosthetics.

24. (B) forgetting to turn off the stove burner. The progression of dementia of the Alzheimer's type is often described by its phases of impairment in functioning. Whereas behaviors linked to memory impairments usually occur in the early stages, social and motor impairments occur later. See reference: Trombly (ed): Bonder, BR, and Goodman, G: Preventing occupational dysfunction secondary to aging.

25. (C) at age level. At 3 years of age, a child is expected to know when he or she has to use the toilet and be able to get on and off the toilet. Three-year-old children may need assistance to cleanse themselves effectively and to manage fasteners or difficult clothing. Complete independence in using the toilet (answer D) is usually achieved by the age of 4 to 5 years. By the age of 2 years (answer B), most children have daytime control over elimination, with occasional accidents, so they still need to be reminded to go to the toilet. One-year-old infants (answer A) indicate discomfort when wet or soiled. See reference: Case-Smith (ed): Shepherd, J: Self care and adaptations for independent living.

26. (C) Moderate assistance Moderate assistance is defined as having the ability to complete the task with supervision and cueing while requiring physical assistance for 20 to 50% of the task. The individual who requires minimal assistance (answer B) is able to complete a task with supervision and cueing while requiring physical assistance for less than 20% of the task. An individual who needs supervision, cueing, and physical assistance for from 50 to 80% of the task is performing at the maximal assistance level (answer D). An individual is rated dependent (answer A) when he or she is able to perform less than 20%, or a few steps, of the activity independently. This individual may require elaborate equipment, may perform the activity extremely slowly, and may fatigue easily. See reference: Pedretti (ed): Foti, D, Pedretti, LW, and Lillie, S: Activities of daily living.

27. (D) presence of self-stimulatory behavior. Self-stimulatory behavior is often seen in autistic children and frequently interferes with function. The other answers are less relevant in terms of essential data for intervention planning. An autistic child may be normal in terms of his or her ability to focus at close range (answer A), wrist flexibility (answer B), and hand preference (answer C), but show poor adaptive behavior. See reference: Neistadt and Crepeau (eds): Florey, L: Psychosocial dysfunction in childhood and adolescence.

28. (A) dual diagnosis. Examples of dual diagnostic

categories are mental health and mental retardation and mental health and substance abuse. Multiply handicapped is the coexistence of physical and mental health types of problems. Answers C and D are not terms commonly used in health care. See reference: Cottrell (ed): Jacobs, B: Dual diagnosis: A parent's perspective.

29. (D) at the midrange of the joint. Proprioception (or position sense) is demonstrated when an OT practitioner passively positions the joint being tested and the individual is able to imitate the position with the opposite extremity. The joint should not be moved through range to an extent that would elicit a stretch or pain response, which would be at the end ranges of the joint. Movement should be at a rate of approximately 10 degrees per second to prevent the stretch reflex from being elicited. The end points of the range are used as the starting positions from which proprioception testing is started because it is in these positions that the stretch or pain response would occur. See reference: Trombly (ed): Bentzel, K: Evaluation of sensation.

30. (C) clothing care, cleaning, and volunteering. Doing laundry, cleaning, and volunteering are all examples of work and productive activities. Answers A and B are examples of ADL. Reading, watching television, and doing small handicrafts (answer D) are examples of play and leisure activities. See reference: Neistadt and Crepeau (eds): Neistadt, ME: Introduction to evaluation and interviewing.

31. (C) 8 months. This is correct because 3 months (number of months premature) are subtracted from the child's chronological age to adjust for prematurity. This child is then given the benefit of time lost because of a shorter gestation period. See reference: Case-Smith (ed): Hunter, JG: Neonatal Intensive Care Unit.

32. (A) -15 degrees to 140 degrees. Negative range of motion documentation may vary from one setting to another. However, this range may be written as a negative (minus) sign preceding the degree (-15 degrees) or as a positive number preceding the neutral position (15 degrees to 0 degrees to 140 degrees). Therefore, answers B, C, and D are incorrect. See reference: Pedretti (ed): Pedretti, LW: Evaluation of joint range of motion.

33. (B) flexion righting reaction. The flexion righting reaction (answer B) is correct because "the development of antigravity neck strength is first associated with the ability to maintain the head aligned with the body when pulled to a sitting position" (p. 273). Answer A is incorrect because protective reactions are elicited through displacement (such as falling forward), and these reactions protect infants from falls. Answer C is incorrect because the body righting on body reaction is represented by the rotation between trunk segments (also a rotational righting

reaction). Answer D is incorrect because the optical righting reaction incorporates vision and allows the child to right the head against gravity (this is also referred to as a vertical righting reaction). See reference: Case-Smith (ed): Nichols, DS: Development of postural control.

34. (D) anosognosia. Anosognosia is a form of neglect in which an individual denies any deficits. Compensation techniques cannot be taught to someone who has no awareness of his or her deficits. A person with a visual field cut (answer A) has a loss of a specific area of vision related to an area of the visual system that has been damaged. When there is an awareness of the loss, compensatory techniques can be taught. A person who has apraxia (answer B) is unable to perform a purposeful movement on command, but is able to understand a loss of ability and can perform activities spontaneously or follow some cues. Aphasia (answer C) is an impairment of receptive or expressive communication verbally, but a person with this is able to comprehend gestures or pictures and use them as a compensatory technique. See reference: Trombly (ed): Quintana, LA: Evaluation of perception and cognition.

35. (C) dysphagia evaluation. A dysphagia evaluation usually consists of a client's mental status; oral motor structure; and head, trunk, and extremity motor functions. Answer A, TMJ does not typically include an evaluation of one's mental status and extremities. Answer B, cranial nerves, does not involve assessment of the extremities and trunk. Answer D, dysmetria (the ability to estimate how much motion is required to reach a target) is not typically included in the assessment of the oral structures. See reference: Pedretti (ed): Nelson, KL: Dysphagia: Evaluation and treatment.

36. (A) measures the skill or function it claims to measure. There are several kinds of validity, including logical, content, and construct validity; however, they all indicate whether the test measures what it claims to measure. Answers B and C describe reliability, which indicates the strength of the test's consistency. A test based on a normative population (answer D) is not necessarily valid, because it has collected statistics on only that group. Scores obtained on a sample population are usually compared with scores on tests measuring similar functions in order to establish validity. See reference: Case-Smith (ed): Richardson, PK: Use of standardized tests in pediatric practice.

37. (C) 9 and 12 months. Children usually begin to cruise (walk sideways holding onto furniture) between 9 and 12 months. See reference: Case-Smith (ed): Nichols, DS: The development of postural control.

38. (C) fair plus (3+). A person with strength of fair or fair minus would be unable to tolerate resistance.

A person with strength of fair plus during a MMT can tolerate minimal resistance. A person whose strength is good minus can tolerate less than moderate resistance but more than minimal resistance. See reference: Trombly (ed): Evaluation of biomechanical and physiological aspects of motor performance.

39. (B) Dressing habits Certain dressing habits may indicate tactile defensiveness; for example, the child may show poor tolerance of certain textures or avoid wearing turtlenecks, socks, or shoes. Conversely, some children may never take off their shoes in order to avoid tactile overstimulation. Reading skills (answer A), friendships (answer C), and the choice of hobbies (answer D) could be affected secondarily, as a result of intolerance of certain textures or human touch or the inability to concentrate. However, because of the close connection between dressing and tactile tolerance, knowledge of the child's dressing habits (answer B) will give the OT practitioner the most reliable information. See reference: Case-Smith (ed): Parham, LD and Mailloux, Z: Sensory integration.

40. (B) demonstrate the procedure on the unaffected extremity, then occlude the individual's vision. The presentation of stimuli in sensory evaluation is extremely important. Because of the compensation that may occur with vision, it is necessary to occlude the individual's vision. Also, the unaffected extremity should be assessed before the affected extremity, the opposite of answer A, to reduce anxiety in the individual. Stimuli should be presented in a random proximal-to-distal pattern. A rapport (answer C) should be established before beginning any of the evaluation procedures, also to reduce anxiety. An individual may not be aware of any deficit areas (answer D), so the whole extremity should be assessed to ensure accuracy. Picture cards are helpful in assessing individuals with expressive aphasia. See reference: Trombly (ed): Bentzel, K: Evaluation of sensation.

41. (D) Read the social worker's report The social worker's report includes details about the patient's family situation, occupational, educational, and cultural background, and expected environment. Referring to this document eliminates the need to duplicate this information. Interviews with the patient and family by OT practitioners (answers B and C) are designed to obtain information concerning role and task performance and performance levels in work, self-care, and leisure. It would be a waste of time to review the entire medical record (answer A) just to obtain information about an individual's social status. See reference: Early: Data gathering and evaluation.

42. (D) A child with spina bifida with lower extremity paralysis Usually, a child in this condition has enough upper extremity coordination and

strength to propel himself on a scooter on which the lower extremities are supported. Such a child also has the cognitive and sensory awareness to negotiate a scooter in its environment. Prone scooters may be contraindicated for the children described in answers A, B, and C. The neck hyperextension required for exploratory play on a prone scooter could cause further increase in the abnormal tone of the child with CP (answer A). A child with low tone who is easily fatigued (answer B) may be unable to maintain this very exhausting position for very long and is likely to become even more tired. Because the child lacks the sensory feedback and cognitive skills, the child with cognitive limitations and poor sensory awareness (answer C) would be at risk of injury. See reference: Case-Smith (ed): Wright-Ott, C, and Egilson, S: Mobility.

43. (D) Support Answer D is correct because the term "support reaction" refers to the ability to co-activate muscle groups of the appropriate extremity or about the midline in order to support the body weight or posture in a certain position. Answer A is incorrect because protective reactions follow the development of support reactions in the arms (which protect the child when falling) and require that the body is free from support. Answer B is not correct because equilibrium reactions are compensatory movements used to regain stability, not to maintain stability. Answer C is not correct because rotational righting reactions involve turning of the head or trunk in order to maintain body alignment. See reference: Neistadt and Crepeau (eds): Kohlmeyer, K: Evaluation of sensory and neuromuscular performance components.

44. (C) A heavy handbag held by handles. The hook grasp is strongly based on the use of digits two to five. The thumb is not always required for the hook grasp and can remain inactive. A needle would be held with two-point pinch while being threaded. A glass would be held with a cylindrical grasp. Finally, a key being placed in a lock would be held by a lateral pinch. See reference: Smith, Weiss, and Lehmkuhl: Wrist and hand.

45. (B) ability to grade movement. The "grading of movement" goal best addresses the difficulty with control of the midrange of a movement pattern (common in children with athetosis). Answer A is incorrect because this goal would be appropriate for a child who cannot break up a flexion or extension pattern during a movement. Answer C is not correct because this goal is appropriate for a child who has difficulty with an arm or hand movement's being too fast or too slow (graded movements are also too fast). Answer D is incorrect because this goal is appropriate for a child who has difficulty bringing both arms to midline and using them effectively together. See reference: Case-Smith (ed): Exner, CE: Development of hand skills.

46. (B) writing a soap opera. Although answers A, C, and D would benefit the self-confidence and stress management needs of women struggling with the issues associated with emotional and physical abuse, they are not expressive group activities. Writing a soap opera would most likely be a creative approach implemented to assist individuals in expressing their inner thoughts, feelings, anxieties, and beliefs. See reference: Early: Group concepts and techniques.

47. (A) learn to type. Typing would allow the individual to communicate legibly in writing, while circumventing the individual's poor handwriting skills. Answer B, fine motor coordination exercises, and answer C, practicing letter or shape formations, are both ways to improve control of the writing utensils by improving coordination through exercises that will provide a greater smoothness to the writing. Answer D, exercises or activities for strengthening flexors and extensors in the finger, also allows improved use of the writing utensil by providing enough strength to properly position the writing tool. However, answers B, C, and D do not bypass the individual having to perform handwriting with a pen or pencil. See reference: Fisher, Murray, and Bundy (eds): Cermak, S: Somatodyspraxia.

48. (C) A client with a C6 injury An individual with C6 quadriplegia has some use of the abductor pollicis longus, extensor pollicis longus, extensor digitorum communis, and extensor carpi ulnaris. The extensor tone of the muscles in conjunction with the splint will operate the power for prehension force. Individuals with Cl or C3 injuries have higher level lesions and lack the wrist extension strength needed to operate the wrist-driven flexor hinge splint. An individual with a T1 injury is able to grasp and manipulate utensils without difficulty or need for assistance. See reference: Trombly (ed): Hollar, LD: Spinal cord injury.

49. (C) Avoid resistive materials For a child with acute juvenile rheumatoid arthritis, the OT practitioner should always use techniques for joint protection and energy conservation. Activities requiring the manipulation of highly resistive materials such as clay, leather, and copper sheets should be avoided; the pressure applied to the joints could exacerbate the condition. Avoiding light touch (answer A) is a precaution more relevant in the treatment of a child with tactile defensiveness. Rapid vestibular stimulation (answer B) is contraindicated for a child who is prone to seizures. The need to avoid above-normal body temperature (answer D) is more relevant to a client with multiple sclerosis because high temperature exacerbates the symptoms. See reference: Case-Smith (ed): Rogers, SL, Gordon, CY, Schanzenbacher, KE, and Case-Smith, J: Common diagnosis in pediatric occupational therapy.

50. (D) Create a comfortable foundation for

fostering parent skills through parent-therapist collaboration All four answers describe possible ways for an OT to impact an infant's developmental outcome. However, the most permanent action would capitalize upon developing family-centered mutual collaboration. With this approach, communication is the key to creating a relationship that will foster parental skill development and expertise. This then provides the parents with effective tools to best nurture and care for their infant at any time and in any environment, and has a permanent impact on the developmental outcome for the infant. See reference: Case-Smith (ed): Hunter, JG: Neonatal Intensive Care Unit.

51. (C) applying grout to a tile trivet and waiting for it to dry. Activities provide a variety of opportunities for therapeutic gains. The process of grouting a tile trivet involves covering the individual's tile design with a grout mixture (which tends to be very liquid in consistency) before setting up the material to dry. Waiting for the grout to dry requires an individual to delay gratification. Working in a group (answer A) promotes cooperation. Selecting a tile design (answer B) involves decision making. Cleaning off the table (answer D) may promote the experience of success after a mess but does not involve the concept of delaying gratification. See reference: Neistadt and Crepeau (eds): Crepeau, EB: Activity analysis: A way of thinking about occupational performance.

52. (B) High contrast and defined borders Answer B is correct because it provides the only combination of features when adapting visual material that assist children with visual discrimination problems. High contrast of the stimuli (shape, letter, numbers, and so on) in relation to the background and defining important areas of the stimuli with a border attract the eye and provide clear input. Answer A is incorrect because low contrast of the stimuli, such as blue ditto lettering, is difficult to discriminate. Answer C is incorrect because undefined borders around the important stimuli make for less clear input. Answer D is incorrect because both features of the visual stimulus would make it difficulty to discriminate See reference: Kramer and Hinojosa (eds): Todd, VR: Visual information analysis: Frame of reference for visual perception.

53. (C) vestibular processing, postural control, and muscle tone. Vestibular processing and postural control are required for maintaining balance. Muscle tone that is too high or too low will limit the individual's ability to move the lower extremities for ambulation; hence, these three components are important for successfully walking in the pool. Fine motor coordination (answer A) is not required to walk across the pool. In addition, while walking in the water requires some strength, it can still be successfully performed with significantly decreased strength because the body weighs significantly less when submerged. Answer B includes postural control and gross motor coordination, which are both important to walking in the pool, but it also includes visual motor integration, which is not. Answer D includes range of motion and praxis, both of which are required to some degree for walking in the pool, but it also includes crossing the midline, which is not required. See reference: AOTA: Uniform Terminology for Occupational Therapy, third edition.

54. (B) holding a class about job-seeking strategies. The purpose of applying remedial strategies is to enhance underlying abilities. Teaching and training methods are commonly used techniques. Answer A, an interest checklist, is a tool used to identify the degree of an individual's interest in a variety of leisure areas. Answer C is an example of a compensatory strategy. Answer D provides opportunities for exploration and expression. See reference: Early: Data collection and evaluation.

55. (B) start by having the members make a collage or drawing which symbolizes how they handle anger. Providing an initial activity encourages group members to become involved in the process more quickly. Having a concrete product related to the topic provides group members with something to talk about and refer to during discussion. Beginning with an activity helps the group members to focus on the topic and on each other. Answers A, C, and D are attempts to facilitate discussion without the use of an activity (a technique used by psychotherapists) and may not provide sufficient structure or interest to generate participation in this type of activity group. See reference: Posthuma: Group activities.

56. (C) demonstrates any reliable, controlled movement. As long as the child can produce any such movement, switches can be adapted to meet positioning and mobility needs. Accurate reach and pointing (answer B) or isolated finger control (answer D) are not necessary to use simple pressure switches. An upright sitting position (answer A) would not be required if the child needed to be positioned in a reclining or sidelying position. See reference: Case-Smith (ed): Swinth, Y: Assistive technology: Computers and augmentative communication.

57. (B) Pass around a scent box and ask each patient to smell the contents Sensory integration theory holds that individuals can learn by receiving, processing, and responding to sensory stimulation. Starting a group for regressed individuals with sensory stimuli such as touch and smell helps to get the individuals' attention and arouse their interest. Asking individuals in this type of a group to introduce themselves (answer A) can be confusing and time consuming, especially when dealing with regressed individuals with limited attention spans. Reading favorite poems (answer C) and discussing lunch menus (answer D) are activities more suited to patients functioning on higher levels than the group de-

scribed here. See reference: Early: Group concepts and techniques.

58. (A) Plaster cylindrical splint A plaster cylindrical splint would encourage a static stretch of the PIP joint contracture. Answer B is a form of PIP extension and is considered to be a dynamic splint. Answer C is used to isolate tendon and joint range of motion, and answer D is also a form of dynamic splinting. See reference: Pedretti (ed): Belkin, J, and English, CB: Orthotics.

59. (C) Patient will be independent in grooming in 1 week, in upper and lower extremity dressing in 2 weeks, and in toileting in 3 weeks. OTRs must be careful to establish goals in all performance areas that will be addressed and permit progress to be documented. For instance, if the therapist expects a patient to achieve independence in grooming, dressing, and toileting simultaneously, then a goal of "independent in grooming, dressing, and toileting in 3 weeks" would be appropriate (answer B). However, this therapist expects the patient to achieve independence at different times, so combining performance areas or lumping the performance areas into one group (answer A) delays the accomplishment of goals. If a patient is expected to achieve independence in these areas at different times, then writing three separate goals permits the record to reflect these incremental improvements. See reference: Piersol and Ehrlich (eds): McGuire, M: The "write" stuff.

60. (B) labeling and calendars. An external memory device uses environmental adaptations or structure to assist the person in remembering specific information. Examples include setting an alarm clock to wake up in the morning, labeling drawers according to contents, and using a log or calendar to keep track of events and activities. An internal memory device would be the use of internalized memory techniques to structure information. Examples would be rehearsal, visual imagery, mnemonics, or elaborating on the information. See reference: Zoltan: Executive functions.

61. (C) Provide enjoyable activities in a safe and accepting environment Children who learn to enjoy activities alone will be more likely to cooperate with peers in a group activity. It is unlikely that the child will initiate and develop social interaction in an environment that inhibits independence (answer A). Children with peer interaction problems need to be taught some basic social skills (answer B) in order to increase successful peer interaction. Children will more likely learn and accept rules and limits established by their group than by an authority figure (answer D). See reference: Kramer and Hinojosa (eds): Olson, LJ: Psychosocial frame of reference.

62. (A) Ballet To promote the development of anticipatory control, movement should be slow, predictable, and controlled from a stable base. Participation in a dance class would involve controlled movement from a stable base. Answers B, C, and D are activities that feature faster-moving objects whose speed and direction of movement cannot be controlled by the player and require quick reactions to unpredictable stimuli. See reference: Case-Smith (ed): Nichols, DS: The development of postural control.

63. (B) Hammering a nail into a piece of wood
Hammering a nail into a piece of wood requires the individual to stabilize the object against the palm and fingers while the thumb is positioned to perform as an opposing force. Answer A is a form of prehension commonly referred to as tip prehension. Answer C, carrying a pail of bolts, requires a hook grasp; this requires the MCP joints to be placed in extension, and the PIP and DIP joints to be flexed and may not include the use of the thumb. Answer D is considered a spherical grasp pattern that requires the fourth and fifth digits to assume a more flexed position for enhanced cupping of the palm. See reference: Pedretti (ed): Belkin, J, and English, CB: Orthotics.

64. (A) increasing self-awareness through expressive activities. Increasing self-awareness would be an initial goal area because people with eating disorders are often out-of-touch with their bodies as well as their psychological and social needs. Expressive activities address psychosocial needs to increase self-awareness by providing opportunities for emotional self-expression and self-assertion. Answer B is incorrect because preoccupation with "good" versus "bad" nutrition may be part of the eating disorder. Answer C is incorrect because people with eating disorders tend to function in school unless physically ill. Family therapy referrals are typically performed by other disciplines on the team at the time of discharge, so answer D is also incorrect. See reference: Neistadt and Crepeau (eds): Ward, JD: Psychosocial dysfunction in adults.

65. (C) Biomechanical According to Colangelo, "The biomechanical frame of reference is applied when a person cannot maintain posture through appropriate automatic muscle activity because of neuromuscular or musculoskeletal dysfunction" (p. 257). This child's physical status has changed with decreasing postural control. Adaptive support devices need to be considered, and a biomechanical frame of reference provides this approach. Answer A is not correct because the neurodevelopmental treatment frame of reference is concerned with improving posture and movement, and supportive equipment is prescribed for that purpose. Answer B is not correct because the sensory integration frame of reference is concerned with sensory input in relation to posture and movement in children with sensory integration disorders (specifically, Duchenne's disease is a neuromuscular disorder). An-

swer D is not correct because the visual perceptual frame of reference is concerned with guiding and compensating for visual perceptual problems, not postural delays. See reference: Kramer and Hinojosa (eds): Colangelo, CA: Biomechanical frame of reference.

66. (D) "The child will correctly identify, by feel only, five out of five common objects". Identifying an object by touch is termed "stereognosis" or "identification of solids." Stereognosis is a tactile discrimination skill needed for the development of fine hand manipulation. Answer A demonstrates localization of tactile stimuli, answer B demonstrates graphesthesia, and answer C is an example of the tactile discrimination of textures. See reference: Case-Smith (ed): Exner, CE: Development of hand skills.

67. (C) Avoid having these individuals in close proximity to others to reduce opportunities for physical contact Avoiding close proximity situations is the recommended environmental modification for sexual acting-out behaviors. Advising the client of your expectations (answer D) is an appropriate use of self in such situations. Standing to the side (answer B) is a recommended environmental modification for highly aggressive and hostile behavior risks. Providing real-life activities in a stimulating environment (answer A) has been found to be helpful with reducing some delusions. See reference: Early: Safety techniques.

68. (B) folding laundry and putting it in a basket while standing. Work-hardening programs prepare individuals to return to work by combining work simulation, strengthening, and behavioral components. A cashier stands during the job; removes clothing from hangers; folds it; puts it in a bag; runs price tags through a scanner; and operates a cash register and makes change. Putting price tags on clothing while seated (answer D) does not include standing, a critical component of the job. Washing dishes while standing (answer C) incorporates the standing aspect of her job but not the other aspects. Moving piles of clothing from one end of the clinic to the other (answer A) involves walking, not standing. The activity that incorporates the MOST components of her job is folding laundry and putting it in a basket while standing. See reference: Pedretti (ed): Burt, CM, and Smith, P: Work evaluation and work hardening.

69. (A) decrease joint stress and pain. It is very important to preserve joint integrity in individuals with arthritis by using adaptive equipment to avoid or reduce the wear and tear stresses on fragile joints. Adaptive equipment would not correct deformities (answer B) because deformities are only corrected by surgery or with orthotic devices that reposition the joints in correct alignment. Adaptive equipment allows activities to be completed but would not simplify work by eliminating steps to an activity (answer C). Another reason adaptive equipment is used is to increase (not decrease) independence (answer D). See reference: Pedretti (ed): Hittle, JM, Pedretti, LW, and Kasch, MC: Rheumatoid arthritis.

70. (B) An activity exploring leisure opportunities and problems In the process of making choices about activities, the first step is developing awareness and knowledge. OT practitioners "… assist the clients in developing awareness of options and limits" (p. 387). This individual's leisure interests are already known, so answer A would be a duplication of information you already have. Magazine picture collages could be adapted to further examine interests and values, but this answer (answer C) does not describe such an adaptation. Answer D is premature at this point because the individual has not identified any goals around which to plan future leisure activities. See reference: Neistadt and Crepeau (eds): Knox, SH: Treatment through play and leisure.

71. (B) Developing vocational interests, social skills, and community mobility skills Answer B is correct because these skills are essential in functioning in the environment after school. Answer A, leisure interests, is not correct because, although they are important to the student's life, leisure skills and interest knowledge are not as essential. Answer C is not correct because, although it describes the student's motor control function, which may influence the type of job the adolescent performs, adaptation can be made in this area of need. Although developing fine motor skills (answer D) is a traditional OT role in school settings, it would not be an appropriate focus for transition planning intervention, of which the case described is an example. See reference: Case-Smith (ed): Rogers, SL, Gordon, CY, Schanzenbacher, KE, and Case-Smith, J: Common diagnosis in pediatric occupational therapy practice.

72. (B) wear noisy bracelets on the wrist or ankle as a reminder to visually scan toward the affected side. Although hazards may be removed from the environment, or padded to prevent injury to an individual, use of these interventions is only feasible in a person's home. It is best to teach the individual visual scanning of the affected area and the environment, a technique that the person may use anywhere. An individual may avoid using sharp tools or extreme water temperature, but this avoidance does not teach him or her how to monitor the affected side visually, because it is a precaution that addresses only the problem with sensation. Noisy bracelets are one technique that may be used to accomplish compensation for both unilateral neglect and absence of sensation. Visual impairments that are not accompanied by sensory or perceptual deficits are more readily overcome with retraining. See reference: Trombly (ed): Quintana, LA: Remediating perceptual impairments.

73. (D) a weighted pen and weighted wrists. Weighting body parts and utensils (or writing tools)

are effective for individuals with ataxia in improving control during performance of a task. Hitting the keys on a keyboard (answer A) would be difficult for such a client, although weighting the wrists could make performance of the activity possible. A keyboard is a good alternative for individuals with difficulty writing due to weakness, limited range of motion, or incoordination. A universal cuff with a pencil-holder attachment (answer B) would be appropriate for an individual with hand weakness who uses a universal cuff for other tasks. A balanced forearm orthosis (answer C) is appropriate for individuals with severe muscle weakness. In addition, individuals with muscle weakness find felt-tip pens easier to write with than ballpoint pens. See reference: Pedretti (ed): Schlageter, K, and Zoltan, B: Traumatic brain injury.

74. (B) labels with white print on a black background. White print on a black background is easier to see for individuals with poor vision. Using Braille labels (answer A) is not appropriate for individuals with peripheral neuropathy because they have decreased tactile sensation in their fingertips. A pill organizer box (answer C) is useful for taking pills on schedule and is particularly helpful for individuals who have memory deficits or complex medication regimens. If the pills were presorted in the box, the client could safely take them without actually identifying them. Using the pill organizer, however, does not address the stated issue of medication identification. Brightly colored pills (answer D) would make it easy for an individual to identify different medications; however, the therapist has no control over how pills are manufactured and what colors are used. See reference: Ryan (ed): Practice Issues in Occupational Therapy: Hansvick, B, and Saxon, MC: The elderly with hearing and visual impairments.

75. (A) Ask group members to discuss how they feel about taking their medications. "Any effort to help a client manage medication independently should begin with a discussion of his or her feelings about it" (p. 421). Clients can often benefit from hearing about the experiences of others. Using diaries (answer B), timers (answer C), lists, and other environmental supports can also increase success in independent medication management. Knowledge of the medication schedule is critical, but the FIRST; action the OT should take is leading the discussion on feelings about taking medications. See reference: Early: Activities of daily living.

76. (B) practicing the whole task of putting on a shirt in a setting similar to the real environment. Retention of a skill will be enhanced if the task is practiced in its entirety during each performance trial because whole task performance is easier to recall than separate steps. Generalization of skills is enhanced when an activity has been acquired in a setting that resembles the natural environment where the skill will be performed. Answer A, practice of each segment of the process, may be useful for improving performance of the activity segments practiced, but will not enhance retention and generalization of the skill. Providing simulation activities may improve some performance components involved in the dressing process, but will not enhance learning of the whole task of putting on a shirt. Answer D, showing a videotape and providing written directions are useful instructional techniques for client education from a cognitive perspective, but they do not provide the motor component necessary for learning a motor skill. See reference: Gillen and Burkardt (eds): Application of learning and environmental strategies to activity-based treatment.

77. (C) Stabilizing the pelvis, hips, and legs Answer C is correct because when the pelvis, hips, and legs do not provide a good central base of support, the child resorts to compensatory movements. Stabilizing the trunk (answer A) is not correct because unless the pelvis is stabilized, arm movements may still be compromised. Answer B is not correct because use of a lap board or chair arms for weight bearing of the upper extremities will compromise the use of the arms and hands to stabilize the body. Stabilizing the head and neck (answer D) is not correct because the pelvis continues to be unstable and therefore is not a good base for arm movements. See reference: Case-Smith (ed): Nichols, DS: Development of postural control.

78. (C) Implement compensatory strategies "The compensation approach focuses on using remaining abilities to achieve the highest level of function possible ... " (p. 370). Compensatory strategies include modifying the environment and are most appropriate for this patient because his prognosis is poor and he is unlikely to improve. An example would be placing the food all on the right side of his meal tray. "The focus of remediation (answer A) is to improve or restore the client's performance.... This approach is used when a client's condition or diagnosis ... are likely to improve enough to allow pretreatment levels of task proficiency" (p. 369). Whereas patient education (answer B) about a visual-field deficit is likely to have little benefit, educating the family is important so that they can implement compensatory strategies. Adaptive equipment (answer D) is a compensatory strategy; however, it would provide little benefit in this situation. See reference: Neistadt and Crepeau (eds): Culler, KH: Treatment of work and productive activities: Home and family management.

79. (D) Present only a few blocks at a time Similar to other children with this diagnosis, this child most likely has poor impulse control and experiences great difficulty completing a task. By presenting a few blocks at a time, the OT practitioner can help the child focus on a few relevant stimuli and make it possible to complete a short-term task successfully. This experience will then help the child increase his

attention span. Soft foam blocks (answer A) are less likely to cause injury if thrown, but their use is not likely to help increase his attention span. Providing blocks of only one color (answer B) may reduce visual stimulation somewhat, and using interlocking blocks (answer C) may make manipulation of the pieces easier, but the overwhelming stimulus caused by presenting all the blocks at once would make these strategies irrelevant. See reference: Case-Smith (ed): Cronin, AS: Psychosocial and emotional domains.

80. (B) Discuss precautions necessary for sex when an indwelling catheter is present Individuals with an indwelling catheter may safely participate in sexual intercourse when certain precautions are observed. If the catheter becomes kinked or closed off, pressure on the bladder must be avoided and the length of time urine flow is restricted should remain under 30 minutes. It is also advisable to avoid drinking fluids for 2 hours before intercourse and to void the bladder before sexual activity. Sexuality is a part of human performance that therapists should be knowledgeable about and comfortable in discussing. When uncomfortable discussing the topic, the therapist may refer the patient to another team member, which may include the physician (answer A). It is not necessary to remove an indwelling catheter for participation in sexual activity and it is not within the scope of OT practice to teach an individual how to remove one (answer C). See reference: Pedretti (ed): Burton, GU: Issues of sexuality with physical dysfunction.

81. (C) express disagreement with coworkers in a productive manner. Assertiveness is the ability to express feelings in an appropriate and productive manner. Answers A, B, and D are examples of other types of social interaction skills. Answers A and B are examples of good conversation, and answer D is an example of proper social conduct. See reference: Early: Psychosocial skills and psychological components.

82. (D) swivel spoon. A swivel spoon allows the head of the spoon to rotate as the individual moves the handle into varying positions, thus compensating for poor supination. An individual who is unable to reach her mouth due to limitations in shoulder or elbow flexion would benefit from a spoon with an elongated handle (answer A). An individual who is unable to hold a spoon because of difficulty with grasp would benefit from a spoon with a built-up handle (answer C). A spork (answer B) is helpful for those who need to use one utensil as both fork and spoon. See reference: Trombly (ed): Feinberg, JR, and Trombly, CA: Arthritis.

83. (A) head pointer and slanted keyboard. The use of a head pointer on a slanted keyboard would be the best solution because it requires no hand use. Answer B, a typing splint, which can be used if there is adequate wrist control but inadequate finger control, and answer D, using a built-up pencil, are incorrect because they both require some upper extremity or hand function. Answer C, an adapted mouse would not improve ability to access keys and would also require some UE movement. See reference: Angelo and Lane (eds): Angelo, J: Low-technology interface devices.

84. (A) Postural hypotension A frequent side effect of neuroleptic drugs is a decrease in blood pressure in response to sudden movements, specifically up and down movements, resulting in faintness or loss of consciousness. The parachute activity involves significant up-and-down body movements and therefore warrants the therapist's attention with this patient population. Answers B, C, and D are also potential side effects of antipsychotic medications but would usually not be problematic with parachute activities. See reference: Early: Psychotropic medications and other biological treatments.

85. (C) Oversized t-shirts and elastic-top pants For a child with difficulty in self-dressing due to incoordination (as seen in athetoid CP), clothing should be loose fitting with simple or no fasteners. Oversized clothing is preferred to tight-fitting garments (answers A and B). Garments with elasticized waist bands are better than those using zippers (answer B) or snaps and buttons (D). See reference: Neistadt and Crepeau (eds): Erhardt, RP, and Merrill, SC: Neurological dysfunction in children.

86. (A) Independent with a sliding board An individual injured at the C7-8 level should be able to perform sliding board transfers independently. Stand-pivot transfers (answer B) are appropriate for individuals who can come to a standing position and bear some weight on the lower extremities. Individuals with injuries C4 or higher are unable to provide physical assistance during transfers but may provide verbal direction (answer C). Individuals with paraplegia can usually perform level transfers without adapted equipment (answer D). See reference: Pedretti (ed): Adler, C, and Tipton-Burton, M: Wheelchair assessments and transfers.

87. (B) show acceptance and understanding to the individual. Paraphrasing is used to clarify and relay acceptance of what an individual has communicated. The OT practitioner paraphrases by repeating in her or his own words what the client has said. Redirection (answer A) is used to promote healthier thoughts and behaviors. Forcing the individual to make a choice (answer C) may be accomplished by providing a question that includes two possible choices. A client is encouraged to provide additional information (answer D) when the OT practitioner asks open-ended questions. See reference: Denton: Treatment planning and implementation.

88. (A) Perform pursed lip breathing when doing activities Pursed lip breathing is a technique that narrows the passage of air during expiration. This technique helps individuals with COPD to keep the airway open and improve breathing efficiency. The overall effect is improved endurance and tolerance for activities. Taking hot showers and avoiding air conditioning during warm weather are incorrect in that both activities are contraindicated for individuals with COPD. Using a long-handled bath sponge may be helpful but is not the MOST likely tip to be on a home program for an individual with COPD. See reference: Neistadt and Crepeau (eds): Ferraro, R: Cardiopulmonary dysfunction in adults.

89. (B) Handing out trays and utensils in a food service group This individual demonstrates limitations in the area of interpersonal skills. Handing out trays and utensils requires minimal interaction, and would provide an opportunity for this individual to practice interacting with others at a limited level. None of the other options provide the opportunity to develop interpersonal skills. See reference: Early: Work, homemaking and childcare.

90. (A) Stop the activity Activity should be stopped immediately when symptoms occur during evaluation of an acute cardiac patient. Symptoms, including confusion; shortness of breath; profuse sweating; cold, clammy skin; chest pain; nausea; and lightheadedness, should be reported to the physician. After the session is over, symptoms should be documented (answer B). Continuing the activity, whether seated or with the patient's permission (answers C and D), is dangerous and may result in further cardiac damage. See reference: Dutton: Introduction to biomechanical frame of reference.

91. (C) ask another OT practitioner for help. Trying to attempt this transfer alone could result in injury to the patient and/or the OT practitioner, even if she uses proper body mechanics (answer A). It is often necessary to get assistance when transferring obese individuals. Asking someone else to do a difficult task for you (answer B) is not professional. If the patient needs to be transferred, not transferring him (answer D) is not an option. See reference: Pedretti (ed): Adler, C, and Tipton-Burton, M: Wheelchair assessment and transfers.

92. (A) jogging. Forceful gross motor activities that involve no physical contact, such as exercising, wedging clay, and woodworking, can provide a physical outlet for sexual tension. Macramé (answer B) is predominately a fine motor activity that would provide no such outlet. Reading *Playboy* magazine (answer C) would only serve to increase sexual tension. This individual would not have the tolerance or self-control for ballroom dancing (D), which involves close physical contact with members of the opposite gender. See reference: Early: Responding to symptoms and behaviors.

93. (D) The individual traces letters through a pan of rice with her fingers. This method involves greater input of sensory information to the brain by performing a gross movement in a more stimulating environment. A verbal description of how to make a letter (Answer A), watching her grip (answer B), or performing strengthening exercises (Answer C) would not give the individual proprioceptive feedback on her letter formation through tactile input. See reference: Trombly (ed): Bentzel, K: Remediating sensory impairment.

94. (D) electronic augmentative communication device. An augmentative communication keyboard is a high-technology aid that can compensate for expressive deficits and assist a student with communication. Answer A is incorrect because an environmental control unit is a device that allows a person with severe disabilities to operate appliances or devices. It may be used to turn on a tape recorder for note taking, but it would not be used as the primary method for conversation and graphics in the classroom. Answers B and C are incorrect because both the Wanchik's writer and a head pointer are low-technology aids for communication, rather than high-technology devices. See reference: Angelo and Lane (eds): Angelo, J: Written and spoken augmentative communication.

95. (D) hand controls for acceleration and braking. Hand controls use hand motions to control the accelerator and brake mechanisms, eliminating the need for lower extremity function. The palmar cuff and spinner knob (answers A and B) are steering options for individuals who need to steer single-handed and allow individuals to maintain constant contact with the steering wheel. Pedal extensions (answer C) can be installed on accelerator and brake pedal for individuals with limited lower extremity reach. See reference: Pedretti (ed): Lillie, SM, in Driving with a physical dysfunction.

96. (B) a cup of instant soup. The most basic level of meal preparation is accessing a prepared meal, which involves tasks such as opening a thermos and unwrapping a sandwich. When an individual becomes proficient at this level, he or she should progress to a higher level. More advanced meal preparation activities can be structured to increase in complexity in the following sequence: prepare a cold meal (answer B); prepare a hot one-dish meal (answer C); and prepare a hot multi-dish meal (answer D). See reference: Neistadt and Crepeau (eds): Rogers, JC, and Holm, MB: Evaluation of activities of daily living (ADL) and home management.

97. (B) project group. The next level of group interaction is termed project group, since the group members are now able to share the completion of a group project; however, they still require strong group leadership to guide them. Following a project group, the next level of group interaction is the ego-

centric cooperative group (answer A), followed by the cooperative group (answer C), and the mature group (answer D), which is the most advanced. See reference: Ryan (ed): The Certified Occupational Therapy Assistant: Blechert, TF, and Kari, N: Interpersonal communication skills and applied group dynamics.

98. (D) Conduct a group discussion about responsibilities people have when living in a group home A cognitive approach is most appropriate with individuals "who must learn to do situational problem solving…when the individual has deficits in attention span, memory, or other cognitive abilities…or when the skills being learned need to be generalized." Discussion that heightens awareness in an attempt to modify behavior is one example of a cognitive intervention. Rewards and praise (answers A and B) are used when a behavioral approach is desired. Posting a schedule (answer C) is an example of an environmental adaptation that may facilitate compliance with chores but does not represent a cognitive approach. See reference: Christiansen (ed): Self-care strategies in intervention for psychosocial conditions.

99. (A) summary feedback, given at the end of the patient's attempts. According to learning theory, providing summary feedback after several trials aids retention and learning by encouraging the person to rely on inner or intrinsic feedback to self-correct errors in performance, rather than the extrinsic feedback given by the therapist. Continuous feedback (answer B) can impede learning because it interferes with the person's ability to use intrinsic feedback to correct errors in performing motor activities and encourages the learner to be dependent upon the therapist's feedback. Giving feedback about mistakes in performance (answer C) is more appropriate in the earlier stages of learning so that the learner can correct performance errors. No feedback (answer D) would not enhance learning. See reference: Pedretti (ed): Pedretti, LW, and Uphred, DA: Motor learning and teaching activities in occupational therapy.

100. (D) instruct her to perform only gentle active range of motion. Gentle active range of motion allows the individual to control the movement and avoid overstretching of inflamed joint tissues. Brisk active range of motion (answer A) and the addition of resistance (answer B) are likely to cause further damage to the joints by increasing stress, which results in increased inflammation. The individual must be taught in therapy of the importance of joint protection during exercise. Eliminating all range of motion exercise (answer C) would result in further joint stiffness and loss of range of motion. See reference: Trombly (ed): Feinberg, JR, and Trombly, CA: Arthritis.

101. (C) I think baking would be a helpful activity

to try. **Baking something you like offers you several choices and decisions. These choices and decisions can help you feel more positive about making other decisions. You can choose a cake mix or a cookie mix. Which would you like?** Answer C limits options as well as provides the rationale for the choices. Answer A is a leading question that really offers only one choice. Answer B does not provide any options. Answer D is a closed question, offering no real choice for the individual. See reference: Denton: Effective communication.

102. (B) 1 foot of ramp for every inch of rise in height. According to the ADA Accessibility Guidelines for Buildings and Facilities, the maximum slope for a ramp should be 1:12. A foot of ramp for every inch of rise in height would be the maximum amount of incline to allow for independent and safe navigation by an individual using a wheelchair. Answers A, C, and D would all make extremely short and steep ramps, which would be either unsuitable or unsafe for an individual independently entering or exiting a home. See reference: Americans with Disabilities Act: Accessibility Guidelines for Buildings and Facilities.

103. (A) Shoulder flexion and protraction Answer A is correct because the infant changes from extensor influences on posture to development of flexion in the supine position. This requires the ability to flex and protract the shoulders against gravity in order to reach forward and upward to grasp toys. Answer B is not correct because shoulder extension and retraction would not be encouraged during supine activities when the toys are placed overhead. Answers C and D are not correct because most activities of looking and reaching can be accomplished without using head or trunk control against gravity in the supine position. See reference: Kramer and Hinojosa (eds): Colangelo, CA: Biomechanical frame of reference.

104. (B) perform desired activities in a simplified manner, to conserve energy. One method used to extend a person's occupational performance as Parkinson's disease progresses is to introduce task simplification. This allows conservation of energy which can then be expended on desired activities. In a person with long-standing Parkinson's disease, encouragement to "work through" fatigue (answer A) and to perform additional exercises (answer B) would further deplete available energy. Recommendations to decrease activity level as much as possible (answer D) would also be detrimental to maintaining occupational performance levels. See reference: Neistadt and Crepeau (eds): Pulaski, KH: Adult neurological dysfunction.

105. (A) Store the most frequently used items on the shelves just above or below the counter When an individual experiences difficulty reaching because of limited range of motion, convenient placement of commonly used items will facilitate home management. Using the largest joint available (answer B) is an important principle of joint protection and although it may be an appropriate suggestion if this individual has arthritis, it would not address the specific problem of reaching high shelves. Although it is possible that range of motion exercises and reaching for high shelves (answers C and D) may eventually improve this individual's shoulder function, neither answer provides a home management solution. See reference: Pedretti (ed): Foti, D, and Pedretti, LW, in Self-care/home management.

106. (D) use active listening techniques. Active listening (answer D) is an effective listening response that enables the patient to know that his or her message has been communicated. Behaviors listed in answers A, B, and C can be counterproductive to developing a therapeutic relationship. Answers A and B may be perceived as enhancing a friendship, rather than a therapeutic relationship, and answer C may be considered inappropriate for someone who does not have adequate social skills. See reference: Ryan (ed): The Certified Occupational Therapy Assistant: Blechert, TF, and Kari, N: Interpersonal communication skills and applied group dynamics.

107. (B) A key guard A key guard is a device that covers the keys and provides a guide for a finger or stick without punching extra keys. A moisture guard (answer A) is a flexible plastic cover that protects the keys from drool, moisture, or dirt. An auto-repeat defeat mechanism (answer C) stops repetition of letters or numbers caused by overlong or involuntary depression of keys. One-finger-access software (answer D) allows the user to lock out keys such as the "shift" or "enter" keys. This enables an individual who uses only one finger or a stick to type capital letters or perform other keyboard functions that require simultaneous depression of more than one key. See reference: Angelo and Lane (eds): Low technology interface devices.

108. (B) corner chair with head support and padded abductor post. A corner chair provides hip, knee, and ankle flexion of 90 degrees, and the abductor post keeps the legs separated when or if extensor tone increases. The corner shape of the chair facilitates shoulder protraction or prevents shoulder retraction, which can prevent the child's hands from coming forward to assist with eating. The prone stander (answer A) would place the child in a standing or extended position, which would reinforce undesirable extensor tone. A supine position (answer C) is not appropriate for eating if other positions are available. The child would not be able to sit in a bolster chair without support (answer D) because of poor head control and extensor tone. See reference: Case-Smith (ed): Case-Smith, J, and Humphry, R: Feeding intervention.

109. (A) Have the patient use stress reduction

using meditation, yoga, and energy conservation techniques Individuals with AIDS should implement a form of exercise to provide mobility and reduce stress without draining his or her physical resources, in addition to using energy conservation techniques during ADL. It would not be appropriate for an individual to participate in an aerobics program because of the high energy demands, and video lectures would provide information about AIDS but not provide support to reduce anxiety. See reference: Reed and Sanderson (eds): Immunologic disorders.

110. (B) to routinely inspect the skin closely for signs of skin breakdown. Teaching the person with a residual limb to compensate for the lack of sensation with visual inspection is essential to prevent injury from skin breakdown. Answer A is incorrect because tapping, rubbing, and application of textures is used when a residual limb is hypersensitive. Answer C, deep massage is a technique used to loosen and prevent scar adhesions. Answer D, teaching procedures of skin hygiene is important, but would not, by itself, prevent skin breakdown, which is the primary concern when the residual limb lacks some or all sensation. See reference: Pedretti (ed): Rock, LM, and Atkins, DJ: Upper extremity amputations and prosthetics.

111. (C) tell the client it is okay to work where he is until he feels comfortable in joining the group. The paranoid client frequently isolates himself or herself from the rest of the group as a self-protective measure. Such a client should be allowed to do this until he or she feels comfortable in joining the group. Although it is a good idea to encourage the person to join the group (answer A), the OT practitioner should not insist when he is uncomfortable (answer B). The paranoid client may attempt to take control of an uncomfortable group situation by demanding that the OT practitioner stay with him, away from the group (answer D). In this instance it is important to be supportive of the patient's need but to remain with the group. See reference: Early: Responding to symptoms and behaviors.

112. (C) Safety razor with extended handle The extended handle is the necessary component that allows this individual to overcome limited shoulder and elbow range of motion in order to reach his face. Attaching a safety razor or electric razor to a universal cuff (answers A and D) would benefit an individual who is unable to grasp a razor but would not enable this individual to reach his face to shave. A safety razor with a built-up handle (answer B) would benefit an individual with limited finger flexion or strength, but it would also be ineffective in enabling this individual to reach his face with the razor. See reference: Neistadt and Crepeau (eds): Holm, MB, Rogers, JC, and James, AB: Treatment of activities of daily living.

113. (C) flange the area around the ulnar styl- **oid.** Reddened areas indicate the splint is too tight in a particular spot. To reduce pressure, it is often helpful to flange splint edges. Lining the splint with any material, whether moleskin or foam (answers A and B), will only make a tight area tighter. Remaking the splint (answer D) is unnecessary and a waste of the OT practitioner's time. See reference: Neistadt and Crepeau (eds): Fess, EE, and Kiel, JH: Neuromuscular treatment: Upper extremity splinting.

114. (A) Gentle, nonresistive activities The initial phase of treatment for the individual with Guillain-Barré syndrome includes PROM and splinting, and positioning to protect weak muscles and prevent contractures. This should be followed by gentle, nonresistive activities and light ADL, as tolerated. Resistive exercises and activities (answers B and D) should be implemented later after strength begins to improve. Activities within later treatment sessions should alternate between gross and fine motor, and resistive and nonresistive types to avoid fatigue. See reference: Pedretti (ed): McCormack, GL, and Pedretti, LW, in Motor unit dysfunction.

115. (B) having the worker put only the last piece into the game package. Working backwards from the last (successful) step of a sequence is known as "backward chaining." Answer A represents the opposite of backward chaining. Answer C is more descriptive of shaping behaviors, and answer D is more descriptive of modeling behaviors. See reference: Pedretti (ed): Pedretti, LW, and Umphred, DA: Motor learning and teaching activities in occupational therapy.

116. (B) a switch-adapted battery-operated toy car that knocks down a block tower. A switch-adapted battery-operated car would be most age appropriate activity that would allow a young child to experience how his or her actions affect the environment. Listening to music on a tape recorder (answer A), unless the tape recorder was specially adapted for the child to turn on, would be a passive activity. Storybook computer software (answer C) would facilitate early learning and a powered wheelchair is a high-technology application for facilitating mobility. See reference: Angelo and Lane (eds): Lane, SJ, and Mistrett, SG: Can and should technology be used as a tool for early intervention?.

117. (A) Work simplification and energy conservation In the first stage of the disease, mild limitations in function and endurance begin to develop. The individual becomes easily fatigued, so work simplification and energy conservation techniques are beneficial. Progressive resistive exercises (answer B) may cause cramping and fatigue, and are not recommended for individuals with ALS. Splinting (answer C) will be required in the later stages to prevent contractures, support weak muscles, and assist with function. Active range of motion and PROM activities will also be required in the later stages as the disease progresses, to prevent contractures and maintain strength. See reference: Pedretti (ed): Pedretti, LW, and McCormack, GL: Amyotrophic lateral sclerosis.

118. (B) Verbal and gestural cues The next least intrusive level of cues consists of the combination of verbal and gestural cues. Physical cues (answers C and D) are the most intrusive, and purely verbal ones (answer A) the least intrusive. See reference: Case-Smith (ed): Shepherd, J: Self-care and adaptations for independent living.

119. (D) lordosis. Lordosis, a concave posterior curvature of the spine, is a result of excessive anterior pelvic tilt. Scoliosis (answer B) is a result of a lateral curve of the vertebral column and is unaffected by anterior pelvic tilt. Kyphosis (answer C), a concave anterior curvature of the spine, may develop in response to exaggerated lordosis. Stenosis (answer A) is a disease of the spine resulting in narrowing of the spinal column. See reference: Norkin and Levangie: The vertebral column.

120. (B) awareness, minimal deficits, and learning potential. The client most likely to benefit from remedial activities would be one with minimal deficits, awareness of limitations, and learning potential. Answer A is incorrect because remedial approaches attempt to change skill levels and this is less likely to be accomplished to a short time frame. Answer C, difficulty transferring skills to new situations, is incorrect because the rationale for using remedial techniques is that practice of the impaired skill will then result in improved performance in functional activities, requiring ability to transfer learning. A remedial approach for a client who has a long history of cognitive deficits, answer D, would not be warranted unless the client exhibited some potential for further improvement. See reference: Neistadt and Crepeau (eds): Toglia, JP: Cognitive-perceptual retraining and rehabilitation.

121. (D) picking up raisins with a pair of tweezers. While all answers describe methods to promote some aspect of handwriting skills, this activity is the only one that targets isolated finger use. Drawing on sandpaper (answer A) can be used to increase kinesthetic awareness and finger strength. Copying shapes (answer B) is primarily a perceptual-motor task. Rolling out Play Doh (answer C) is an activity that can promote bilateral hand use and the development of palmar arches. See reference: Case-Smith (ed): Amundsen, SJ, and Weil, M: Pre-writing and handwriting skills.

122. (B) pain as a result of disease or injury that persists for long segments of time that has not resolved itself in the anticipated time. Chronic pain, such as pain related to the low back, exists for long periods of time and is present for much of the individual's day. Answers A and C are examples of

acute pain, and answer D is an example of an "overt" motor behavior that might be seen in a patient with a chronic or acute condition. See reference: Neistadt and Crepeau (eds): Engel, JM: Treatment for psychosocial components: Pain management.

123. (C) teach use of mirror feedback to make the person aware of his or her facial expression. Teaching the use of a mirror to make the person aware of his or her facial expressions can help the person to understand how he or she appear to others. It can also help the person learn to smile and use more facial expression, which can be accomplished with concentration. Answers A, B, and D are useful strategies for improving communication, rather than facial expression. See reference: Trombly (ed): Newman, EM, Echevarria, ME, and Digman, G: Degenerative diseases.

124. (C) Making a checklist of steps in the process, then consulting the list while doing laundry in the actual setting Making a checklist and having the person use the checklist during the activity would provide an external memory aid during practice of the functional activity. This would provide compensation for cognitive deficits during task training in the specific context where it will be performed. Answers A, B, and D are methods that require a person to be able to transfer learning of skills from one context to another. See reference: Pedretti (ed): Wheatley, CJ: Evaluation and treatment of cognitive dysfunction.

125. (D) loose-fitting clothing. Individuals with paraplegia can dress independently. The process is somewhat easier when loose-fitting clothing and dressing loops are used. Buttonhook zipper pull devices and clip-on ties (answers A and B) are useful for individuals without the hand function required to button, pull up a zipper, or tie a tie. Individuals with C6 through C8 quadriplegia usually require assistance to put on shoes but may be able to put on specially adapted shoes independently. See reference: Christiansen (ed): Garber, SL, Gregorio, TL, Pumphrey, N, and Lathem, P: Self-care strategies for persons with spinal cord injuries.

126. (B) Provision of foot support Adequate foot support is probably the first concern of the practitioner for the child to feel secure on the toilet and to be positioned for bowel control. Answer A is not correct because management of fasteners can be developed later, after positioning for stability has been achieved. Answer C is not correct because provision of a seatbelt may not be necessary if foot support (or back support) is provided. Answer D is not correct because climbing onto the toilet independently may be developed later (as it in fact occurs with normal developmental progression). See reference: Case-Smith (ed): Shepherd, J: Self care and adaptations for independent living.

127. (C) Divide the laundry into several small loads for carrying "Several small loads place less stress on the back than one or two larger ones" (p. 724). Folding laundry from a basket on the floor next to the chair (answer A) would require bending and twisting, two movements that people with low back pain should avoid. Pain should be avoided when possible (answer D), and preventive strategies should be urged to help the person avoid getting to the point of severe pain. See reference: Pedretti (ed): Smithline, J: Low back pain.

128. (B) provide the cold packs followed by purposeful activity. Purposeful activity should follow, not precede (answer A) a cold pack. Answer C, providing the cold packs as the main focus of intervention is incorrect because "physical agent modalities may be used by occupational therapy practitioners when used as an adjunct to or in preparation for purposeful activity by a practitioner who has demonstrated service competency" (p. 1075). OT practitioners may use physical agent modalities (PAMs) according to the guidelines noted above so answer D is also incorrect. See reference: AOTA: Registered occupational therapists and certified occupational therapy assistants and modalities.

129. (B) have the resident dress in bed with garments which are stretchy and one size larger than usual; preview each step of the process with the resident. The resident who is resuming the activity has low endurance as well as cognitive deficits so would benefit from an adapted, structured approach. Dressing in bed will require less energy initially; the larger, stretchy garments will make dressing easier, and reviewing each step before it occurs will provide cognitive cues. Answer A, having the client select clothing then dressing him or her, does not provide enough participation to be therapeutic. Answers C and D are too demanding and do not provide the structure necessary to ensure safety and successful performance. See reference: Hellen: Daily living care activities.

130. (A) neck flexion. Answer A is correct because this method decreases the abnormal extension pattern that is influencing the oral motor patterns. Jaw and tongue thrust are part of an overall extension pattern. Answers B, C, and D would only increase the abnormal pattern in the mouth because they are part of an extension pattern. See reference: Case-Smith (ed): Case-Smith, J, and Humphry, R: Feeding intervention.

131. (B) flexion. Flexion at the wrist, especially while grasping or pinching, should be avoided. Repetitive flexion and extension movements also cause compression of the median nerve. Answers A, extension, C, ulnar deviation, and D, radial deviation, do not cause inflammation to the area surrounding the median nerve by repetitive compression or a static hold to that area of the wrist. See reference:

Hunter, Schneider, Mackin, and Bell (eds): Baxter-Petralia, P: Therapist's management of carpal tunnel syndrome.

132. (B) Obtain a raised toilet seat The individual will most likely continue to require a raised toilet seat for several months in order to avoid flexing the hip past the designated range. A handheld shower (answer D) is not usually necessary and would be an expensive temporary measure; however, a shower chair with adjustable legs and grab bars could be helpful. High-contrast tape (answer C) may help to make ascending and descending stairs safer for individuals with limitations in vision. Moving items from low cabinets to higher locations may help this individual comply more readily with the necessary hip precautions, but moving objects from high cabinets to lower spots (answer A) would not. See reference: Pedretti (ed): Morawski, D, Pitbladdo, K, Bianchi, EM, Lieberman, SL, Novic, JP, and Bobrove, H: Hip fractures and total hip replacement.

133. (A) group size of fewer than five members. Group size strongly influences how members relate to one another. In general, an ideal group size is 7 to 10 members for the most interaction among members. Groups with fewer than five members tend to increase the focus on the leader in their interactions. Group membership of similar goals improves cohesiveness more than interactions. Differing ages is not known to have an impact on interactions. See reference: Neistadt and Crepeau (eds): Schwartzberg, SL: Group process.

134. (B) upright. For a child with increased tone, the upright position appears to give the best postural control. A forward (answer A) or backward tilt (answer C) increases the effect of gravity and thus adds to the difficulty of maintaining posture. At all times, the child should sit squarely with even weight distribution on both buttocks, never tilted asymmetrically (answer D). See reference: Case-Smith (ed): Wright-Ott, C, and Egilson, S: Mobility.

135. (A) A lightweight folding frame A lightweight folding frame is needed when a wheelchair will be frequently lifted in and out of a car trunk or back seat and folded to fit into the space. This is much easier on the individual or family member who will be lifting the wheelchair. Answers B, C, and D will add a great deal of weight and bulk, which makes the wheelchair much more difficult to lift in and out of the car. This in turn may cause an individual or family member to be more reluctant to go on a community outing. See reference: Angelo and Lane (eds): Taylor, SJ: Evaluation for wheelchair seating.

136. (B) have the individual work at the keyboard for 30 minutes. Increasing the duration the individual is able to tolerate working on the computer is the most appropriate way to progress this individual. A heavier mouth stick (answer A) would make the task more difficult and yield no benefit. An individual with C4 quadriplegia would not have the potential to use a typing device that inserts into a wrist support (answer C). Teaching the individual how to correctly instruct a caregiver in use of the keyboard (answer D) would be downgrading the activity. See reference: Christiansen (ed): Garber, SL, Gregorio, TL Pumphrey, N, and Lathem, P: Self-care strategies for persons with spinal cord injuries.

137. (B) self-assessment. Self-assessment of the each individual's stressors and stress reactions is the first step in designing a stress management program. Time management techniques (answer A), which help individuals schedule, prioritize, and develop appropriate attitudes about daily task requirements, may comprise one of the following sessions. Aerobic exercise (answer C) is an appropriate method for reducing stress in individuals with MS, but care should be taken in designing a program that will not lead to overheating. Progressive relaxation exercises (answer D) involve systematic tensing and relaxing of muscles and are not appropriate for individuals with hypertension, cardiac disease, upper motor neuron lesions, or spasticity. See reference: Neistadt and Crepeau (eds): Giles, GM, and Neistadt, ME, in Treatment for psychosocial components: stress management.

138. (C) the sidelying position. The sidelying position reduces the influence of reflexes, extensor tone, and gravity, all of which make protraction of the shoulders and forward reach difficult. Answer A is incorrect because the standing position will not reduce extensor tone, which encourages shoulder retraction and makes forward reaching of both arms to midline more difficult. Answer B is also incorrect because in the prone position the upper extremities are involved in weight bearing; however, this position may help facilitate forward reach by developing shoulder protraction. Answer D is not correct because in the quadruped position, the upper extremities are involved in weight bearing; if, however, the position is attainable, shoulder protraction and forward reach may be facilitated. See reference: Kramer and Hinojosa (eds): Colangelo, CA: Biomechanical frame of reference.

139. (A) Perform PROM and then position and elevate the affected extremity. Positioning, the use of a compression glove, edema massage, and PROM exercises are all effective methods for reducing edema and preventing further edema. The goal is to promote the movement of fluid back into normal circulation rather than allowing it to collect in one area or body part. Gentle PROM is necessary to help maintain joint structure and provide nutrients to the joint. The actual movement of the extremity may serve as a "pump" to assist in moving excess fluid back into the body. These techniques are contraindicated for individuals who have deep vein thrombosis. Edema is caused in part by the loss of movement in

an extremity because there is no contraction of muscles, which helps to pump the fluid to the heart. Splinting (answer B) is effective in preventing deformity, but compression gloves are more effective in reducing edema. Taking no action (answer C) could result in permanent damage to the tissue of the involved extremity. Having the individual attempt to squeeze a ball (answer D) would be futile because the left arm is flaccid. See reference: Trombly (ed): Woodson, AM: Stroke.

140. (B) wearing permanent-press clothing. Using a wrinkle-resistant fabric eliminates or decreases the amount of ironing needed. The side-loading washer (answer A) is an example of household equipment adapted to eliminate excessive reaching from a wheelchair. An extended-handle dustpan (answer C) eliminates bending or stooping from a standing or sitting position. Neither the dustpan nor the washer, however, eliminates or reduces the amount of work needed for the tasks. Good body mechanics (answer D) are necessary to protect or maintain physical health, but they do not eliminate or reduce the amount of work. See reference: Trombly (ed): Trombly, CA: Retraining basic and instrumental activities of daily living.

141. (A) Replace the spoon with a blunt-ended fork For a child with incoordination and tremors, stabbing food with a blunt-ended fork is often more effective for feeding than using a spoon. The food will not fall off the fork, and the blunt tines will prevent any injury to the child. Building up the spoon handle (answer B) is more appropriate for a child with a weak grasp. A swivel spoon (answer C) and bending the handle 45 degrees (answer D) are more appropriate for a child with limited forearm and wrist motion. See reference: Case-Smith (ed): Case-Smith, J, and Humphry, R: Feeding and oral motor skills.

142. (C) further decline. Because MS is a degenerative disease, it is likely that the individual receiving a wheelchair will eventually decline further in functional performance. Improved wheelchair mobility and gains in strength (answers A and D) are not characteristic of progressive degenerative diseases. When ordering a wheelchair for a pediatric or adolescent client, it is important to anticipate growth of the individual (answer B). See reference: Neistadt and Crepeau (eds): Pulaski, KH, in Adult neurological dysfunction.

143. (A) skin inspection. Visual inspection of an insensate area is essential for preventing pressure sores, which may develop when there are no sensory cues to alert a person to skin breakdown. Nail trimming (answer B) is an important issue to address with individuals with diabetes but is secondary to skin inspection in importance; moreover, the nursing staff may address this issue with the patient. Many individuals with diabetes have abnormalities in nail growth, and instead of trimming their own nails they have them trimmed by a podiatrist. Retirement planning (answer C) and returning to work (answer D) are issues that may be addressed when discussing discharge plans. See reference: Trombly (ed): Bentzel, K: Remediating sensory impairment.

144. (D) Chaining Chaining is frequently used when teaching a multiple step task because it is easier to teach only one step at a time than it is to teach a complete activity. Repetition and rehearsal involve repeating the whole activity until the activity is learned. Cueing uses an external source to remind a person of the next step or part of that step. See reference: Pedretti (ed): Pedretti, LW, and Umphred, DA: Motor learning and teaching activities in occupational therapy.

145. (B) Functional-position resting splint Bedridden individuals are often provided with splints to prevent the development of flexion contractures in the hand that can lead to problems with hygiene. A functional-position resting hand splint is most appropriate because it will prevent flexion contractures from developing and allow the caregiver access to his hand for cleaning. Neither the dorsal nor volar wrist splints (answers A and C) would keep the fingers in extension, which is necessary to prevent development of finger contractures. Dynamic finger-extension splints (answer D) are appropriate for individuals who have active finger flexion but limited active finger extension. See reference: Neistadt and Crepeau (eds): Fess, EE, and Kiel, JH: Neuromuscular treatment: Upper extremity splinting.

146. (B) Sip and puff switch A sip and puff switch (answer B) is operated by breath control and is unaffected by random movements of the extremities. An infrared switch (answer A) sends an infrared beam from the switch to a surface that reflects the light back to the switch. When the beam is broken, the switch is activated. The switch may be activated by an eye blink or finger twitch. Random movements of the extremities may misalign the person's head or body, causing false activation. A P switch (answer C) is a piezoelectric sensor that is activated by tensing a muscle so that a signal is relayed to a switch. A rocking lever switch (answer D) activates a device when one side of the switch is pushed, and turns the device off when the other side of the switch is pushed. Infrared switches, P switches, and rocking lever switches could all be activated accidentally by random movements. See reference: Angelo and Lane (eds): Switches.

147. (B) adult day care. This environment (answer B) provides programming for an elderly patient that is psychosocial in nature and focuses on vocational skills and social activities. Partial hospitalization (answer A) is a type of outpatient program that serves as a transition to community living. It offers most of the structure and services available on an inpatient unit while allowing individuals to live in the community

and to receive services by visiting the program. Home health care (answer C) provides treatment services to individuals in their own homes who have chronic or debilitating illnesses in order to increase their functional independence. Although most individuals who receive home health services have disabilities that are primarily physical, secondary psychiatric disorders are quite common. Psychosocial rehabilitation centers (answer D) focus on the social rather than the medical aspects of mental illness. Psychosocial clubs and rehabilitation centers provide socialization programs, daily living skills counseling, prevocational rehabilitation, and transitional employment. See reference: Early: Treatment settings.

148. (B) continue the same positioning and splinting program that was indicated before discharge. It is necessary to continue positioning and splinting after discharge because active scar development continues for many weeks, depending on the severity of the burn. The same positioning and splinting devices used at the hospital are used at home, with changes made as needed during follow-up visits. Individuals stay in the hospital until their conditions can be managed at home with outpatient visits to maintain status. Individuals are not kept until they are completely healed, which would be the only situation in which a home program would not be necessary. If an individual follows the home program only as he or she deems appropriate during the day or night instead of as scheduled by the therapist, the position time may not be sufficient to prevent deformity from occurring. See reference: Trombly (ed): Alvarado, MI: Burns.

149. (D) refer him to her OTR supervisor, who has attended a workshop on sexuality and spinal cord injury. Anyone providing sexuality counseling must not only be comfortable with his or her own sexuality but must have certain competencies as well. These competencies include awareness of personal and societal attitudes concerning sexuality, knowledge of male and female reproductive systems and how different disabilities affect sexuality, and the interpersonal skills to communicate with patients about sensitive and personal issues concerned with sexuality. When an OT practitioner has developed these skills through continuing education and is available to the patient (answer D), it is not necessary to refer the patient to his psychiatrist (answer C). The OT practitioner in this situation, who is unknowledgable and embarrassed by the patient's question (answers A and B), should not be the one to counsel him on these issues. See reference: Neistadt and Crepeau (eds): Freda, M: Treatment of activities of daily living: Sexuality and disability.

150. (B) give praise for completed dressing; do not help the child get dressed. Since the child has achieved dressing independence, he does not need assistance (answer A), clothing adaptations (answer C), or verbal prompts (answer D) to complete the task. In fact, assisting him now may cause him to lose his independence and regress to relying on his parents again. See reference: Ryan (ed): McFadden, SA: The child with mental retardation.

151. (D) managing stigma. More stigma is attached to issues surrounding mental health than physical health, and individuals with mental illness frequently experience prejudice. It is important for individuals reentering the community to be prepared for this with strategies that will enable them to cope with stigmatization. Self-esteem, assertiveness, and anger management (answers A, B, and C) are qualities an individual will need to effectively deal with stigma. See reference: Cottrell (ed): Van Leit, B: Managed mental health care: reflections in a time of turmoil.

152. (B) Methods of accommodation in the classroom The MOST essential information for parents and teachers to receive from the OT is is how to provide accommodations for the child in the classroom, along with information on juvenile rheumatoid arthritis and how the various symptoms may affect the child's ability to participate in school activities. Information on the OT evaluation (answers A and C) and progress in OT (answer D) are of lesser importance and may in fact be unimportant in terms of the child's current functional problems. See reference: Case-Smith (ed): Rogers, SL, Gordon, CY, Schanzenbacher, KE, and Case-Smith, J: Common diagnoses is pediatric occupational therapy practice.

153. (B) Outpatient OT "It is no longer expected that patients discharged to home will be totally independent…These patients are frequently capable of achieving further gains and could appropriately be followed…in an outpatient setting" (p.682). A patient with such high levels of function is not an appropriate candidate for a home health referral (answer A). Work-hardening programs (answer C) are for individuals who are severely deconditioned as a result of disease or injury or those who have significant discrepancies between their symptoms and objective findings. If the patient has potential for further functional improvement, continuation rather than discontinuation (answer D) of services is indicated. See reference: Trombly (ed): Woodson, AM: Stroke.

154. (C) to get up slowly from a standing, sitting, or lying position. This strategy can be used to avoid postural hypotension, a sudden decrease in blood pressure resulting in feeling faint or loss of consciousness when moving from lying or sitting to standing. Photosensitivity, an increased sensitivity to the sun, is another side effect often associated with neuroleptic medications that can be addressed by limiting sun exposure (answer A). Individuals experiencing extrapyramidal syndrome, which may cause muscular rigidity, tremors, or sudden muscle spasms, should avoid using power tools or sharp instruments (answer B). Dry mouth is a common side

effect of many drugs and can be intensified by the dehydrating effects of caffeinated drinks and alcohol (answer D). All of the above are possible side effects of neuroleptic medications, but answer C is most important because it is the only one the client has experienced. See reference: Early: Psychotropic medications and other biological treatments.

155. (C) supervision. At this level, the child performs the task on his or her own but cannot be safely left alone, or the child may need verbal cueing or physical prompts for 1 to 24% of task. At the independent level (answer A) the child performs the complete task, including the set-up. At the independent-with-setup level (answer B) the child performs the task after someone sets it up. Minimal assist (answer D) signifies that the child performs 50 to 75% of the task independently, but needs physical assistance or other cueing for the remainder of the task. See reference: Case-Smith (ed): Shepherd, J: Self-care and adaptations for independent living.

156. (B) use moderately heated water. Hot water may contribute to fatigue in individuals with MS and should therefore be avoided. Moderate water temperature is recommended. Bathing in cool water (answer A) is unnecessary and may cause chilling and increase spasticity. Bathing rather than showering (answer C) may be recommended for individuals with poor balance or standing tolerance, such as those with MS or COPD. Bathing at the sink (answer D) may be recommended for individuals who experience difficulty bending, such as those with hip or knee replacements or back pain, but durable medical equipment is typically available for all of these diagnoses so that bathing in the tub would be possible through the use of a tub bench and hand held shower. See reference: Ryan (ed): Practice Issues in Occupational Therapy: Jensen, D, and Linroth, R: The adult with multiple sclerosis.

157. (C) Coping strategies for continuing medication compliance Medication noncompliance is a primary factor related to frequent readmissions for individuals with psychiatric conditions. The other strategies listed are also important but are not the primary issue. See reference: Early: Activities of daily living.

158. (B) Boy Scouts. While answers A, C, and D describe activities that may help build his sense of competence, only participation in Boy Scouts includes the necessary interaction with peers. Noncompetitive activities, a uniform to signify belonging, predictable routines, and exposure to role models are all elements of the Boy Scouts that can help him develop social competence. See reference: Case-Smith (ed): Cronin, AF: Psychosocial and emotional domains.

159. (A) wrist cock-up splint. Carpal tunnel syndrome is a condition that results from compression of the median nerve at the wrist. A wrist cock-up splint positions the wrist in 10 to 20 degrees of extension to alleviate symptoms and prevent further damage. Answer B refers to splints made out of thermoplastic materials and does not indicate a splint type specific to carpal tunnel syndrome. Resting hand splints (answer C) are typically used to prevent development of deformity in individuals with arthritis or quadriplegia. Dynamic MP flexion splints (answer D) are used to assist flexion at the MP joints when this motion is weak or absent. See reference: Trombly (ed): Trombly, CA, and Linden, CA: Orthoses: Kinds and purposes.

160. (D) A clustered independent living arrangement These are usually composed of "apartment clusters or other types of housing in close proximity to each other, in which groups of residents with disabilities share services such as attendants and transportation" (p. 362). Cradle-to-grave homes (answer A) are houses designed and built with accessibility in mind. If a resident of a cradle-to-grave home begins to use a wheelchair later in life, the home will already be wheelchair accessible. Transitional living centers (answer B) "provide temporary living arrangements for individuals who are in a transitional phase between hospital or institution and independent community living" (p. 362). Adult day programs (answer C) are rehabilitation-oriented day programs for clients who live in the community; they are not residential. See reference: Trombly (ed): Law, M, Stewart, D, and Strong, S: Achieving access to home, community, and workplace.

161. (C) Bring the seat in for reevaluation within 6 months Fit and function of seating and mobility should be reassessed within 6 months to account for the child's growth as well as any changes in posture. Parents should not make unsupervised adaptations (answer A) because improper positioning could harm the child. Weekly adjustment (answer B) is usually not necessary, and transporting the seat every week would be an unnecessary inconvenience to the parents. The end of the IEP (answer D) may be more than 6 months away and too long to wait. See reference: Case-Smith (ed): Wright-Ott, C, and Egilson, S: Mobility.

162. (D) 5 feet by 5 feet An outward opening door needs a space of 5 feet by 5 feet to allow for the wheelchair to be maneuvered around the door. A standard wheelchair requires 5 feet of turning space for a 180- or 360-degree turn. An area that is 3 feet by 5 feet (answer A), 4 feet by 4 feet (answer B), or 4.5 feet by 3 feet (answer C) would not provide enough space to allow the wheelchair to be turned. See reference: Pedretti (ed): Smith, P: Americans with disabilities act: accommodating persons with disabilities.

163. (B) aftercare. Aftercare is the arrangement for postdischarge services, which may be needed by the individual after he or she is discharged from an OT program. For individuals having received services in a rehabilitation unit, this may include linkages with the Bureau of Vocational Rehabilitation in order to prepare for gainful employment. Another example would be a psychiatric patient being referred to a community center to continue the program that has been established on an inpatient unit. Answer A is a follow-up plan. This is different in that these services are provided by the same program. An example of this is when an individual on a rehabilitation unit is asked to return for a visit 1 month after discharge. This is generally done to verify that issues or problems have not arisen and that the individual's health status is not declining. Answer C is a treatment program that may be prescribed to an individual to do during treatment or after discharge so that the health status may be maintained or progress will be enhanced. Home health services, answer D, is the provision of health care in the patient's home. These services are provided for those who are physically unable to commute to an outpatient center for treatment. See reference: Reed and Sanderson (eds): Practice with the elderly populations.

164. (C) righting reactions. Righting reactions develop after the integration of primitive reflex patterns, which are thought to be necessary for survival in the normal newborn. Righting reactions allow children to right their heads against gravity and to realign their bodies around the movement of the head in that process. Prehensile reactions refer to grasping patterns and reach, which differentiate humans from other primates. Equilibrium reactions develop after righting reactions and allow the child to maintain a standing and walking posture. See reference: Neistadt and Crepeau (eds): Kohlmeyer, K.: Evaluation of sensory and neuromuscular performance components.

165. (B) a tub bench and toilet rails. A tub bench and toilet rails make bathroom transfers easier and safer and allows the person with a unilateral LE amputation to transfer independently. Lightweight cooking utensils (answer A) are recommended for those with weakness or joint involvement of the upper extremities. Answers C and D are incorrect because long-handled dressing devices and reachers are more likely to be recommended when compensation for hip or trunk flexion is needed, and use of these devices might discourage the normal bending activity in the person with LE amputation. See reference: Pedretti (ed): Pasquinelli, S: Lower extremity amputations and prosthetics.

166. (B) objective. Measured results based on an individual's performance are included in the objective section. The subjective portion (answer A) of the SOAP note contains information provided by the patient or family. Analysis of the measurements is recorded in the assessment area (answer C) of the SOAP note. Plans for future sessions are included in the plan section (answer D). See reference: Sabonis-Chafee and Hussey: Treatment planning and implementation.

167. (D) facilitate effective treatment. The primary purpose of documentation is to facilitate the treatment process. By defining the problem, goals and objectives, and a treatment plan, the practitioner's thoughts are organized in order to carry out goal-directed services. Additional purposes of documentation are to serve as legal documentation; report services provided for reimbursement; and provide communication among the team, patient, or family. Answers A, B, and C are incorrect in that they are not part of the primary reasons for documentation. However, some forms of documentation may be necessary to meet accrediting agencies guidelines or be used in research. See reference: AOTA: Effective documentation for occupational therapy.

168. (B) "The client will initiate one request to one other group member for sharing or using group materials within a 1-week period." Reducing the number of requests and the variety or number of individuals the client is expected to interact with is the best way to simplify the initial goal. Extending the amount of time to accomplish the goal (answer A) does not make the goal easier to achieve. Increasing the number of individuals (answer C), and subsequently the number of requests, to five also makes the goal more difficult to achieve. Changing interactions to the group leader (answer D) moves the goal away from the original problem area of peer social conversation to authority conversations. See reference: Early: Analyzing, adapting, and grading activities.

169. (B) walking as part of a walking club. Walking as part of a walking club throughout a facility can provide an outlet for the movement needs of some people with dementia. Walking in a structured way can be calming, provide an activity of exploration, and help to refocus the resident. Answers A (reminiscing about previous jobs), C (singing oldies in a group), and D (a craft activity) are good activities but would not provide the element of movement to the same degree. See reference: Hellen: Meaningful activities: Daily life stuff.

170. (D) the Americans with Disabilities Act of 1990. Also referred to as the ADA, this act provides civil rights protection for disabled individuals in five specific areas. These areas include telecommunications, transportation, public accommodations, employment, and the activities of state and local government. Answer A, the Architectural Barriers Act of 1969, literally opened doors for changes to occur in gaining access for disabled individuals. Answer B, the Federal Rehabilitation Act of 1973, expanded service intervention for those individuals who were more severely disabled. Answer C, the Fair Housing

Amendment Act of 1988, expanded the coverage of Title VIII. See reference: Christiansen and Baum (eds): Trefler, E: Assistive technology.

171. (C) Tai Chi. Tai Chi would be the best activity because it incorporates slow stretching movements. This type of movement can help improve balance which is often affected when muscles become rigid, particularly muscles of the neck and trunk. Answer A, weight training would not be recommended because resistive activity can increase rigidity. Answer B, walking, is a good general exercise, but would not provide stretching movement. Answer D, gardening, would not be particularly useful because it can be performed without requiring stretching movements. See reference: Pedretti (ed): Hooks, ME: Parkinson's disease.

172. (D) Sitting in a circle and reciting a short poem The purpose of a closure activity in a Five-Stage group is to provide a familiar activity to end the group on a positive, affirming note. Answer A is an orientation activity (stage I). Answer B is typical of an activity that would be used to transition from visual perceptual (stage III) to cognitive activities (stage IV). Answer C is a movement activity (stage II). See reference: Ross and Bachner (eds): Ross, M: A five-stage model for adults with developmental disabilities.

173. (B) Improved verbal and nonverbal communication skills Improved verbal and nonverbal communication skills would be the most relevant behavioral outcome indicating program effectiveness. Answers A, C, and D may all indirectly benefit as a result of improved social and communication skills, but these would not directly reflect positive outcomes for measuring effectiveness of social skill training programs. See reference: Cottrell (ed): Salo-Chydenius, S: Changing helplessness to coping: An exploratory study of social skills training with individuals with long-term mental illness.

174. (C) Preparing and consuming nutritional and normal-sized portions of food Individuals with eating disorders are generally well versed in weight loss techniques (answer A), as well as making food look appealing for others to eat (answer D). "They have extensive knowledge of the caloric content of foods (answer B) but little knowledge of other aspects of food content, such as vitamin and nutritive value.... A cooking group would support the experience of preparing and consuming normal-sized portions of food" (page 143). See reference: Early: Understanding psychiatric diagnosis: The DSM-IV.

175. (D) suggesting furniture and accessories that promote better positioning at work. The best recommendation is for ergonomically correct furniture and accessories. Additional adaptations may include tool modification and the training of workers in appropriate positioning. Answers A and C, setting up stress management and smoking cessation programs, are not considered to be ergonomic adaptations. Answer B is not an example of an ergonomic adaptation but is a treatment intervention. See reference: Pedretti (ed): Kasch, MC: Hand injuries.

176. (D) collaboratively develop an IFSP. The service plan required by federal law (I.D.E.A. 99-457, Part H) and provided through early intervention programs is called an individual family service plan. Answers A and B refer to the IEP (individual education plan), a service plan required for school-aged children. Answer D is not correct because the IFSP must be developed collaboratively with other team members. See reference: Case-Smith (ed): Stephens, LC, and Tauber, SK: Early intervention.

177. (D) Obtain the same results as another OT practitioner who has demonstrated service competency In order to establish service competency, it is necessary to obtain the same results as a competent OT practitioner when performing a treatment technique or evaluative procedure. Demonstrating service competency often requires more than one trial in order to refine techniques to obtain the same results. Answers A, B, and C do not provide the opportunity for the OT practitioners to compare and contrast their techniques and measurements in order to obtain similar results. See reference: Neistadt and Crepeau (eds): Sands, M: Practitioners' perspectives on the occupational therapist and occupational therapy assistant partnership.

178. (C) Advanced supervision Advanced levels of supervision occur on an as-needed basis. Individuals being supervised at this level have demonstrated skill and expertise in the area of OT in which they are working. They may also serve as a resource person and assist in continuing education or research as it relates to their expertise. Answer A describes close supervision, which is direct daily contact between the supervisor and the employee. This form of supervision is recommended for entry-level therapists and therapists reentering the OT profession. Answers B and D describe routine supervision and general supervision. These forms of supervision are for the therapist who can function independently and have mastered basic role functions of OT. See reference: AOTA: Occupational therapy roles.

179. (D) Explain to the administrator this is not an appropriate solution and then develop an alternate solution. OT departments frequently are understaffed and need to operate as efficiently as possible. The collaborative teamwork between an OTR and a COTA is vital in treatment planning and implementation. When a collaborative relationship is operational, the COTA may participate in evaluation and treatment planning, provide treatment, and carry out documentation. Complying with the administrator's instructions (answers A, B, and C) would result in inadequate supervision and would violate both

the Standards of Practice and Code of Ethics. It is not within the OTA's scope of practice to carry out treatment planning and implementation without supervision. See reference: Neistadt and Crepeau (eds): Sands, M: Practitioners' perspectives on the occupational therapist and occupational therapy assistant partnership.

180. (C) frequent handwashing. Handwashing is the primary prevention against infection from blood-borne pathogens in the health care environment. Handwashing is one of four workplace strategies that aid in the prevention of exposure. Other strategies include using engineering controls, protective equipment, and universal precautions. Answers A, B, and D are examples of protective equipment. However, the primary prevention method is handwashing. See reference: Sabonis-Chafee and Hussey: Service management functions.

181. (B) providing staff education, recommendations, and support for restraint alternatives. Providing education on the effects of restraints and recommendations and program support for alternatives to the use of restraints, such as activities, distraction techniques, and environmental adaptations would be the MOST appropriate functions for the OT. Answers A, C, and D would be elements of a facility's restraint reduction efforts, but would not be likely to be performed by the OT. See reference: Hellen: Physical wellness: Mobility and exercise.

182. (D) call 911. The OT practitioner should be knowledgeable of situations that may be potentially dangerous for patients. This question requires that the practitioner be knowledgeable about the appropriate ranges for heart rate and blood pressure. Both of the measures are above safe ranges and indicate that the patient is medically unstable. Therefore, immediate medical services would be necessary. Answers A, B, and C do not recognize the seriousness of the situation and could delay the necessary medical attention. See reference: Neistadt and Crepeau (eds): Ferraro, R: Cardiopulmonary dysfunction in adults.

183. (C) home health care. Home health care provides treatment services to individuals in their homes who have chronic or debilitating illnesses in order to increase their functional independence. Although most individuals who receive home health services have primarily physical disabilities, secondary psychiatric disorders are quite common. Partial hospitalization (answer A) is a type of outpatient program that serves as a transition to community living. It offers most of the structure and services available on an inpatient unit while allowing individuals to live in the community and to receive services by visiting the program. Adult day care (answer B) provides psychosocial programs for elderly patients that focus on avocational skills and social activities. Psychosocial rehabilitation centers (answer D) focus on the social rather than the medical aspects of patients with mental illness. Psychosocial club and rehabilitation centers provide socialization programs, daily living skills counseling, prevocational rehabilitation, and transitional employment. See reference: Early: Treatment settings.

184. (B) The source of the referral, the reason for the referral, and the date the referral was received The initial note is used to record basic information, results of initial evaluations, and, often, the treatment plan. In addition to documenting the items in (answer B), the COTA may also contribute data collected from assessments she or he has performed. The OTR is responsible for analyzing an individual's assets and deficits and for projecting the outcome of treatment (answers C and D). See reference: Early: Medical records and documentation.

185. (C) evidence of interrater reliability. Interrater reliability is a measure of the variation among various observers' perceptions of a subject's performance or some other characteristic. Supervisory feedback (answer A) and evidence of competence in the ability to competently administer the evaluation (answer B) may also be reasons for a student or new practitioner to ask the supervisor to check her results, but not for an experienced therapist. Answer D, evidence of incompetence in performing this skill, would be unlikely. See reference: Bailey: Collecting and analyzing qualitative data.

186. (B) Complete a tool count of departmental sharps. Although answers A and C are required and necessary, the only activity that would be done daily is a tool count. It is recommended that tool counts be completed before and after patient activities. This ensures that sharps are not removed by patients that may provide them the opportunity to harm themselves or others. Strictly monitoring clients with suicidal ideations (answer D) must be mandatory but denying these individuals the opportunity to participate in therapy is an appropriate choice of treatment. See reference: Early: Safety techniques.

187. (A) allows the therapist to obtain facts. Fact gathering is the primary advantage to closed questions. The OT practitioner should be aware that posing mostly closed questions can lead to biased information gathering, as with answers B and D. Although you can generally ask more closed questions in a short amount of time, this is generally not a patient-focused goal. See reference: DePoy and Gitlin: Design classification.

188. (B) the OTR must assume responsibility for all OT services delivered. An OTR is always responsible for services provided by the COTA under his or her supervision. The AOTA does not require that the patient have a referral for provision of services. However, it is important to note that state licensure laws and accrediting agencies may require a formal refer-

ral. Answer A is incorrect because the OTR is operating within AOTA standards. A written letter of consent (answer C) is not required by either state or accrediting agencies. A COTA would not initiate contact with the physician (answer D) without discussing the case with the supervising OTR. See reference: Ryan (ed): Practice Issues in Occupational Therapy: Ryan, SE: Therapeutic intervention process.

189. (D) merit increases. A merit increase is based on demonstrated ability and performance. A merit increase typically is awarded after a performance review or assessment of an employee's demonstrated work skill (answer B). Disciplinary action (answer A) is a formal reproach taken in the occurrence of a violation of departmental, facility, or professional standards. Clinical education (answer C) is the responsibility of each OT and may be offered through employment as a benefit. See reference: Neistadt and Crepeau (eds): Perinchief, JM: Management of occupational therapy services.

190. (C) analyzed the work flow. An organized work flow is one in which the employees and patients can move smoothly through the department. Environments with poor work flow may have areas that are "bottlenecks" or cause a congestion of individuals at one or more areas. Identifying the patterns in which work may most efficiently be completed is helpful in designing a new floor plan so that all areas may be optimized. Answers A, B, and D all occur in the space planning process but are not correct based on the description. Elements critical to identifying a location (answer A) may include proximity to other physical medicine disciplines. However, the question indicated that the department was reallocating current space. Determination of equipment needs (answer B) may be accomplished by taking an inventory of current equipment compared with anticipated equipment. This procedure will identify items that may need to be purchased. Determining functional areas (answer D) is based on identification of the activity areas (e.g., clinic, offices, storage areas). See reference: Jacobs and Logigian (eds): Developing a new occupational therapy program.

191. (C) workers' compensation. Workers' compensation is a state-supported program into which employers pay. Beneficiaries receive coverage for services that are identified to be covered within their respective state. Medicare (answer A) is a federal program for health coverage for individuals 65 years or older, disabled individuals, or people in the end stages of renal disease. Medicaid (answer B) is a joint state and federal program that provides coverage for the poor and medically indigent. The Education for All Handicapped Children Act (answer D) is assisted through the provision of state and federal grants and was amended 1990 to the Individuals with Disabilities Education Act (IDEA). See reference: Neistadt and Crepeau (eds): Bailey, DM: Legislative and reimbursement influences on occupational therapy: Changing opportunities.

192. (C) Interpret the results based on data collected by the COTA Once the OTR has assigned performance of an evaluation to a COTA, the OTR is responsible for analyzing and interpreting the results. Service competency (answer A) would need to be established prior to the COTA administering the evaluation. Collecting data (answer B) is the responsibility of the COTA in this scenario. Developing the treatment plan (answer D) would follow analysis of the data. See reference: Early: Data collection and evaluation.

193. (A) collecting chart review information. After a certified OT has demonstrated service competency, it is appropriate for him or her to complete data collection through record reviews, interviews, general observations, and behavior checklists. Answers B, C, and D require interpretive and analytical skills in which OTs have received additional training. A certified OT assistant can collaborate with an occupational therapist, but it is inappropriate to have a COTA complete these portions independently. See reference: AOTA: Occupational therapy roles.

194. (B) Universal precautions Health-care personnel should follow universal precautions when blood or body fluids are present. Suicidal, escape, and medical precautions are guidelines developed for individuals identified with risks that are not noted in this question. See reference: Early: Safety techniques.

195. (B) The patients' written consents to take the photographs and use them for publicity A photograph of a person who is being treated at a health care facility would release privileged information and would violate confidentiality just as much as releasing the individual's name or diagnosis (answers A and D). No information about a person may be released without a written consent. It is not necessary to obtain permission of the department head to use a photograph to promote a positive image for the facility (answer C). See reference: Bailey: Final preparation before implementing the research plan.

196. (C) complete a review of the literature. Review of the written material is necessary in preparing the design of the research project. The literature review helps the researcher to state the purpose

clearly and establish boundaries. Stating the purpose and the hypothesis follows the identification of the research question; therefore, answer A is incorrect. The design of the research and the establishment of the boundaries are affected by information from the literature review; therefore, answers C and D are incorrect. See reference: DePoy and Gitlin: Developing a knowledge base through review of the literature.

197. (D) not to use PAMs in the new state. Although AOTA policy supports the use of PAMs by qualified practitioners as an adjunct to or in preparation for purposeful activity, state laws supersede AOTA policies. Answers A, B and C all violate state law as well as the OT Code of Ethics and could result in loss of licensure, loss of NBCOT certification, a fine, or imprisonment. See reference: AOTA: Occupational therapy code of ethics.

198. (C) notify the OTR. Regardless of the source of the referral or the anticipated length of stay, the COTA must first notify the OTR of the referral, who is ultimately responsible for any action taken. Under the supervision of the OTR, that COTA may then initiate screening, chart review, or ADL evaluation (answers A, B, and D). See reference: Ryan (ed): Practice Issues in Occupational Therapy: Ryan, SE: Therapeutic intervention process.

199. (C) unacceptable because it violates the Code of Ethics. Whether or not an alternate date has been arranged (answer A) or the agency the practitioner works for allows it (answer B), stating services were provided on a day when they, in actuality, were not, is falsification of documentation and violates the OT Code of Ethics. The client's inability to participate in therapy the next day because of illness (answer D) would only serve to further complicate an already compromised situation; however, this is not the reason why the action is unacceptable. See reference: Neistadt and Crepeau (eds): Hansen, RA: Ethics in occupational therapy.

200. (A) Community newsletter Community newsletters are examples of external marketing, commonly used to educate consumers about OT. Answers B, C, and D are all examples of internal marketing strategies. See reference: Jacobs and Logigian (eds): Jacobs, K: Marketing occupational therapy services.

SIMULATION EXAMINATION 4

Directions: Circle the correct answer to the following questions. When you have completed this examination, check your answers against the answer key that follows. As you will see, an explanation is given for each answer along with a reference for further study. The book author is listed as well as the chapter author. See the bibliography for complete references. Study the areas in which your comprehension was low, then test yourself again by taking Simulation Examination 5.

Pediatrics

1. Results of an OT evaluation show that a young child has many tactile defensive behaviors. The MOST appropriate beginning activity for intervention to normalize sensory processing would require that:
   A. the therapist has the child play "sandwich" between heavy mats.
   B. the therapist applies a feather brush lightly to the child's arms and legs.
   C. the child is blindfolded and must guess where he or she is touched on the body.
   D. the therapist has the child play the "duck, duck, goose" circle game.

2. A preteen with a diagnosis of spastic cerebral palsy (CP) is enjoying computer-assisted learning while making significant progress in written communication, but he complains of general fatigue, body aches, and eye strain. Based on this information, which area would be MOST relevant for the OT practitioner to reassess?
   A. The time he spends at the computer
   B. The size of the computer screen
   C. The challenge level of the learning program
   D. His control of the keyboard

3. In assessing the dressing skills of a 5-year-old child, the OT practitioner observes that the child is able to put on a jacket, zip the zipper, and tie a knot in the draw string but needs verbal cueing to tie a bow. The OT practitioner would

MOST likely determine that the child's dressing skills are:
   A. age appropriate.
   B. delayed.
   C. advanced.
   D. limited.

4. A young child has been wearing a left upper extremity prosthesis for 3 weeks. When consulting with the child's preschool teacher, the OT practitioner recommends:
   A. offering toys that the child can manipulate with one hand.
   B. stressing bilateral activities incorporating the prosthesis.
   C. teaching the child one-handed manipulation techniques.
   D. involving the child in activities that do not require manipulation, such as sing-alongs.

5. To develop the MOST relevant goals and objectives for a child's OT program, the OT practitioner should focus goals on:
   A. the child's priorities.
   B. the priorities of the parents or caregivers.
   C. the therapist's priorities for solution of problems identified in the OT evaluation.
   D. child, caregiver, and therapist priorities.

6. The OTR is assessing the muscle tone of a child with athetoid CP. In documenting the assessment results, the therapist would MOST likely describe the quality of the muscle tone as:
   A. fluctuating.
   B. spastic.

C. flaccid.

D. rigid.

7. **An OT practitioner is instructing a family how to observe for sensory overload when carrying out a sensory integration home program. The MOST important autonomic response to watch for is:**

A. nausea and dizziness.

B. self-stimulation.

C. head banging.

D. flushing, blanching, or perspiration.

8. **An OT practitioner is working with a 3-year-old who has spastic diplegia. The mobility device which would be MOST appropriate to use in assisting this child to explore space would be:**

A. a body length prone scooter.

B. an airplane mobility device.

C. a tricycle.

D. a power wheelchair.

9. **A child has poor visual attention, which affects the child's school work. To improve the child's attention during a visual task, the OT is MOST likely to recommend:**

A. increasing competing sensory input—work with lively background music.

B. increasing competing visual input—work against a patterned background.

C. reducing competing sensory input—use headphones during work.

D. reducing visual input—use dim lighting.

10. **Through the evaluation process, the therapist may consider many possibilities for intervention; however, the specific plan for implementation of intervention is MOST often developed at which point in the OT process?**

A. After observation or screening

B. After the interview

C. After the evaluation

D. After the development of the goals and objectives

11. **A school-age child demonstrates aggressive and disruptive behavior in school, which is a result of a low sensory threshold. Which of the following suggestions would be MOST useful to discuss with the teacher regarding an upcoming class trip by bus to the zoo?**

A. Review the bus rules with the child and apply consequences consistently

B. Let the child sit at the front of the bus and use a tape player and earphones

C. Give the child the responsibility of monitoring classmates as "bus patrol"

D. Let the child set the criteria for a successful trip and provide a reward if the criteria are met

12. **A mother of a child who is medically indigent and does not have health insurance is concerned about payment for laboratory work and OT services in the hospital. The OT practitioner explains that federal and state programs exist that fund health care for the poor and medically indigent. This program is referred to as:**

A. Medicare.

B. Medicaid.

C. workers' compensation.

D. Education for All Handicapped Children Act.

13. **The OT practitioner has just completed observation of a child eating lunch. Which of the following statements BEST describes the OBJECTIVE observations?**

A. "The child did not appear to like the food presented."

B. "The child demonstrated tongue thrust."

C. "The child was uncooperative and kept pushing the food out of her mouth."

D. "The child was obviously not hungry at the time."

14. **A student is unable to focus on a blackboard 20 feet away and then refocus on the book on her desk to copy a mathematics problem. This MOST likely indicates a problem with:**

A. ocular motility.

B. binocular vision.

C. convergence.

D. accommodation.

15. **The OT practitioner has written the following statement: "Continue social skills training program and encourage client to attend one new after-school club activity within the next week." The MOST appropriate section to place this statement is the:**

A. subjective section.

B. objective section.

C. assessment section.

D. plan section.

16. **Which of the following is the BEST position for promoting isolated head control in a child with very limited postural control and significant upper and lower extremity weakness?**

    A. Standing in a standing frame with knee and hip support

    B. Quadruped with chest supported in a sling

    C. Prone over a wedge

    D. Sitting on a therapy ball with hips supported by the therapist

17. **A child is lacing a series of geometric beads from a stimulus card and is unable to identify a moon-shaped bead when it is turned sideways on the table. This MOST likely indicates difficulty with:**

    A. figure-ground perception.

    B. form constancy perception.

    C. position in space perception.

    D. visual sequencing.

18. **A therapist is discussing discharge plans with the parents of a 7-year-old child with sensory defensiveness problems. The OT practitioner is recommending additional activities for a "sensory diet" to provide proprioceptive input. The MOST appropriate activity for this child would be to:**

    A. walk barefoot on textured surfaces.

    B. rock over a large therapy ball.

    C. play in a large box full of styrofoam pellets.

    D. perform slow push-ups against the wall.

19. **The MOST appropriate device to use for promoting development of upper lip control is a:**

    A. straw.

    B. spork.

    C. deep spoon.

    D. shallow spoon.

20. **OTs working in the area of early intervention have frequent contact with a child's parents. Which of the following statements BEST describes how parents should be involved in the OT program?**

    A. Parents should not be present during OT sessions.

    B. Parents should be trained as substitute therapists.

    C. Parents should be considered as part of a collaborative partnership with therapists.

    D. Only one parent needs to be present when the OT program is discussed.

21. **A child with a learning disability has significant problems with visual memory. An OT practitioner may use which of the following to better enhance visual memory?**

    A. Provide memory tasks that are of low interest to the child.

    B. Decrease visual attention before doing memory tasks.

    C. Combine task with additional sensory input (tactile, proprioceptive, and auditory).

    D. Repeat the visual memory task once.

22. **The BEST position that the OT practitioner can place a 15-month-old child in to provide the opportunity to further develop trunk rotation is the:**

    A. supine position.

    B. prone position.

    C. sidelying position.

    D. sitting position.

23. **When teaching children with moderate mental retardation to feed, groom, and dress themselves, the OT is MOST likely to use which technique?**

    A. Chaining

    B. Practice and repetition

    C. Demonstration

    D. Role modeling

24. **Poor impulse control has been identified as the primary deficit in a 12-year-old boy with conduct disorder. Which of the following is the MOST effectively written functional OT goal?**

    A. Within 6 months, the client will participate in classroom activities for 1 hour without disruptive outbursts, twice a day.

    B. Within 6 months, the client will attend to an activity for 30 minutes, demonstrating improved impulse control.

    C. The client will show a 50% reduction in the frequency of disruptive outbursts within 6 months.

    D. When presented with a new activity, the client will follow directions without protest, four out of five times, within 6 months.

25. **A child has poor sitting balance, which interferes with seated tabletop activities. Which of the following treatment recommendations is MOST appropriate for promoting the development of ongoing postural adjustments in sitting?**

    A. Use a sturdy chair with lateral trunk supports while the child is doing homework

B. Use a corner floor seat with built in desk surface while the child is self-feeding

C. Provide a bolster for back support while the child is coloring

D. Provide a therapy ball to sit on while the child is playing a game of checkers

26. During assessment of a 10-month-old child with Down syndrome, the OT notes hyperextensibility of all joints, which MOST likely reflects:

A. increased muscle tone.

B. decreased muscle tone.

C. anterior horn cell disease.

D. muscle and joint disease.

27. An OT practitioner is planning discharge and follow-up via a consultant-only basis for a child with paraplegic spina bifida who has just started using a powered wheelchair. The community resource that the OT recommends as MOST critical for this child is:

A. the local social service agency.

B. a local wheelchair equipment vendor.

C. the family physician.

D. an early intervention program.

28. A child has difficulty controlling food in her mouth when swallowing. In helping the parents to plan snacks, the OT practitioner would be MOST likely to recommend:

A. chicken noodle soup.

B. peanut butter.

C. carrot sticks.

D. applesauce.

29. A school-age child with visual perceptual deficits is being discharged from OT. Which compensatory technique for dealing with visual figure-ground problems should the OT practitioner recommend to the child's teacher?

A. Place a red line on the left side of the paper

B. Use a timer for certain activities

C. Teach the child to use lists and color coding of books and folders

D. Block out all areas of the page except important words

30. An OT manager is developing a proposal for OT services in the neonatal intensive care unit (NICU). Using the developmental support care approach as the basis for services, how would the OT BEST de-
scribe OT's scope of practice in the NICU?

A. Modifying the environment to protect the infant from overstimulation and inappropriate stimuli

B. Providing passive range of motion (PROM), positioning and handling, fabrication of splints, and referral to early intervention

C. Educating parents and hospital staff

D. Implementing motor and behavioral skill acquisition through developmental milestone positioning

31. An OT practitioner is speaking with parents who believe that their child with CP could benefit from OT consultation at school. In order for a school-age child to receive OT services within a school system, which of the following forms must be completed FIRST?

A. UB-82

B. FIM

C. IEP

D. HCFA-1500

32. When preparing a home program with the goal of independent toileting for a young child with postural instability, the MOST important adaptation the OT practitioner can recommend is:

A. replacing zippers and buttons with Velcro closures.

B. mounting a safety rail next to the toilet.

C. introducing toilet paper tongs.

D. placing a colorful "target" in the toilet bowl.

33. During a coloring activity, an OT practitioner observes a preschooler stabilizing a crayon between the thumb and fingers. The practitioner MOST accurately documents this grasp as:

A. pincer grasp.

B. radial-digital grasp.

C. palmar grasp.

D. lateral pinch.

34. The OT treatment goal for a child with athetoid CP is self-feeding. Which of the following adaptations would BEST solve the problem of food sliding off the plate when the child attempts to pick it up with a spoon?

A. Swivel spoon

B. Nonslip mat

C. Mobile arm support

D. Scoop dish

35. **A child with learning disabilities that have resulted in low frustration tolerance and poor self-esteem is learning how to tie shoelaces. Which of the following methods would be MOST appropriate for this child?**

    A. Physical guidance
    B. Verbal cues
    C. Backward chaining
    D. Forward chaining

36. **Working with a preschooler in the home, the OT practitioner observes the child climb into a highchair and jump up and down on a toy trampoline. When presented with a new rocking horse as a birthday present, however, the child is unable to determine how to mount the horse. This MOST likely indicates a problem in the area of:**

    A. fine motor skills.
    B. gross motor skills.
    C. reflex integration.
    D. motor planning.

37. **An individual with underreactive sensory processing has been referred to OT. Based on a sensory integration frame of reference, activities for this individual should have which of the following facilitory characteristics?**

    A. Arrhythmic and unexpected
    B. Arrhythmic and slow
    C. Sustained and slow
    D. Unexpected and rhythmic

38. **A sixth grade student has a diagnosis of juvenile rheumatoid arthritis. Which of the following leisure activities would BEST suit this child for helping him maintain range of motion?**

    A. Swimming
    B. Basketball
    C. Soccer
    D. Aerobics

39. **While observing a child for the first time, the OT practitioner notes that the child responds to a loud noise by abducting and extending the arms. The reflex, or reaction, observed in this child is documented by the OT as a:**

    A. rooting reflex.
    B. Moro reflex.
    C. flexor withdrawal reflex.
    D. neck righting reaction.

40. **Setting up an obstacle course that provides several options for allowing a child to choose the direction he will take (unstructured) would be MOST appropriate if the OT practitioner wished to encourage:**

    A. exploratory play.
    B. symbolic play.
    C. creative play.
    D. recreational play.

41. **A child displays poor postural stability because of low muscle tone. To promote beginning antigravity control, the FIRST activity that should be performed is:**

    A. pull-to-sit, leaning back against therapy ball.
    B. prone scooter obstacle course.
    C. hippity-hop races.
    D. batting a balloon while the child is suspended in net.

42. **An OT practitioner is preparing the family of 5-year-old child diagnosed with developmental delay for discharge. The child has just achieved independence in self-feeding with a spoon. The BEST suggestion for the parents to help the child maintain her skill level at home is to:**

    A. use hand-over-hand technique to reinforce correct technique.
    B. consistently point out incorrect hand placement and or movement patterns.
    C. let the child's older sister feed her occasionally as a reinforcement.
    D. praise her for what she does well; reinforce her independence.

43. **During the interview with the parents of a 3-year-old child with mild CP, the OT practitioner learns that the child is regularly fed by his grandmother and does not have any independent feeding skills. The FIRST issue the OTR needs to explore further is:**

    A. the degree of abnormal muscle tone in the UEs.
    B. the possibility of developmental delay.
    C. the cultural context and family interaction patterns.
    D. the need for adapted equipment.

44. **A 12-year-old will be discharged after having received treatment for anxiety disorder. Which would be the MOST appropriate recommendation for an extracurricular school activity:**

    A. competitive gymnastics team.

B. debating club.

C. school newspaper.

D. basketball team.

45. A child with CP tends to flex forward while riding her adapted tricycle even though her lower extremities are correctly positioned. The adaptation that would BEST enable her to maintain a more upright position is:

A. raising the seat height.

B. raising the handlebars.

C. lowering the seat height.

D. lowering the handlebars.

46. Direct OT services are being discontinued for a student with attention deficit disorder, but consultation will be provided to help the child adjust to the new classroom. Which of the following recommendations is MOST appropriate?

A. Use dim lighting and reduce glare by turning down lights

B. Remove all posters and visual aids to reduce visual distractions

C. Provide a screen to reduce peripheral visual stimuli

D. Restructure classroom activities into a series of short-term tasks

47. A 6-month-old child, when pulled into sitting with several trials, demonstrates a head lag. The OT practitioner evaluating this child should MOST accurately conclude that head control is:

A. developing in a typical manner.

B. slightly delayed by 1 month.

C. significantly delayed by several months.

D. advanced.

48. An OT practitioner working for the school system has identified a general need to enhance the fine coordination skills of the elementary school students to facilitate better writing skills. The BEST population-based intervention would be to:

A. screen students for writing problems and provide in-depth assessment of those identified.

B. provide remedial activities for those students identified having fine coordination deficits.

C. recommend activities to develop fine coordination that teachers can incorporate into classroom programming.

D. recommend additional OT staff to provide direct services for students.

49. On completion of an evaluation of a child with CP, the OT has identified the primary objective of inhibition of flexor spasticity in the hand. The activity that would be MOST appropriate in meeting this objective would be:

A. building a block tower.

B. active release of blocks into a container.

C. traction on the finger flexors.

D. weight bearing over a small bolster in prone.

50. An OT practitioner is working with a preschooler with spina bifida who is about to transition to a fully inclusive kindergarten. Lower extremity weakness and postural control are primary concerns, along with bilateral and fine motor coordination. Knowing there will be significant emphasis on writing activities, which of the following should the OT practitioner recommend?

A. Send the child to the OT room for fine motor activities when the class is working on writing skills

B. Arrange for the child to work in an area of the classroom where distractions can be minimized

C. Arrange for the child to have a flat desk to work on, in either standing or sitting positions

D. Provide a vertical work surface where writing and other hand skills can be practiced

51. An OT practitioner is working with an individual who is about to be discharged from OT after rehabilitation for a hand injury. The client has not been able to work for 3 months and is still unable to perform the job requirements as a sales manager in a clothing store. Which of the following recommendations should the OT practitioner recommend concerning OT services?

A. The client should continue to perform a home program at time of discharge.

B. The client should receive home health OT.

C. The client should enroll in a work-hardening program.

D. The client should discontinue OT services at the time of discharge.

52. An individual begins therapy with a blood-thinning medication after surgery

for an endarterectomy. Which would be the BEST grooming tool for the OT practitioner to recommend for use in the hospital and after discharge?

A. An electric razor
B. A single-blade safety razor
C. A straight razor
D. A double-blade safety razor

53. **A patient with Parkinson's disease has particular difficulty with both starting movement and stopping movement. The BEST strategy for the OT to teach the person and the person's caregivers is to:**

A. encourage the person to perform deep breathing exercise when movement is "frozen."
B. have the person practice the starting phase of the movement repeatedly.
C. have the person mentally identify the series of steps needed to initiate the movement.
D. provide a sensory cue, such as saying "stop!"

54. **According to proper body mechanics, the BEST way for an OT practitioner to perform a stand pivot transfer with a patient is to:**

A. move slowly, twisting the body from the trunk.
B. keep feet a shoulder width apart, lifting with the arms.
C. keep knees bent and feet planted when moving.
D. maintain a normal curve of the back, slowly shifting feet as the turn is completed.

55. **While performing endurance training activities, an individual on a cardiac rehabilitation unit begins to slow down, using progressively smaller movements to perform the activity. Which of the following is the most appropriate action for the OT practitioner to take?**

A. Stop the activity.
B. Upgrade the activity for the next session.
C. Modify the activity to make it less challenging.
D. Replace the activity with isometric exercises.

56. **A client with a history of chronic obstructive pulmonary disorder (COPD) has limited endurance. The long-term goal for this client is to prepare three meals a week. The MOST relevant short-**

term goal the for OT practitioner to focus on is:

A. the use of energy conservation.
B. work-hardening activities.
C. graded activities to increase strength.
D. safety in the kitchen.

57. **To practice transfers using a transfer board with a patient, the OT practitioner must have the patient use a wheelchair that has:**

A. detachable footrests.
B. detachable armrests.
C. antitip bars.
D. brake handle extensions.

58. **A family would like to place grab bars around the toilets in the house for easy access during transfers by the mother, who uses a wheelchair. At what height should they be placed?**

A. 28 to 32 inches
B. 33 to 36 inches
C. 38 to 41 inches
D. 43 to 46 inches

59. **An individual with left hemiparesis and impaired balance wishes to vacuum the floors upon return home. The BEST type of vacuum cleaner for the OT practitioner to recommend is a(n):**

A. canister vacuum cleaner.
B. upright vacuum cleaner.
C. self-propelled vacuum cleaner.
D. handheld cordless vacuum cleaner.

Mental Health

60. **Which of the following is the BEST example of the subjective section of a discharge summary?**

A. "Pt. reports overall pain levels are lower and ability to perform ADL has improved."
B. "Pt. continues to c/o back pain with activity."
C. "Pt. has improved from minimal assistance to independence in ADL performance."
D. "My back hurts when I get in and out of the tub, and when I lift bags of groceries."

61. **An individual who has been receiving treatment for an overuse syndrome is about to be discharged. Which of the following is the BEST example of the assessment section of a discharge summary?**

A. "Pt. can work for up to 3 hours at the computer using periodic stretch breaks."

B. "Pt. will take stretch breaks every 30 minutes when working at the computer."

C. "Pt. reports being able to work at the computer much longer and more comfortably than initially."

D. "Pt. has improved significantly in his ability to work at the computer by using periodic stretch breaks."

62. A OT practitioner is educating a family member whose sibling was admitted to the intensive care unit after sustaining an inhalation injury and full-thickness dorsal hand burns while lighting a campfire. The family member does not understand why the client would benefit from hand splints. Which of the following would be the MOST appropriate response to the family member?

A. Burn hand splints decrease pain and allow for active range of motion.

B. Burn hand splints prevent hypertrophic scarring.

C. Burn hand splints prevent the need for skin grafting.

D. Burn hand splints prevent stress on the tendons and ligaments, decreasing edema.

63. Each morning, an OT practitioner performs ADL training with a teenage client who has quadriplegia. On the first day, the practitioner works with the client, arranging the shirt on the lap. When the client masters that particular skill, they work on sliding both arms into the sleeves and pushing the shirt up past the elbows. When this skill is mastered, they will work on gathering the shirt up at the collar and pulling it on over the head. This technique is BEST known as:

A. repetition.

B. cueing.

C. rehearsal.

D. chaining.

64. Following a heart attack, an individual reports to the OT practitioner that his wife overreacted and that there is really nothing wrong with him. The nurse reports poor compliance with cardiac precautions. Which of the following is the MOST important action for the OT practitioner to take?

A. Monitor the individual's response to activi-

ties to prevent him from performing at activity levels that are too high and unsafe.

B. Instruct the individual in energy conservation techniques to minimize energy expenditure.

C. Emphasize the consequences of not observing cardiac precautions and provide concrete proof of the myocardial infarction (MI) to the individual.

D. Refer the individual for psychological services.

65. A middle-aged client with paraplegia is learning to perform wheelchair-to-car transfers with an OT practitioner. Which is the BEST way for the OTR to recommend independent car transfers?

A. By teaching a family member to assist with all car transfers

B. By teaching the client to use public transportation in place of practicing car transfers

C. By learning to use a sliding board with car transfers

D. By learning to use tenodesis functions when transferring to the car

66. An OT practitioner is assisting an individual with mild hemiparesis in transferring from the wheelchair to a mat table using a stand pivot transfer technique. The FIRST verbal cue the OT gives to the individual is:

A. "Stand up."

B. "Scoot forward to the edge of the wheelchair."

C. "Unfasten the wheelchair brakes."

D. "Position the wheelchair so that it directly faces the mat table."

67. An OT practitioner applies weights to the wrists of a woman who is making a macramé planter to improve strength in her shoulders. The MOST accurate description of this treatment approach is:

A. neurophysiological.

B. neurodevelopmental.

C. biomechanical.

D. rehabilitative.

68. An individual with a high-level spinal cord injury is returning home. Which type of adaptive technology would the client MOST likely require to ensure safety in the home?

A. An environmental control unit (ECU)

B. A call system for emergency and nonemergency use

C. A remote control power door opener

D. An electric page turner

69. **To improve written communication, an OT practitioner would be MOST likely to recommend a large keyboard to enhance computer access when the client:**

    A. has limited UE range of motion but adequate fine coordination.

    B. fatigues rapidly when reaching for the keys.

    C. uses only one hand to access the keyboard.

    D. has good UE range of motion but difficulty accessing small targets.

70. **The BEST way to instruct an individual with hemiparesis to button a shirt is to:**

    A. button all the buttons before putting the shirt on.

    B. get the shirt all the way on, then line up the buttons and holes and begin buttoning from the top.

    C. get the shirt all the way on, then line up the buttons and holes and begin buttoning from the bottom.

    D. use a buttonhook with a built-up handle.

71. **An OT practitioner is working with a patient with a high-level spinal cord injury who has no functional movements to determine the best method of input access for a powered wheelchair. The MOST likely recommendation for this patient to activate the wheelchair would be to use a:**

    A. joystick.

    B. sip-and-puff switch.

    C. single-switch digital control.

    D. mouth stick.

72. **An OT practitioner making a bedside visit finds her patient poorly positioned with an edematous upper extremity caught between the mattress and the bed rail. The MOST appropriate intervention to address the edema in the upper extremity is to:**

    A. elevate the arm on pillows so it rests higher than the heart.

    B. massage the arm gently, stroking toward the fingers.

    C. instruct him to avoid active range of motion.

    D. instruct him to avoid PROM.

73. **An individual covered by Medicare who has been receiving OT and PT in the home is now able to transfer in and out of the car with supervision of a caregiver. The individual has visited a friend who lives 30 minutes away. OT services are still required to improve mobility, upper extremity function, and home management skills. Which of the following actions should the OT practitioner take FIRST?**

    A. Provide a home program and discharge the patient.

    B. Explain to the patient and caregiver that one must be "homebound" in order to be eligible for home care services.

    C. Refer the patient for outpatient therapy and provide a comprehensive discharge summary to the outpatient setting.

    D. Communicate with the PT and inform her of the patient's status.

74. **A student OT practitioner needs to design an adaptation and decides to focus on gardening for a client with a back injury. The MOST appropriate adaptation for him to design would be:**

    A. ergonomically correct hand tools.

    B. a wheelbarrow with elongated handles.

    C. a 12-inch-high seat with tool holders.

    D. a raised-bed garden.

75. **An OT practitioner is working on keyboarding activities with a client with asymmetrical muscle tone who keeps falling to the side while sitting in a wheelchair. What is the MOST appropriate wheelchair adaptation the practitioner can use to stabilize the upper body in a midline position?**

    A. Change to a reclining wheelchair

    B. Use an arm trough

    C. Provide lateral trunk support

    D. Provide lateral pelvic support

76. **An OT practitioner is working on transfer training with a young client who recently underwent bilateral below-knee amputations. Which of the following should the OTR FIRST suggest for independent transfers from the wheelchair to the bathroom tub seat?**

    A. Stand pivot transfers

    B. Sliding board transfer

    C. Dependent lift transfer

    D. Transfers should not be initiated until receiving prosthetics

77. The technique of stabilizing a person's forearm on the table when writing would MOST likely be used by the OT practitioner if the person exhibited:

A. decreased vision.

B. poor endurance.

C. limited fine movement.

D. incoordination.

78. A resident in a long-term care facility is being treated by the OTR to regain self-feeding skills. The MOST effective strategy for beginning self-feeding with a resident who is tactilely defensive around the facial area is to:

A. have the therapist clear food pocketed in the resident's cheeks.

B. use a guiding technique: place food in the resident's hand and bring it to the mouth.

C. wipe food particles off a person's mouth and chin as he or she eats.

D. allow resident to select whatever food or beverage he or she prefers.

79. An elderly patient who was hospitalized for a right cerebrovascular accident (RCVA) with left upper extremity flaccidity and decreased sensation is beginning to experience sensory return in the left upper extremity. The OTR should recommend modifying the treatment plan to include:

A. remedial treatment, such as rubbing or stroking the involved extremity.

B. remedial treatment, such as the use of hot mitts to avoid burns.

C. compensatory treatment, such as testing bathwater with the uninvolved extremity.

D. compensatory treatment, such as using a one-handed cutting board to avoid cutting the insensate hand.

80. An OT practitioner is preparing an outpatient who has received a resting hand splint for discharge. It is MOST important that the patient and caregivers understand the need to:

A. bend the splint if it doesn't fit comfortably.

B. discontinue use of the splint if it isn't cosmetically pleasing.

C. care for the splint with special washing directions.

D. observe for signs of pain, redness, and irritation, then discontinue use and report to therapist.

81. An OT practitioner is working with a group of patients who have orientation deficits resulting from head injuries. Using an adaptive or compensatory approach, the MOST appropriate intervention would be to:

A. provide verbal cues, external aids such as calendars and family pictures, and opportunities to practice using the external aids.

B. reduce the number of distractions; move the group to a quiet room.

C. present information in short units, spaced with time between each segment.

D. connect new information to previously learned knowledge and skills.

82. During a cooking evaluation, an individual with a history of traumatic brain injury (TBI) exhibits moderate upper extremity incoordination. Which of the following recommendations would be MOST beneficial for this individual?

A. Use built-up utensil handles

B. Use heavy utensils, pots, and pans

C. Use a high stool to work at counter height

D. Place the most commonly used items on shelves just above and below the counter

83. An OT practitioner is assessing hand sensation in an older adult with diabetic neuropathies who frequently complains of hand pain. It appears that the client would benefit from a desensitization program. The OT informs the client that hypersensitivity training is typically graded from:

A. soft to hard to rough.

B. tap to rub to touch.

C. light to medium to heavy.

D. rough to hard to soft.

84. An individual has sustained a large, full-thickness burn to both upper extremities while running a fireworks display. The client is in the acute care phase of treatment. Which of the following BEST represents an acute care rehabilitation goal?

A. Prevent loss of joint and skin mobility

B. Provide adaptive equipment

C. Provide compression and vascular support garments

D. Prevent scar hypertrophy through scar management techniques

85. An OT practitioner provides a leatherworking activity to an individual with C7

quadriplegia in order to increase grip strength. Which component of this activity would be **MOST** effective in promoting this goal?

A. Holding the hammer
B. Holding the stamping tools
C. Squeezing the sponge to wet the leather
D. Lacing with a needle

86. **An individual demonstrates a left visual field cut as a result of a TBI, and demonstrates difficulty crossing the midline during many self-care activities. Which of the following activities would MOST effectively promote this individual's ability to cross the midline?**

A. Making a coil pot out of clay
B. Making a macramé planter
C. Stringing a bead necklace
D. Weaving on a frame loom

87. **An OT practitioner is selecting foods for an initial treatment session with a client with dysphagia. In general, which of the following foods would BEST represent an adequate selection for intervention?**

A. Vegetable soup
B. Salad
C. Watermelon
D. Eggs

88. **An OT is planning to provide a program to address the needs of persons with Alzheimer's disease and their families as part of a hospital outreach program. One of the areas of intervention which would be MOST beneficial to maintaining safety and supporting function at home in the advanced stages of Alzheimer's is:**

A. strength and endurance activities.
B. cognitive rehabilitation techniques.
C. environmental modification.
D. assertiveness skills.

89. **While observing a client who has just been admitted to the rehabilitation unit after a right CVA with left hemiplegia, the OT practitioner notices that the patient's right arm lays limply by the patient's side. In documenting this observation, the OT will MOST likely use the term:**

A. paralysis.
B. flaccidity.
C. subluxation.
D. spasticity.

90. **An individual with an upper extremity fracture has asked an OT practitioner how to maintain strength in her arm until the cast is removed. The activities that would BEST accomplish this goal are those which incorporate:**

A. isometric muscle contractions.
B. isotonic muscle contractions.
C. progressive resistance.
D. passive movement.

91. **While assessing dressing skills with a patient who recently had a stroke, the OT practitioner notes that the individual is unable to see buttons on a printed fabric. This MOST likely indicates that the client may be having difficult with:**

A. spatial relations.
B. figure-ground perception.
C. body image.
D. visual closure.

92. **An OT practitioner is making a home visit to an elderly client who lives alone. The client exhibits severe hand weakness. When addressing safety in the home, the OTR should be MOST concerned with the client's ability to:**

A. work locks and latches on doors and windows.
B. use built-up utensils while eating.
C. use energy conservation techniques.
D. manipulate fasteners on clothing.

93. **An OT practitioner is working with a homemaker who sustained a partial-thickness burn 6 months ago. Which scar management technique is MOST appropriate for the OTR to introduce during the rehabilitative phase of treatment?**

A. Preventing scar development through static splinting
B. Controlling edema to prevent loss of range of motion
C. Minimizing scar hypertrophy through compression garments and proper skin care
D. Promoting self-care skills in order to resume the role of homemaker

94. **A 45-year-old client with COPD has the long-term goal of being able to shop independently for groceries. The client has achieved the short-term goal of going to a convenience store and purchasing three items. Which statement is the**

BEST example of a revised short-term goal?

A. "Client will purchase 10 items at the supermarket with supervision."

B. "Client will cook a one-dish meal."

C. "Client will shop independently for a birthday present for her daughter."

D. "Instruct client in energy conservation techniques that apply to grocery shopping."

95. After evaluation, a short-term goal for an individual who had a total hip replacement was to dress with minimal assistance, using adaptive equipment and verbal cues to follow hip precautions. After 1 week of treatment, the individual is able to dress with standby assistance, using adaptive equipment and verbal cues to follow hip precautions. What skills does this person need to demonstrate before changing the goal?

A. Less time needed to perform dressing

B. Improved concentration

C. Ability to consistently follow hip precautions

D. Ability to use adaptive devices appropriately

96. An OTR is working with a client who sustained an injury to the right upper extremity while rollerblading. The referral states that the client sustained a Colles' fracture. The OTR explains to the client that a Colles' fracture is a:

A. fracture to the pisiform.

B. fracture to the ulnar styloid.

C. fracture to the carpometacarpal joint.

D. fracture to the distal radius.

97. A patient's weight has changed during the course of hospitalization, and the wheelchair seat is now 2.5 inches wider on each side of the patient's hips. Which is the BEST recommendation the OT practitioner can make regarding proper wheelchair fit?

A. Obtain a wider wheelchair because this one is too narrow.

B. The patient should be encouraged to lose weight.

C. The sides of the chair should be padded to improve the fit.

D. Obtain a narrower wheelchair because this one is too wide.

98. An OT practitioner is working on a feeding program for an individual with amyotrophic lateral sclerosis (ALS) who is in the late stages of the disease process.

Which of the following is the MOST appropriate intervention for this individual?

A. Provide a rocker knife, plate guard, and nonskid mat

B. Implement a pureed diet and allow adequate time for eating

C. Emphasize upper extremity strengthening

D. Minimize the use of adaptive equipment

99. An OT practitioner is fabricating a splint for a client with swan-neck deformities. This splint is designed to maintain the client's fingers in a position which prevents further:

A. hyperextension of the PIP and DIP joints.

B. hyperextension of the PIP joint and flexion of the DIP joint.

C. flexion of the PIP joint and hyperextension of the DIP joint.

D. hyperextension of the MP joint and flexion of the PIP joint.

100. An OT practitioner is working in a outpatient upper extremity and hand clinic. The practitioner's case load consists of clients who have tendinitis, nerve compression syndromes, and myofascial pain. The OT practitioner can assume that these diagnoses are MOST commonly associated with:

A. osteoarthritis conditions.

B. peripheral vascular diseases.

C. cumulative trauma disorders.

D. neuroma-related conditions.

101. While measuring the active range of motion of a patient's metacarpophalangeal (MCP) joints, it is MOST important for the OT practitioner to provide stabilization:

A. above the MCP joints.

B. below the MCP joints.

C. at the wrist.

D. on top of the MCP joints.

102. When an OT practitioner makes or issues splints, the PRIMARY criterion common to all splints is that the:

A. fingers should be flexed in a functional position.

B. thumb is opposed and abducted.

C. splint should be worn at all times.

D. pressure marks or redness from the splint should disappear after 20 minutes.

103. The OT practitioner who is measuring the strength of a patient's three-jaw-chuck grasp pattern must know how to use a(n):

A. aesthesiometer.

B. pinch meter.

C. dynamometer.

D. volumeter.

104. An OT practitioner is educating a level-I OT student about the various types of splints primarily used in burn units. Which of the following BEST represents these splints?

A. Resting splints and ankle foot orthotics

B. Dynamic and posterior neck splints

C. Below-the-knee amputation and burn wrist cock-up splints

D. Airplane and burn hand splint

105. An elderly client, who has had several falls at home and ambulates with a cane, is preparing for discharge to the home of an adult child who is renovating some rooms for the parent. The OT has been asked to recommend flooring for the client's rooms. The BEST recommendation for the OT to make is:

A. carpeting with low or looped pile.

B. wood floor.

C. area rugs.

D. carpeting with deep pile and padding.

106. An OT practitioner is assessing hand function in a man with arthritis by observing him as he makes a peanut butter sandwich. The individual is unable to remove the lid from a 28-ounce peanut butter jar but is able stand at the counter, spread peanut butter on the bread with a knife, and replace the lid when he has finished making the sandwich. These observations would MOST accurately reflect deficit in the performance component:

A. range of motion.

B. coordination.

C. endurance.

D. strength.

107. An OT practitioner is working on feeding with an individual with a C3 spinal cord injury. The strategy that will enable the HIGHEST level of independence is for the individual to:

A. clearly direct a caregiver in preferred head

position, food portion size, and choice of food to eat.

B. use a mobile arm support.

C. use a wrist support with a utensil inserted into the cuff.

D. use a universal cuff with a utensil inserted into the cuff.

108. During a perceptual evaluation, an OT practitioner determines that an individual exhibits constructional apraxia, body scheme disturbances, and unilateral neglect. During the functional part of the evaluation, these deficits are MOST likely to contribute to self-care difficulties related to:

A. spatial relations.

B. dressing apraxia.

C. anosognosia.

D. figure-ground discrimination.

109. An OT is planning intervention for an individual who recently experienced a left CVA resulting in right-sided hemiplegia and motor apraxia. To BEST facilitate the individual's attempts to perform morning ADL the OT should plan to:

A. provide the individual with detailed, step-by-step commands for each task throughout the ADL process.

B. make the environment as simple and uncluttered as possible and use sharp contrast to make objects clearly stand out.

C. have the individual visualize the task first and then provide general statements such as "Let's get ready."

D. teach the individual to move slowly through the environment and encourage touching of objects during the task.

110. A home health OT is working with an individual who is ambulatory but demonstrates poor balance. The individual has a walker, a standard cane and a wheelchair at home, but financial constraints have prevented any home modifications. Which of the following ambulatory methods would be MOST appropriate for use during meal preparation training?

A. Use a standard cane

B. Use a walker

C. Use a wheelchair

D. Hold on to counters and walls

111. A client that the OT practitioner is treating brings an order from his physician requesting treatment for epicondylitis.

Which of the following adjunct activities should be used to treat the ACUTE symptoms of tennis elbow?

A. PROM, weight bearing, and mobilization
B. Resistive exercises, heat application, and work simulation
C. Heat application, PROM, and strengthening
D. Ice application, immobilization, and splinting

112. An adult with polymyositis and dermatomyositis, is able to complete full range of shoulder flexion while in a supine position during an evaluation with an OT practitioner. However, against gravity, the client is only able to achieve 50% of the range for shoulder flexion. The practitioner grades this muscle as:

A. good (4).
B. fair (3).
C. fair minus (3-).
D. poor plus (2+).

113. An individual who recently experienced an MI is now medically stable and has been referred to OT. In order to determine the individual's current endurance level, the OT practitioner plans to monitor performance of self-care activities. The FIRST step is to:

A. take the individual's vital signs after performance of self-care activities.
B. observe the individual for signs and symptoms during self-care activities.
C. take the individual's vital signs at rest.
D. take vital signs 5 minutes after the individual has completed self-care activities.

114. When administering an evaluation of upper extremity function to a newly admitted patient with Guillain-Barré syndrome, it is MOST important to:

A. test proximal muscle strength first.
B. perform the evaluation over several sessions.
C. include sensory testing.
D. evaluate range of motion.

115. An OT practitioner is working with a client who demonstrates the inability to swallow when attempting to self-feed water ice. The OTR should interpret the inability to swallow as:

A. deglutition.
B. dysmetria.
C. dysphagia.

D. dysarthria.

116. A client requests a drink of water after working on upper extremity exercises during therapy. The OT practitioner reads in the patient's chart that "Mr. J is on a nonoral feeding program." The OTR interprets that:

A. the client is on thin liquid only feedings.
B. the client is on stage I foods only.
C. the client is receiving nasal tube feedings.
D. the client is eating pureed only foods.

117. During a stress management group, an individual recently diagnosed with multiple sclerosis (MS) complains that his teenage children are resistive to helping with chores that were previously his responsibility, such as mowing the lawn and taking out the trash. The stress management technique that would MOST successfully address this concern is:

A. using effective communication skills.
B. applying time management techniques.
C. deep breathing.
D. laughter.

118. An individual diagnosed with Guillain-Barré syndrome exhibits good upper extremity strength. The activity that would be MOST appropriate for further strengthening is:

A. peeling potatoes.
B. vacuuming.
C. polishing furniture.
D. washing windows.

Physical Disabilities

119. An artist recently diagnosed with MS is interested in pursuing a leisure activity that will promote physical fitness. Because the individual's symptoms are limited to mild UE numbness and slight weakness in the dominant hand at this point, the BEST activity to recommend is:

A. volleyball.
B. painting with the dominant hand.
C. swimming in a cool water pool.
D. jogging on a track or treadmill.

120. A long-term goal for an individual with progressive weakness is for the family to carry out his feeding program. They

have achieved the short-term goal of understanding how the individual's disability affects his ability to feed himself. Which statement is the BEST example of a revised short-term goal?

A. "Pt. will participate in feeding program."
B. "Pt. will feed himself with moderate assistance."
C. "Family will feed patient safely and independently 100% of the time."
D. "Family will demonstrate independence in current positioning and feeding techniques."

121. **When evaluating the somatosensory system, the OTR would have to include testing procedures for?**

A. Taste
B. Smell
C. Vision
D. Touch

122. **According to Signe Brunnstrom, a person who demonstrates developing spasticity on the hemiplegic side of the body with weak, associated movements in synergy and little active finger flexion would be in which stage of recovery?**

A. One
B. Two
C. Three
D. Four

123. **An OT practitioner is planning a program for an individual who needs to increase shoulder strength, range of motion, and endurance. Which of the following activities is MOST suitable for periodic upgrading?**

A. Blowing up and tying balloons of various sizes
B. Playing a game of balloon darts
C. Painting faces on balloons
D. Playing balloon volleyball

124. **An adult with MS has decreased sensation of the buttocks and bilateral lower extremities. When educating an individual with absent sensation, the OT practitioner should include:**

A. training to inspect for pressure sores on bony prominences and affected areas.
B. instructions pertaining to careful trimming of fingernails and toenails.
C. padding to areas of a splint that cause redness on the individual.
D. hypersensitivity training.

125. **The goal for an elderly client with lower extremity weakness is to be independent with bathing, but this requires the tub to be more accessible to the client who uses a walker. Which environmental adaptation would be BEST to achieve this?**

A. Place the light switch outside the door so the bathroom is lit before entering
B. Provide long-handled adaptive devices to facilitate lower extremity dressing
C. Provide transfer tub bench and install grab bars
D. Place nonskid decals in the tub and mats on the floor to prevent slipping on the wet floor

126. **An OT practitioner is training an individual in the principles of joint protection. The principles that the OT would MOST likely include would be:**

A. using the strongest joint, avoiding positions of deformity, and ensuring correct patterns of movement.
B. massaging a joint before exercise.
C. practicing vivid imagery and relaxation exercises during difficult functional activities.
D. application of heat before treatment and application of cold after range of motion treatment.

127. **An OT practitioner is teaching several older adults with COPD energy conservation techniques in home management skills. Following learning principles for older adults, the MOST effective way to present the information would be for the OT to:**

A. present all the important principles to be covered together in a single presentation.
B. keep the presentation loosely structured, rather than highly organized.
C. attempt to persuade clients about the importance of those points on which the clients don't seem to agree.
D. present important principles in small units that are spaced at a slower than normal pace.

128. **A nonspeaking person who uses a wheelchair is suddenly making many errors on the augmentative communication device but experienced no difficulty the previous day. Which of the following is the FIRST step the OT practitioner should take in responding to this problem?**

A. Refer the person to physician for evaluation.

B. Reposition the person in the wheelchair to allow optimal range of motion.

C. Reassess the person's communication abilities.

D. Replace the communication device.

129. An OT practitioner is working with a patient who has mild difficulties swallowing, The OT instructs the patient that the BEST position for him to maintain during feeding activities is:

A. 30 degrees of neck extension.

B. 10 degrees of head extension past the midline.

C. 10 degrees of head flexion from the midline.

D. 30 degrees of head flexion.

130. An individual who is s/p total hip arthroplasty (posterolateral approach) is working on independence in lower extremity dressing. Which of the following instructions is MOST important to convey to this individual?

A. Sit during dressing activities

B. Avoid internal rotation and adduction of the involved hip

C. Use a long-handled shoe horn and dressing stick

D. Wear shoes with elastic laces

131. A patient who has had a CVA has difficulty using his left upper extremity for reaching activities because of fluctuating muscle tone. According to the Neurodevelopmental Treatment (NDT) approach, one of the MOST effective ways to teach a person to normalize high muscle tone in affected extremities prior to functional activities is by:

A. placing a weighted cuff on the extremity.

B. weight bearing through the upper extremity in sitting or standing.

C. using the unaffected arm for all reaching activities.

D. "forced use" of the affected extremity.

132. A therapist is working with a patient who has had an UE amputation to determine whether a hook terminal device (TD) or a functional prosthetic hand would be most appropriate for the patient. The patient's primary concern is his ability to return to work and function as a carpenter. The MOST important factor in the OT's recommendation would be that:

A. a functional prosthetic hand has a better cosmetic appearance.

B. a hook provides better prehensile function and allows greater visibility of objects.

C. a hook weighs less than a hand.

D. a functional hand is covered by a rubber glove that stains easily.

133. Which of the following devices will be required by an individual with C7-8 quadriplegia when performing oral hygiene activities?

A. Mobile arm support with utensil holder

B. Universal cuff

C. Toothbrush with built-up handle

D. Wrist support with utensil holder

134. An elderly patient, who lives alone, has been briefly hospitalized following a car accident and is being discharged from the acute care setting. The patient continues to need rehabilitative services to maximize functional independence and eventually return home. This person is medically stable, motivated, and cognitively intact and has rehabilitation potential. But the person tires quickly, is weak, and tolerates only brief periods of therapy. The MOST appropriate recommendation for the OT to make regarding this patient is:

A. attending an inpatient physical dysfunction rehabilitation program.

B. extending the patient's stay in the familiar acute care hospital to receive additional therapy.

C. attending a rehabilitation program in a skilled nursing or extended care facility.

D. seek nursing home placement for this patient.

135. An individual has been instructed to place towels, one at a time, on a high shelf in order to increase shoulder flexion. The individual is able to easily place 10 towels. Which of the following modifications would MOST effectively improve endurance in the shoulder flexors?

A. Place the towels on a higher shelf

B. Increase the number of towels from 10 to 20

C. Place the towels on a lower shelf

D. Add a 1-pound weight to each arm

136. A newly referred patient complains of frequently dropping lightweight items and reports a numb feeling in both

hands. **Which of the following instruments is MOST important for evaluating this individual?**

A. Goniometer
B. Dynamometer
C. Pinch meter
D. Aesthesiometer

137. **An OT practitioner is working with an individual with impaired memory. When the client is unable to follow verbal instructions, the practitioner changes the approach to demonstration. This is an example of:**

A. activity analysis.
B. activity adaptation.
C. grading the activity.
D. clinical reasoning.

138. **Which of the following is the MOST appropriate goal to address when working with clients diagnosed with cognitive disorders?**

A. Improve their social skills in relating to others
B. Create new habits of time use
C. Implement compensatory strategies to manage the environment
D. Facilitate resumption of previous life roles

139. **An individual alternately exhibits laughing and crying throughout a treatment session. This behavior should be documented as:**

A. mania.
B. emotional lability.
C. paranoia.
D. denial.

140. **An OT practitioner is working as a consultant to a long-term care facility that is designing a dementia care unit. The OT would MOST likely recommend which type of environmental attributes as therapeutic?**

A. Controlled stimulation with meaningful sensory cues
B. High sensory stimulation, to encourage active engagement
C. Subdued, low sensory stimulation environment, to prevent agitation
D. Stimuli that are very similar to that found in the residents' home environments

141. **A patient needs assistance with memory problems. The strategy which BEST re-**

flects an external compensation method of intervention is:

A. teaching the person to retrace steps mentally to stimulate memory.
B. teaching the person to use a diary or log.
C. training the person to repeat important pieces of information aloud to aid memorizing.
D. working with a memory training computer program.

142. **An individual with mental illness wants to travel to the library independently but keeps getting lost. Which of the following actions should the OT practitioner take FIRST?**

A. Take the individual to the library and obtain a library card.
B. Assess the individual's ability to read.
C. Identify the bus that goes to the library and obtain a bus schedule.
D. Assess the individual's topographical orientation skills.

143. **An OT practitioner is assessing a client who has schizophrenia and appears to be experiencing acute symptoms of the disease. Which of the following is considered to be an acute or positive symptom of schizophrenia that the OT might document in her assessment?**

A. Flat affect
B. A lack of pleasure
C. Hallucinations
D. Withdrawal from others

144. **An OT practitioner treats most clients under the behavioral frame of reference. The activity feature that is MOST consistent with a behavioral frame of reference is:**

A. the level of skill required is appropriate for the generally expected skills for that age.
B. the symbolic potential of the activity.
C. the combined activity demands of sensations, perceptions, and motor skills.
D. the measurability of activity performance.

145. **The therapist needs to identify an activity that will address psychosocial goals by (1) allowing the individual to experience success using a messy process and (2) requiring the individual to delay gratification. The activity process that is the BEST for providing this experience is:**

A. working in a group of three other individuals.

B. selecting the design pattern for a tile trivet.

C. applying grout to a tile trivet and waiting for it to dry.

D. encouraging the individual to clean off the table at the end of the group session.

146. While evaluating a middle-aged individual, the therapist asks the client about the grade school he or she attended. This is an example of the OT practitioner attempting to obtain data pertaining to the individual's:

A. retention.

B. remote memory.

C. orientation.

D. recent memory.

147. An individual with mental illness has accepted a secretarial position but is concerned about high levels of distractibility that may interfere with concentration and job performance. Which of the following interventions is MOST appropriate for this individual?

A. Arrange for the individual to have a job coach

B. Ask the employer to provide more frequent breaks

C. Explain the problem of distractibility to the employer

D. Ask the employer to provide an isolated cubical as the work space

148. During discharge planning, the patient asks the OTR, "What should I do when people at work ask me where I have been all this time?" How can the OTR BEST address this concern?

A. Arrange for the patient to discuss this with the social worker.

B. Suggest that the patient tell the truth.

C. Suggest that the patient report having been on an extended vacation.

D. Arrange for the patient to attend a discharge group to discuss these concerns.

149. The goal of an arts and crafts group for chronically mentally ill individuals is to improve their decision-making abilities. The MOST appropriate approach to initiating a mosaic tile activity would be to:

A. provide each patient with an individual project and have him or her choose a tile color for the project.

B. have the patients choose from a variety of projects.

C. have the patients decide on a design, size,

shape, and colors for a group mosaics project.

D. have each patient decide on a pattern and two tile colors to use in the his or her mosaic project.

150. A client who is an alcoholic is in search of a group to attend upon discharge that will assist with the rehabilitative process. The MOST appropriate self-help group for the OT to recommend to an individual who abuses alcohol is:

A. Mothers Against Drunk Drivers (MADD).

B. Al-Anon.

C. Alcoholics Anonymous (AA).

D. group therapy.

151. An OT is participating in the evaluation of an older adult in the early stage of Alzheimer's disease. The deficit MOST likely to be evident is:

A. aphasia.

B. incontinence.

C. memory impairment.

D. the inability to dress and undress.

152. Upon completion of the initial interview and chart review, the NEXT step to be taken by the OT is to:

A. analyze the data.

B. develop a treatment plan.

C. perform selected assessments.

D. select appropriate evaluation procedures.

153. An adult with schizophrenia walks with a shuffling gait and hunched posture. Using a movement-centered frame of reference, which of the following activities would MOST effectively contribute to normalization of this individual's posture?

A. Dancing with rapid alternating movements

B. Playing the game Twister

C. Digging a garden with a shovel

D. Rocking in a rocking chair

154. An OT practitioner is planning a meal preparation activity for an adult client with attentional and organizational deficits secondary to alcohol abuse. The treatment goals address the client's difficulties in properly sequencing tasks. The MOST appropriate activity to use FIRST is:

A. setting the table.

B. planning an entire meal.

C. baking cookies using a recipe.

D. preparing a shopping list.

155. An OT practitioner is developing transition activities for a group of 16-year-old students diagnosed as trainable mentally retarded. Which of the following activities would be **BEST** for addressing goals related to transition?

A. Role-play ordering food in the classroom
B. Go out for lunch to a fast-food restaurant
C. Order a take-out lunch by phone
D. Select lunch items from a picture menu in the classroom

156. An individual tells the **OT** practitioner, "I don't know about going home tomorrow. I wanted to be discharged yesterday and the doctor suggested I stay in the hospital another day." Which of the following responses **MOST** accurately reflects an active listening approach?

A. "It sounds as if you're not sure whether you are ready to be discharged."
B. "You know, your doctor is a very intelligent person."
C. "How about calling your doctor when you get home if you feel a panic attack coming on."
D. "You've been doing extremely well; what are you afraid of?"

157. In evaluating an adolescent with psychosocial problems, an **OTR** would be **MOST** likely to begin the process by screening the adolescent's level of function in which areas?

A. Play and social behavior, overall development, and visual motor skills
B. Socialization, task performance, daily living skills, and time management
C. Interest in work, leisure, and self-care
D. Motor skills, sensory processing, and cognition

158. In carrying out inpatient treatment groups for individuals with schizophrenia, the **OT** practitioner should routinely:

A. use projective media such as clay to facilitate expression of feelings.
B. allow an individual group member to work in an isolated area away from the group.
C. use simple and highly structured activities.
D. discuss the individuals' delusions with them.

159. An **OT** practitioner uses a remediation of functional performance deficits ap-

proach in addressing individuals treated in a psychosocial setting. The activity that is **MOST** consistent with this approach is:

A. an expressive group magazine collage.
B. a class about job-seeking strategies.
C. the modification of the environment to provide familiar visual cues.
D. a review of the individual's balance of time among ADL, work, and leisure activities.

160. An OT practitioner is conducting an ongoing assertiveness training group. Which of the following strategies would be **MOST** helpful in the development of group cohesion?

A. Define assertiveness, passivity, and aggression for the group members
B. Allow and encourage all group members physically and verbally to release their aggressive feelings toward inanimate objects
C. Demonstrate commonly used assertiveness techniques to the group members
D. Encourage group members to share similar experiences and reactions with each other

161. An individual with mental retardation lives in a group home and is expected to participate in laundry activities. The individual is usually successful with routine performance of daily tasks, is able to recognize whether clothing is clean or dirty, demonstrates sequencing skills, and is independent in most self-care activities. What advice should the OT practitioner provide to the group home staff to enable the individual to perform laundry activities at the **HIGHEST** level of independence possible?

A. The staff will probably need to instruct individual to place dirty items in the hamper and remove sheets from the bed.
B. The staff should encourage problem solving when obstacles arise.
C. The individual will be independent in use of a washer and dryer, but the staff may need to demonstrate the use of new products.
D. The staff may need to monitor water temperature and the amount of soap being used.

162. An OT practitioner is working with an individual who demonstrates the inability to begin a task or activity. The practitioner documents that the client **MOST** likely has problems with:

A. attention.
B. concentration.
C. initiation.
D. apraxia.

163. **An OT practitioner has been hired to develop a community-based program for patients with chronic mental illness. The FIRST step in the process which the practitioner must complete is:**

A. program planning.
B. program implementation.
C. needs assessment.
D. program evaluation.

164. **Which of the following statements would BEST explain the purpose of a prevocational evaluation program to a new participant?**

A. "The program will help you to learn about your interests, talents, and skills for assembly jobs."
B. "This program will help you to learn about the skills you have that are needed on MOST jobs and about your potential for work."
C. "This program will help you identify the responsibility you have to your employer while you are in treatment and to inform your employer of these responsibilities."
D. "This program will help you to develop skills for getting a job."

165. **When reporting data collected to the OTR, it is MOST important for the COTA to:**

A. observe everything the patient said and did during the interview and provide extensive notes for the OTR to read.
B. provide the OTR with a comprehensive treatment plan based on the results of the evaluation.
C. provide a summary of observations of the patient's behavior, including what the patient said and did during the interview.
D. provide an interpretation of how the patient behaved during the interview.

166. **Before working in a chronic psychiatric unit, a practitioner must understand the effects that certain medications have on daily function. The extrapyramidal side effect syndrome experienced by individuals receiving antipsychotic medications that impairs swallowing and leads to involuntary jerky arm and leg movements can BEST be described as:**

A. parkinsonian syndrome.
B. antipsychotic medication overdose.
C. tardive dyskinesia.
D. lithium toxicity.

167. **An individual has demonstrated competence in heating canned soup. The OT practitioner recommends modifying the treatment plan and upgrading the cooking activity to:**

A. baking brownies.
B. making an apple pie.
C. making toast.
D. making a fresh fruit salad.

168. **While completing the assessment and treatment planning process, an OT practitioner confers with the client to establish program goals. As the practitioner writes these goals, they should MOST appropriately reflect:**

A. specific measurable statements with time frames.
B. time frames for what will be accomplished.
C. specific measurements of the individual's skill and performance.
D. activities to be completed that correspond with the goals and objectives.

169. **An OTR is using leather stamping as part of a group activity but feels the need to increase the problem-solving processes within the group. The BEST approach for encouraging problem solving in a craft media group is to:**

A. begin with activities that have obvious solutions and high probabilities of success and then gradually increase the complexity.
B. begin with activities that require gross motor responses and progress to activities that require fine motor responses.
C. structure the number and kinds of choices available.
D. gradually increase the time used in the activity by 15-minute increments.

170. **An OT practitioner is working with an individual who has had an injury to the nondominant right cerebral hemisphere. The MOST relevant communication strategy to enhance this person's understanding of directions would be to provide:**

A. written information presented on the left side of the body.
B. exaggerated facial expressions and body gestures rather than words.

C. simply stated, concrete verbal instructions.

D. pictures of instructions presented on the left side of the body.

171. An OTR and COTA are each completing sections of a discharge summary. The section LEAST appropriate for the COTA and MOST appropriate for the OTR to complete is the:

A. discharge recommendations.

B. patient's current level of independence in ADL.

C. patient's most recent strength and coordination measurements.

D. patient's discharge disposition.

172. Which aspects of psychosocial performance are MOST important to emphasize in developing a client's work potential in a prevocational program?

A. Punctuality, accepting directions from a supervisor, and interacting with coworkers

B. Memory, sequencing of the work tasks, attending to work tasks, and making decisions

C. Standing tolerance, eye–hand coordination, and endurance

D. Maintaining personal cleanliness and adhering to safety precautions

173. An OT practitioner in a long-term care facility is working with several residents who seem very isolated and disengaged from the other residents. The OT has identified a need to provide these residents with a group activity that would enhance self-esteem, provide opportunities for social skills and assist residents in integrating past experiences with present life. The BEST type of group to accomplish these goals is a:

A. reminiscence group.

B. meditation group.

C. grooming activities group.

D. movement activities and games group.

174. Which of the following is the BEST activity for reducing the physical symptoms of muscle tension associated with anxiety disorders?

A. Copper tooling

B. Aerobic exercise

C. Line dancing

D. A woodworking kit

175. An OT practitioner is leading a discussion with a group of individuals who are diagnosed with major depression. The MOST helpful approach for the therapist to take is to:

A. be upbeat, positive, and cheerful when encouraging the individuals to discuss their feelings.

B. offer even-tempered acceptance, reflecting back what is heard without agreeing the situation is hopeless.

C. remain silent and still while the individuals are describing their feelings.

D. allow the individuals to structure and lead the group discussion.

176. During a group activity, an OT practitioner observes a client making frequent negative comments pertaining to the collage activity that the group is working on. These comments are MOST likely an indication of:

A. passivity.

B. insecurity.

C. hopelessness.

D. indecision.

177. An OTR with expertise in hand rehabilitation is assessing a COTA's service competency in hand function assessment. At what point is service competency established?

A. When the COTA consistently obtains the same results as the OTR

B. After the COTA passes the NBCOT examination

C. When the COTA has obtained a specified number of continuing education credits in hand rehabilitation

D. After the COTA has practiced for a minimum number of years, as specified by state licensure

Service Management and Professional Practice

178. A senior COTA has been given the responsibility of supervising staff COTAs in an OT department. This means that the:

A. staff COTAs will require only minimal supervision from an OTR.

B. the senior COTA's caseload will be reduced.

C. the senior COTA can redefine the role of COTAs in the department.

D. the senior COTA will evaluate, guide, and teach the staff COTAs.

179. An OTR needs to provide "general supervision" to an experienced COTA in a long-term care treatment setting. As defined by the AOTA, the OTR will have contact with the COTA:

A. once a day.
B. once a week.
C. once a month.
D. as needed.

180. The supervisor of OT is off work and in a local establishment listening to a band with her friends. She observes one of the therapists she supervises at another table being intimate with a gentleman she is currently treating on an outpatient basis. Which of the following actions should the supervisor take in order to be consistent with the OT Code of Ethics?

A. Indicate to the therapist that she may maintain the relationship as long as it does not impair the patient's treatment.
B. Notify the state licensure board and terminate the employee.
C. Notify NBCOT of the situation and reassign the patient to a different therapist.
D. Discipline the employee and refer the patient to another outpatient center.

181. A fieldwork supervisor is completing the final evaluation of a student who is in the last week of level-II fieldwork. In order to successfully complete level-II fieldwork, the supervisor must determine that the student is functioning:

A. slightly below entry level.
B. at or above the minimal entry level of competence.
C. at an intermediate skill level based on the Occupational Therapy Roles.
D. at an advanced skill level based on the Occupational Therapy Roles.

182. An OT practitioner is a member of a treatment team reviewing the treatment options for an individual who is experiencing acute psychiatric symptoms but is not suicidal. This individual has been living with family members. The BEST treatment environment for this individual to receive OT services would be:

A. partial hospitalization.
B. day care.
C. home health care.
D. community mental health center.

183. An individual who has a productive cough is scheduled to have an ADL evaluation by the OTR in an acute care facility. The MOST important action for the OTR to take, according to universal infection precautions, is to:

A. wash hands before and after seeing the client.
B. wear gloves.
C. wash all surfaces the individual comes in contact with before and after.
D. wear gloves, a gown, a mask, and goggles

184. An OT manager in a large department is trying to determine which staff will be able to supervise level-II fieldwork students in the upcoming months. OT practitioners may only be selected to be primary student supervisors if they:

A. are certified OT practitioners with at least 6 months of experience.
B. have at least 1 year of experience as a certified OT practitioner.
C. are certified by the NBCOT.
D. have supervised a level-I student before the level-II student.

185. An OT practitioner is conducting a program evaluation for the quality assurance program in the OT department. The MOST appropriate area for the OT to evaluate would be the:

A. levels of self-care skills attained by clients with head trauma at discharge.
B. number of patient visits in 1 month.
C. pay scale of therapists compared with others in area facilities.
D. annual departmental expenditures on supplies.

186. An OTR is filling out an incident report regarding a patient who was seen on the rehabilitation unit. Which of the following scenarios is the MOST likely to be the subject of an incident report?

A. The patient complained of nausea during a standing activity.
B. A patient with a spinal cord injury indicated that his hand splints were uncomfortable.
C. A patient who had a total hip replacement did not follow precautions while completing dressing activities but did not complain of discomfort.
D. A patient with the diagnosis of a CVA and left neglect caught his left arm in the wheel of the wheelchair, resulting in a cut and bruise.

187. An entry-level OT practitioner wants to know the extent of her liability when providing occupational therapy. Which of the following answers is MOST accurate?

A. Only OTRs need to have liability insurance.

B. Only COTAs need to have liability insurance.

C. Both OTRs and COTAs should have liability insurance.

D. Neither OTR or the COTA need to have liability insurance.

188. A COTA working in outpatient rehabilitation teaches herself how to use paraffin by reading books on physical agent modalities (PAMs), carefully reading the instructions that came with the paraffin bath unit, and practicing on herself for several weeks. Is it now acceptable for this COTA to provide paraffin treatments?

A. No, COTAs may not administer PAMs.

B. No, it violates the OT Code of Ethics.

C. Yes, she has demonstrated service competency.

D. Yes, only when an OTR is on duty in the facility.

189. An individual who has been attending a stress management group led by an OTR/COTA team in a private practice brings along a friend one day. The friend would like to attend the group to learn how to better handle personal stress. This individual, however, does not have a physician's referral. The fee is reasonable, and like the others in the group, this new client will pay out of pocket. Will the OT practitioners be able to accept this new person into the stress management group?

A. No, the OT cannot be provided without a physician referral.

B. Only if the client brings a prescription to the next visit.

C. Yes, because it is a group and not individual treatment.

D. Yes, if the state law does not require a physician referral.

190. Which of the following is the BEST example of the plan section of a discharge summary when using the SOAP note format?

A. "The patient reports intentions to continue to practice proper body mechanics at work."

B. "The patient demonstrates independence in performing the home exercise program."

C. "The patient expressed a desire to return to work but does not yet demonstrate the capacity for the required sitting tolerance."

D. "The patient has been provided with a lumbar support and a written copy of the home program."

191. A home health OT has received a referral for an individual with Medicare coverage. Which one of the following actions must occur before the therapist can initiate evaluation or treatment?

A. Identify the deficits that impair functional abilities

B. Establish short- and long-term goals

C. Obtain a physician's plan of care identifying services to be provided

D. Obtain the individual's history of the current illness

192. An OT practitioner is writing a job description for an aide position in the OT department. According to AOTA guidelines, which of the following is BEYOND the scope of practice of an aide?

A. Cue an individual with schizophrenia to maintain attention to task during a weekly OT-led cooking group

B. Practice use of a sock-aid and shoe-horn in OT department with a patient who has had a hip replacement and is able to perform the task safely but takes an excessive amount of time

C. Help place food on the spoon for a patient practicing the use of a universal cuff in the patient's room at lunchtime, while the OT supervisor runs a lunch group in the dining room

D. Help a child maintain correct positioning during paper and pencil activities while the OT works with the child at the next desk

193. Which of the following inpatient services can be billed as OT services for a client whose hospitalization is covered by Medicare?

A. Treatments from the OT plan provided by an OT practitioner

B. Treatments from the OT plan provided by a music therapist

C. Treatments from the OT plan provided by a recreational therapist

D. Treatments from the OT plan provided by an art therapist

194. An OT practitioner is completing research on patients with hemiplegia and functional return of the upper extremity. The practitioner is attempting to obtain a random sample of patients. Collecting a random sample **MOST** likely means that the therapist will use:

A. the entire population of the facility's stroke patients.

B. all patients who have had a CVA with resulting deficits in the upper extremity function.

C. a numbers table to select the population.

D. a small group of patients who are representative of the population with each individual meeting criteria, which validates that they are a representative subset of the population.

195. At a team planning meeting for a 2-year-old child with multiple handicaps, it is decided that the OT will fulfill the roles of other therapies needed as well. This decision requires a "role release" from the teacher, PT, and speech therapist. Which of the following team approaches for young children does this method describe?

A. Unidisciplinary
B. Multidisciplinary
C. Interdisciplinary
D. Transdisciplinary

196. An OTR and a COTA work in a collaborative relationship. The teamwork between the two professionals is **BEST** exemplified by which of the following examples?

A. The OTR completes the assessment and instructs the COTA to provide a specific intervention.

B. The COTA updates the OTR on the progress a patient has made in the past week, and both provide information to update the goals.

C. The COTA gives a progress note to the OTR and the OTR writes the discharge summary based on the progress note.

D. The OTR tells the COTA what type of equipment to order for a patient and the COTA orders the equipment from a medical equipment company.

197. An advanced-level COTA has expressed interest in taking on some administrative duties in an OT department. Which of the following tasks would be **MOST**

appropriate for the OTR to assign the COTA?

A. Development of a quality-assurance program

B. Supervision of entry-level OTRs and COTAs

C. Supervision of noncertified personnel

D. Development of marketing strategies to promote a new program

198. An instructor from a local nursing school has asked an OTR to speak about OT to a class of first-year nursing students. The OTR feels uncertain about doing the lecture because of a lack of resources. The **MOST** appropriate action for the OTR to take is:

A. recommend to the nursing course instructor that they call AOTA and obtain public relations information to share with her students.

B. decline to do the in-service but send information to the instructor.

C. decline to do the in-service and find an OT to do the lecture.

D. use brochures, posters, videotapes, and films available from the AOTA to enhance the presentation.

199. An OT practitioner has been running a "beauty group" with a group of chronically mentally ill older women. Which of the following is the **MOST** important action to take with the makeup at the end of the session?

A. Put all supplies in a basket to be used next time.

B. Label any supplies used by individuals with communicable diseases with the individual's name and put the rest in a basket.

C. Label lipstick with the individuals' names. Eye makeup and blush can be shared.

D. Label each item with the individuals' names. Cosmetics should never be shared.

200. The OTR is responsible for overseeing the first step in the OT process, which is the referral. Referral practices vary widely from setting to setting, but the OTR needs to know that the type of referrals required are determined by:

A. the AOTA.

B. the American Medical Association.

C. state OT associations.

D. federal, state and local regulations, and third-party payers.

ANSWERS FOR SIMULATION EXAMINATION 4

1. (A) the therapist has the child play "sandwich" between heavy mats. The sandwich activity provides heavy touch pressure over the child's body, which can be inhibitory to a child experiencing sensory defensiveness. Answer B is incorrect because light use of a feather brush stimulates the light touch system, which is already impaired and would be extremely uncomfortable for a child with tactile defensiveness. Answer C is not correct because the use of a blindfold when a child is already reacting to unexpected touch would most likely create a fearful response in a child with tactile defensiveness. Finally, answer D, although not using a blindfold, also has unexpected touch from the back as a characteristic of the game, and this would also be aggravating to the child's existing problem. Answer A, the use of proprioceptive input to break through the protective response to light touch, will initially treat the child's defensiveness problem instead of stimulating further reaction. See reference: Kramer and Hinojosa (eds): Kimball, JG: Sensory integration frame of reference: theoretical base, function/dysfunction continua and guide to evaluation.

2. (A) The time he spends at the computer Because computer work requires very little active movement and the lower extremities, trunk, and neck are generally held in a static position, it is essential to assess how much time the child spends in this position. The OT practitioner needs to instruct the child to take regular breaks and maintain proper positioning while at the computer to avoid further strain. Answers B, C, and D address other relevant factors in computer use but none that would directly produce the symptoms described. See reference: Ryan (ed): The Certified OT Assistant: Ryan SE, Ryan BJ, and Walker, JE: Computers.

3. (A) age appropriate. The child being observed is performing dressing activity which is age appropriate for child of 5 years. A typical child at this age can dress unsupervised and is able to tie and untie knots but generally does not know how to tie a bow independently. See reference: Case-Smith (ed): Shepherd, J: Self-care and adaptations for independent living.

4. (B) stressing bilateral activities incorporating the prosthesis. Two-handed activities for play, school, and self-care should be used to incorporate the prosthesis into the child's body image. Avoiding the use of the prosthesis (as suggested in answers A, C, and D) is counterproductive. See reference: Pedretti (ed): Rock, LM, and Atkins, DJ: Upper extremity amputations and prosthetics.

5. (D) child, caregiver, and therapist priorities. The problems established in the OT evaluation are not the only basis for writing OT goals and objectives. The child's priorities as well as the caregiver's needs

and concerns must be addressed so that immediate needs are met and there is a commitment on everyone's part to the success of the program. See reference: Case-Smith (ed): Richardson, PK, and Schultz-Krohn, W: Planning and implementing services.

6. (A) fluctuating. Children with athetoid CP have fluctuating muscle tone (answer A), which usually fluctuates from low to normal. Spastic muscle tone is characteristic of children with spastic CP (answer B). Flaccid muscle tone (answer C) or low muscle tone is usually seen in young children with CP and usually is later classified as spastic, athetoid, or ataxic. Rigid muscle tone is characterized by tonic muscle activity that does not fluctuate; therefore, answer D is incorrect. See reference: Case-Smith (ed): Rogers, SL, Gordon, CY, Schanzenbacher, KE, and Case-Smith, J: Common diagnosis in pediatric OT practice.

7. (D) flushing, blanching, or perspiration. These responses are autonomic nervous system signs of sensory overload. Answers A, B, and C are not correct because they do not describe autonomic responses to the activity. See reference: Case-Smith (ed): Parham, LD, and Mailloux, Z: Sensory integration.

8. (A) a body length prone scooter. Spastic diplegia is defined as abnormal tone affecting all four extremities but with primary involvement of the lower extremities; therefore, the child may use his upper extremities to propel himself through space while having his lower extremities positioned on the scooter. The airplane mobility device (answer B) is designed for children with good lower extremity function who need support in the upper body. A tricycle (answer C) requires good lower extremity control, including reciprocal movement. A power wheelchair (answer D) is designed for individuals with limited upper and lower extremity function. See reference: Case-Smith (ed): Wright-Ott, C, and Egilson, S: Mobility.

9. (C) reducing competing sensory input—use head phones during work. Reducing competing sensory input is helpful in increasing visual attention. Increasing competing input (answers A and B) or reducing the amount of visual input (answer D) may serve to reduce the ability to attend. See reference: Case-Smith (ed): Schneck, CM: Visual perception.

10. (D) After the development of the goals and objectives "Once short- and long-term goals have been agreed upon, an implementation plan must be made regarding how to provide services to meet these goals most effectively" (p. 256). See reference: Case-Smith (ed): Richardson, PK, and Schultz-Krohn, W: Planning and implementing services.

11. (B) Let the child sit at the front of the bus and use a tape player and earphones A child who is seated in the front of the bus will experience less jostling by peers, resulting in less tactile and visual stimulation. Also, the earphones will serve to reduce auditory overload. The method described in answer A is the only one that addresses the underlying problem of the child's low tolerance for sensory stimulation. Answers A, C, and D are behavioral management techniques that do not take the child's hypersensitivity into account. See reference: Case-Smith (ed): Cronin, AF: Psychosocial and emotional domains.

12. (B) Medicaid. Medicaid is a joint federal and state program. Because it is a joint program, benefits vary widely from state to state. In each state, the Medicaid program must include Aid to Families with Dependent Children (AFDC) and Supplementary Security Income (SSI). Medicare (answer A) is a federal program that funds health coverage for individuals 65 years of age or older, disabled individuals, and people in the end stages of renal disease. Workers' compensation (answer C) is a state-supported program funded by employer contributions. Beneficiaries receive coverage for services identified as covered within their respective states. The Education for All Handicapped Children Act (answer D) mandates programs funded in part through state and federal grants. It does not fund health care but requires any school receiving federal assistance to provide handicapped children with a free, appropriate education in the least restrictive environment. See reference: AOTA: The OT Manager: Thomas, VJ: Evolving health care systems: Payment for OT services.

13. (B) "The child demonstrated tongue thrust." "Tongue thrust" is an objective, well-defined term. The other answers are less objective. Answer A infers the child's emotional reaction. Answer C implies voluntary control and judges behavior. Answer D interprets data based on insufficient evidence. See reference: Early: Medical records and documentation.

14. (D) accommodation. Visual accommodation is the ability to focus efficiently from near to far distance, and vice versa. Answer A, ocular motility, refers to the ability to pursue an object visually in an efficient and smooth manner. Answer B, binocular vision, is the ability to focus the eyes on an object at varying distances and on seeing a single object clearly. Answer C, convergence, is the ability to move the eyes inward or outward with continued focus on the object. See reference: Kramer and Hinojosa (eds): Todd, VR: Visual information analysis: Frame of reference for visual perception.

15. (D) plan section. The plan section of a SOAP note includes statements related to continuing treatment; the frequency and duration of the treatment; suggestions for additional activities or treatment

techniques; the need for further evaluations; and, when needed, recommendations for new goals. The subjective portion of a SOAP note (answer A) refers to what the patient reports or comments about the treatment. The objective portion of the SOAP note (answer B) focuses on measurable and/or observable data obtained by the OT practitioner through specific evaluations, observations, or use of therapeutic activities. The assessment part of a SOAP note refers to the effectiveness of treatment and any changes needed, the status of the goals, and justification for continuing OT treatment. See reference: Borcherding: Writing the "P"—Plan.

16. (C) Prone over a wedge Considering the information given, answer C is the best answer because head control is isolated, with the trunk supported. The child does not have adequate control to stand in a standing frame (answer A). Answer B is not correct because, although the chest is supported by a sling, the child's shoulders, arms, and hips must be able to control the position. Sitting on the therapy ball (answer D) would require both head and trunk control. See reference: Case-Smith (ed): Nichols, DS: Development of postural control.

17. (B) form constancy perception. Form constancy perception is the ability to match similar shapes regardless of change in their orientation in space. Figure-ground perception (answer A) is the ability to distinguish the bead from the background. Position in space perception (answer C) is the ability to determine the spatial relationships of the beads to each other. Visual sequencing (answer D) is an activity that requires the ability to copy the same sequence of beads. Although these abilities are all required for this bead-stringing task, the error described refers to a form constancy error. See reference: AOTA: Uniform Terminology for OT, third edition.

18. (D) perform slow push-ups against the wall. Having the child perform push-ups against the wall is an activity which provides joint compression of the upper extremities with motor activity—a combination which will have a normalizing effect on the nervous system. Answers A and C are not correct because they emphasize additional tactile input. Answer B is not correct because it emphasizes slow vestibular input. See reference: Kramer and Hinojosa (eds): Kimball, JG: Sensory integration frame of reference: theoretical base, function/dysfunction continua, and guide to evaluation.

19. (D) shallow spoon. The use of a shallow spoon encourages the development of upper lip control because it makes it easier for the lip to remove all of the food on the spoon. It would be more difficult for the child to get food off a deep spoon (answer C). Straws (answer A) can be used to develop sucking. A spork (answer B) is a device that combines the qualities of a fork and a spoon and is useful if the child can only manage one utensil. See reference: Case-Smith (ed): Case-Smith, J, and Humphry, R: Feeding intervention.

20. (C) Parents should be considered as part of a collaborative partnership with therapists. "The first interactions of the therapist with a family open the door to establishing a partnership" in which "the family and therapist collaborate using agreed upon roles to obtain agreed upon goals for the child" (p.117). Parents should be encouraged to observe their child in therapy so that they may better understand the program and their child's problems; therefore answer A is incorrect. Answer B is incorrect because although some parents may carry out therapy programs at home, "the goal is not for parents to become quasiprofessionals" (p. 117). It is also recommended that both parents be present when an OT program is discussed (answer D is incorrect), so that one does not become dependent on the other for information and communication. See reference: Case-Smith (ed): Humphry, R, and Case-Smith, J: Working with families.

21. (C) Combine task with additional sensory input (tactile, proprioceptive, and auditory). Answer C is correct because additional sensory input, when combined with a visual memory task, facilitates memory. Answer A is not correct because interest in the task should be high in order to enhance visual memory. Answer B is not correct because visual attention is a prerequisite to visual memory. Answer D is incorrect because serial or varied repetition enhances visual memory. See reference: Kramer and Hinojosa (eds): Todd, VR: Visual information analysis: Frame of reference for visual perception.

22. (D) sitting position. Answer D is correct because the upright sitting position provides the child with the opportunity not only to further control head movement (stability has developed in horizontal positions), weight bearing, and weight shifting, but to rotate the trunk as he or she reaches toward the opposite side of the body. Answers A and B are not correct because head and neck stability have most likely developed primarily in the prone and sidelying positions before the child's attaining a seated position. See reference: Kramer and Hinojosa (eds): Schoen, SA, and Anderson, J: Neurodevelopmental treatment frame of reference.

23. (A) Chaining Chaining with a child who demonstrates a cognitive disability shows the entire process of a task with all sequences. Initially, the child performs only the beginning or end of the task. Thus, the child initially concentrates on only a small part of the task and gradually increases participation in all sequences in their correct order. Answers B, C, and D are other methods that can be used, but forward and backward chaining are instructional methods that have been particularly successful with individu-

als who are mentally retarded. See reference: Early: Medical and psychological models of mental health and illness.

24. (A) Within 6 months, the client will participate in classroom activities for 1 hour without disruptive outbursts, twice a day. A functional goal relates the skill to be developed to a child's environment or life tasks, therefore making it more meaningful to the child and the family. Answers B, C, and D are measurable but not functional goals, because they do not address the context in which the skill is applied. See reference: Case-Smith (ed): Richardson, PK, and Schultz-Krohn, W: Planning and implementing services.

25. (D) Provide a therapy ball to sit on while the child is playing a game of checkers Answer D is the only one that contributes to the development of postural background movement. This is done by requiring the client to continually adjust to the subtle movements of a usable surface on an ongoing basis. Answers A, B, and C provide additional external support—that is, they provide adaptations using a compensatory approach rather than facilitating the development of new skills. See reference: Case-Smith (ed): Nichols, DS: The development of postural control.

26. (B) decreased muscle tone. Decreased muscle tone is usually characterized by joints that are lax and hyperextensible. Low muscle tone and joint hyperextensibility are also frequent characteristics of Down syndrome. Answer A is incorrect because loss of range of motion would be the joint characteristic of increased muscle tone. Answers C and D are incorrect because they are diagnoses that cannot be made on the basis of joint laxness, even though instability at the joint may occur with either of these conditions. The observation of joint hyperextensibility is merely an indication of below normal muscle tone and not necessarily the indication of a specific condition or disease process. See reference: Kramer and Hinojosa (eds): Colangelo, CA: Biomechanical frame of reference.

27. (B) a local wheelchair equipment vendor. Although any community resource may be helpful to a child and family with a severe physical disability, answer B is correct because of the possible breakdown in this piece of equipment, which has already been purchased. The OT practitioner needs to consider this possibility and provide local support for a problem solution. Therefore, although answers A, C, and D may serve as resources for other needs of the child, only a specialist in wheelchair equipment will be able to solve mechanical problems that arise. See reference: Case-Smith (ed): Wright-Ott, C, and Egilson, S: Mobility.

28. (D) applesauce. Foods with even consistency, uniform texture, and increased density such as applesauce are the easiest to control and swallow. Foods with multiple textures like chicken noodle soup (answer A), sticky foods like peanut butter (answer B), and foods that are fibrous or break up in the mouth like carrot sticks (answer C) should be avoided. See reference: Case-Smith (ed): Case-Smith, J, and Humphry, R: Feeding intervention.

29. (D) Block out all areas of the page except important words Answer D is correct because this compensatory technique is a way of dealing with visual figure-ground or visual discrimination problems. The child needs to learn how to rule out extraneous stimuli and focus on the important area of a task, such as reading. Answer A is not correct because this is a technique used to orient the child with left-right visual tracking problems. Answer B is not correct because it is a technique used to deal with visual attention problems. Answer C is not correct because it is a technique used to help children deal with visual memory problems. See reference: Kramer and Hinojosa (eds): Todd, VR: Visual information analysis: Frame of reference for visual perception.

30. (A) Modifying the environment to protect the infant from overstimulation and inappropriate stimuli Answers B and D represent traditional OT rehabilitation with an emphasis on specific diagnoses, developmental delay, immature sleep-wake state acquisition, limited range of motion, and splint fabrication. This approach will continue to be of importance within the NICU. The developmental support care approach, however, has expanded the traditional rehabilitation model to include and focus upon a protective and preventative component, which best defines OT in the NICU at the present time. Therefore, answer A best describes a protective and preventative approach to intervention in the NICU. Answer C, educating parents and staff, is a crucial aspect of both the traditional rehabilitation model and the Developmental Support Care approach to implementing services in the NICU. However, it is not the best descriptor of an OT's scope of practice. See reference: Case-Smith (ed): Hunter, JG: Neonatal Intensive Care Unit.

31. (C) IEP The individual education plan is a form that must be completed for children receiving services in the school system. This documentation standard was defined in the Education of the Handicapped Act (1975 and 1986). The UB-82 form (answer A) is used to process insurance claims. FIM (answer B), which stands for "functional independence measure" is a method used on rehabilitation units to measure an individual's level of independence. The HCFA-1500 form (answer D) is used to bill Medicare and other insurance carriers for health care services. See reference: Neistadt and Crepeau (eds): Perinchief, JM: Management of OT services.

32. (B) mounting a safety rail next to the toilet. In order to sit independently on the toilet and relax

sufficiently to control muscles needed for elimination, the child has to feel posturally secure. Safety rails next to the toilet, low toilets that allow the child to put both feet on the ground, and reducer rings to decrease the size of a toilet seat all help to provide maximal stability for the child with unstable posture. Answers A, C, and D describe adaptations used for other deficits. Replacing zippers and buttons with Velcro closures (answer A) is helpful for a child with reduced strength or fine motor coordination. Introducing toilet paper tongs (answer C) helps increase reach in a child with limited range of motion. Placing a colorful target (answer D) helps boys aim into the bowl, a difficulty associated with perceptual or cognitive limitations. See reference: Case-Smith (ed): Shepherd, J: Self care and adaptations for independent living.

33. (B) radial-digital grasp. Children usually develop a radial-digital grasp at age 9 months; they use the grasp for precision control. A pincer grasp (answer A), or tip pinch, is characterized by opposition of the thumb and index fingertips to allow the child to make a circle with the fingers. The palmar grasp (answer C) is a power grasp, in which the individual flexes the fingers around an object while stabilizing it against the palm. In a lateral pinch (answer D), the individual places the pad of the thumb against the radial side of the index finger near the DIP joint. This pattern is used as a power grip on small objects. See reference: Case-Smith (ed): Exner, CE: Development of hand skills.

34. (D) Scoop dish This is the most correct answer because the sides of the scoop dish provide a shape that aids the scooping movement. A high back to the plate provides a surface to push the food against to aid in getting the food onto the spoon. The swivel spoon (answer A) helps primarily when supination is limited. The nonslip mat (answer B) helps stabilize the plate itself, and the mobile arm support (answer C) positions the arm and helps the weak shoulder and elbow muscles to position the hand. See reference: Case-Smith (ed): Case-Smith, J, and Humphrey, R: Feeding intervention.

35. (C) Backward chaining In backward chaining, the OT practitioner completes all of the steps except the last one. As the child becomes competent, the practitioner completes all but the last two steps and so on, until the child is able to perform the entire activity. This method provides immediate gratification and is particularly useful for children with low frustration tolerance and poor self-esteem. Physical guidance (answer A) requires the least amount of cognitive ability and provides the child the opportunity to learn through a sensory motor experience. Verbal cues (answer B) may be perceived as intrusive and critical by children with low self-esteem. Forward chaining (answer D) begins with the child's completing the first step and the practitioner's completing the rest. When competent, the child progressively takes on more of the steps and the practitioner does fewer. This method is beneficial for individuals who have difficulty with sequencing and generalizing skills. See reference: Case-Smith (ed): Shepherd, J: Self-care and adaptations for independent living.

36. (D) motor planning. Motor planning or praxis problems are often seen in young children when they are dealing with novel equipment. Motor planning requires an adequate body concept and the ability to cognitively plan movements. Fine motor skills (answer A) are required for dexterity and manipulation and are not required for mounting a rocking horse. In order to climb into the highchair and jump on a trampoline, the child must have integrated reflexes (answer C) and adequate gross motor skills (answer B). See reference: AOTA: Uniform Terminology for OT, third edition.

37. (A) Arrhythmic and unexpected Sensory integration treatment is complex and highly individualized and must be monitored carefully to observe the effects of sensory input of varying types on the individual. The characteristics of facilitatory sensory input are unexpected, arrhythmic, uneven, or rapid input. Answer B is not correct because, although arrhythmic input is excitatory, slow sensory input is inhibitory. Sustained and slow sensory input (answer C) is inhibitory, not facilitatory. Answer D is incorrect because, although facilitatory input is unexpected, rhythmic input is inhibitory. See reference: Bruce and Borg: Movement-centered frame of reference.

38. (A) Swimming Swimming provides active movement through wide ranges of motion with minimal impact on the joints. The sports in answers B, C, and D involve bouncing, jumping, and kicking, which place additional stress on the joints. Resistive activities such as these, which place the joints under additional stress, would be contraindicated. See reference: Neistadt and Crepeau (eds): Newman, EM, Echevarria, ME, and Digman, G: Degenerative diseases.

39. (B) Moro reflex. The Moro reflex is characterized by abduction, extension, and external rotation of the arms. The rooting reflex (answer A) is the turning of the head toward tactile stimulation near the mouth. The flexor withdrawal reflex (answer C) is characterized by flexion of an extremity in response to a painful stimulus. The neck righting reaction (answer D) involves body alignment in rotation after turning of the head. Only the Moro reflex causes an extension movement. See reference: Neistadt and Crepeau (eds): Kohlmeyer, K: Evaluation of performance components.

40. (A) exploratory play. Exploratory play provides children with experiences that develop body scheme, sensory integrative and motor skills, and concepts of sensory characteristics and actions on objects. Therefore, the obstacle course is an example of ex-

ploratory play. Symbolic play is associated with the development of language and concepts (use of "dress-up" materials would be an example of this type of play). Creative play and interests are characterized by refinement of skills in activities that allow construction, social relationships, and dramatic play (finger painting is an example of creative play). Recreational play is leisure experiences that allow the exploration of interests and roles such as arts and crafts or sports. See reference: Case-Smith (ed): Morrison, CD, and Metzher, P: Play.

41. (A) pull-to-sit, leaning back against therapy ball. While all answers involve antigravity control, answer A addresses beginning control in neck and shoulders. Since control develops cephalocaudally, neck and shoulder control should be addressed first. By using an incline, the pull of gravity can be reduced, thus facilitating maximum control. See reference: Case-Smith (ed): Nichols, DS: The development of postural control.

42. (D) praise her for what she does well; reinforce her independence. Since the child has just achieved independence in spoon feeding, she may still need frequent reinforcement of the new skill. It is more effective to encourage her for what she does well than to point out her mistakes (answer B). To provide assistance either by using a hand-over-hand technique (answer A) or by feeding her as a reward appears to be counterproductive and may cause her to lose independence in this skill. See reference: Ryan (ed): Practice Issues in OT: McFadden, SA: The child with mental retardation.

43. (C) the cultural context and family interaction patterns. Cultural expectations may determine behavior standards and the expression of family roles. Continued feeding of a young child with a handicap may be the expression of nurturing and caring. Such an expression may be viewed as more important than the promotion of independence and self-reliance. Answers A, B, and D may be valid issues as well, but should be addressed after the OT has familiarized himself or herself with the cultural and familial context of the feeding process. See reference: Case-Smith (ed): Case-Smith, J, and Humphry, R: Feeding intervention. Also, Shepherd, J: Self care and adaptations for independent living.

44. (C) school newspaper. Anxiety disorder is characterized by extreme self-consciousness and anxiety about competence. Public exposure and pressure for on-the-spot performance heighten the anxiety. By becoming involved in the newspaper preparation, the student will have an opportunity to develop a sense of competence without the pressure of a face-to-face audience and judged competition, as represented by activities described in answers A, B, and D. See reference: Case-Smith (ed): Cronin, AF: Psychosocial and emotional domains.

45. (B) raising the handle bars. The correct answer is B because raising the handle bars demands that the arms are raised, thus bringing the child to the upright posture. Answers A and C are not correct because the hips and lower extremities are already positioned correctly and this positioning would be disrupted. Answer D is not correct because the arms would be lowered and trunk forward flexion would be increased. See reference: Kramer and Hinojosa (eds): Colangelo, CA: Biomechanical frame of reference.

46. (C) Provide a screen to reduce peripheral visual stimuli Although all the answers describe techniques that could assist the student, the use of a carrel is most appropriate in a mainstreamed classroom, because the other methods or adaptations (answers A, B, and D) could have a negative impact on the other children's ability to learn. See reference: Case-Smith (ed): Schneck, CM: Visual perception.

47. (C) significantly delayed by several months. Answer C is correct because at 6 months of age, a child should initiate head flexion when pulled into a sitting position. The child assists with pulling of the arms and some trunk flexion or use of the abdominals at this age. Usually by 2 months of age, an infant is beginning to assist with being pulled to sit with some head flexion. Answers A, B, and D are not correct because they do not address the significance of the child's delay in head control. See reference: Neistadt and Crepeau (eds): Kohlmeyer, K: Evaluation of sensory and neuromuscular performance components.

48. (C) recommend activities to develop fine coordination that teachers can incorporate into classroom programming. Recommending classroom activities that will develop the performance component of fine coordination would be the best population-based intervention since it involves addressing the occupational performance needs of many students. Answers A, B, and D focus OT efforts toward individual intervention approaches. See reference: AOTA: Guide To OT Practice.

49. (D) weight bearing over a small bolster in prone. Weight bearing on the arms can help with overall inhibition of tone before participating in hand skill activities. Inhibition of flexor spasticity occurs through slow joint compression from weight bearing, as well as facilitation of ulnar to radial function in the hand. Answers A and B are incorrect because they require voluntary control of release of objects without inhibition. Answer C is incorrect because traction on the finger flexors would increase spasticity in the flexor muscles and make opening of the hand more difficult. See reference: Case-Smith (ed): Exner, CE: Development of hand skills.

50. (D) Provide a vertical work surface where

writing and other hand skills can be practiced A vertical work surface encourages an upright posture, upper body strengthening, and eye-hand coordination. A horizontal work surface (answer C) would result in a hunched posture during writing activities. A distraction-free environment (answer B) is helpful for children who are easily distracted, but there is no indication this child requires such an accommodation. Pulling out the child to an OT room (answer A) when adaptations can be made that allow the child to fully participate would be counterproductive to the philosophy of an inclusive setting. See reference: Neistadt and Crepeau (eds): Erhardt, RP, and Merrill, SC: Neurological dysfunction in children.

51. (C) The client should enroll in a work-hardening program. Work-hardening programs are designed to "incorporate job-specific work tasks that progress the client to the physical demand levels of the actual job" (p. 380). Continuing to perform her home program (answers A and D) or discontinuing OT services would probably not enable the client to return to the work force after a 3-month absence. Home health OT (answer B) is appropriate for individuals who are unable to leave their homes to attend outpatient therapy. See reference: Ryan (ed): Practice Issues in OT: Engh, J, and Taylor, S: Work hardening.

52. (A) An electric razor An electric razor is the safest for shaving because a rotary head or foil, instead of a blade, is in contact with the skin. Any shaving over the incision area or near it would not be recommended until the incision area is healed. The other razors have blades that could nick or cut the skin, which would need to be avoided until the patient is no longer treated with blood thinners and normal blood coagulation can occur. See reference: Trombly (ed): Trombly, CA: Retraining basic and instrumental activities of daily living.

53. (D) provide a sensory cue, such as saying "stop!" The use of auditory, visual, or tactile sensory cues can help the person with Parkinson's disease to change the motor program in which they are engaged. Deep breathing exercises (answer A), practicing of movements (answer B), and mentally reviewing steps in the sequence of movement (answer C) will not provide the sensory information needed at the moment to evoke movement or change a "frozen" movement pattern. See reference: Trombly (ed): Newman, EM, Echevarria, ME, and Digman, G: Degenerative diseases.

54. (D) maintain a normal curve of the back, slowly shifting feet as the turn is completed. A correct transfer is performed slowly with the knees bent and the feet a shoulder width apart, while the normal curve of the back is maintained and the lifting is performed with the legs. The body should not be twisted at the trunk (answer A), as this could injure the back. Lifting with the arms (answer B), instead of the legs could also injure the therapist's back. Another way of injuring the back during a transfer is to keep the feet planted when moving (answer C) because this causes twisting of the back and may damage the knees. See reference: Palmer and Toms: Body mechanics and guarding techniques.

55. (C) Modify the activity to make it less challenging. The practitioner should recognize subtle signs of fatigue, such as frustration, slowing down, hurrying to finish, lessening range of motion, and use of substitution movements, which indicate the training level was too difficult and should be downgraded. Other signs include the heart rate's exceeding the target heart; increase of more than 20 bpm above resting pulse; failure to return to resting heart rate after a 5-minute rest; systolic pressure that does not increase at all or that increases more than 20 mm Hg from baseline. Stopping the activity (answer A) is necessary if the individual experiences symptoms such as dyspnea, chest pain, lightheadedness, or diaphoresis. The activity should be upgraded (answer B) only when the individual is able to perform the activity without signs of fatigue or cardiac symptoms. Isometric exercises (answer D), which interfere with bloodflow through the muscles and create a heightened demand on the cardiovascular system, should not be used in individuals with cardiac conditions. See reference: Dutton: Introduction to biomechanical frame of reference.

56. (A) the use of energy conservation. Energy conservation techniques reduce the amount of energy expenditure an individual requires to perform various activities. For a client with COPD and limited endurance, energy conservation techniques should be taught early so they can be implemented and reinforced while performing other activities, such as preparing meals. Work-hardening (answer B) and graded activities to increase strength (answer C) would not address the need to perform meal preparation in the most energy efficient manner. Safety in the kitchen (answer D) would be more relevant to individuals with sensory or balance loss than limited endurance. See reference: Trombly (ed): Atchison, B: Cardiopulmonary diseases.

57. (B) detachable armrests. Armrests need to be removed to allow the individual to move sideways out of the chair. Footrests (answer A) may be swung away but do not need to be detached to perform a transfer. Antitip bars (answer C) prevent a wheelchair from tipping over backwards (such as when performing a wheelie or when going up or down a step), but not when transferring. Brake handle extensions (answer D) allow the brakes to be locked more easily but would be in the way of a board transfer. See reference: Pedretti (ed): Adler, C, and Titon-Burton, M: Wheelchair assessment and transfers.

58. (B) 33 to 36 inches This is the proper height for grab bars to allow for the upper extremities to lift

the body with enough clearance to transfer onto the toilet seat. A height of 28 to 31 inches (answer A) would be too low to allow the body to clear the toilet seat when the arms are straightened. A height of 38 to 41 inches or 43 to 46 inches (answers C and D) would be too high to effectively push down with the arms to lift the body onto the toilet seat. See reference: Rothstein, Roy, and Wolf: American's with disabilities act and accessability issues.

59. (A) canister vacuum cleaner. A canister vacuum cleaner may be managed by someone with weakness and balance problems while the person is sitting. The hose is light enough to be easily pushed, and the canister is on wheels and may be moved by a seated person pushing it with the foot or having someone move it for him or her. An upright vacuum cleaner is too heavy for repetitive pushing and pulling, and its use can cause exhaustion or pull the person off balance. A self-propelled vacuum cleaner could also pull a person off balance by moving too fast for the person to respond with appropriate postural adjustments. A handheld vacuum cleaner requires too much stooping to do anything but a very small area of the floor, because repetitive bending can cause fatigue quickly and challenges decreased balance. See reference: Trombly (ed): Stewart, C: Retraining housekeeping and child care skills.

60. (A) "Pt. reports overall pain levels are lower and ability to perform ADL has improved." The subjective section of the discharge summary should indicate "whether the patient believes the goals set were achieved and whether the patient feels ready to function at home" (p. 35). Answers B and D are subjective reports but do not indicate the patient's perception of any changes in status. Answer C is an example of a statement that belongs in the assessment section of a discharge summary. See reference: Kettenbach: Writing subjective (S).

61. (D) "Pt. has improved significantly in his ability to work at the computer by using periodic stretch breaks." The assessment section of a discharge summary identifies the functional performance deficits and indicates whether they have been resolved or, if they still exist, to what degree. Answer C is a subjective report. Answer A is an example of a statement that belongs in the objective section of a discharge summary. Answer B belongs in the plan section. See reference: Kettenbach: Writing assessment (A).

62. (D) Burn hand splints prevent stress on the tendons and ligaments, decreasing edema. Burn hand splints prevent stress on the superficial tendons and ligaments, decreasing edema secondary to the avoidance of dependent positioning. Answer A, decreasing pain and allowing for active range of motion, is not correct because of the immobilizing nature of the static splint. Answers B, prevent scarring, and C, prevent skin grafting, are not primary reasons for using burn hand splints. See reference: Neistadt and Crepeau (eds): Rivers, EA, and Jordan, CL: Skin system dysfunction: Burns.

63. (D) chaining. Teaching a task one step at a time, gradually adding more steps as steps are mastered, is called chaining. Chaining is frequently used when teaching a multistep task because it is easier to learn one step at a time than it is to learn a complete activity. Repetition and rehearsal (answers A and C) involve repeating the whole activity repetitively until the activity is learned. Cueing (answer B) uses an external source to remind a person of the next step or part of that step. See reference: Zoltan: Executive functions.

64. (A) Monitor the individual's response to activities to prevent him from performing at activity levels that are too high and unsafe. "Denial is a common defense mechanism in [individuals with] coronary artery disease because of the vague characteristics of symptoms and the hidden nature of the disability. At times, denial is considered a healthy response, and health professionals must be careful not to strip the patient of this coping mechanism by forcing the patient to face reality [answer C] too quickly... Careful monitoring of a patient's activities is important at this time to protect the patient from performing at unsafe, higher activity levels" (p. 698). This individual, because of his denial, is unlikely to be willing to learn or apply energy conservation techniques (answer B), which can benefit him. The OT should attempt to understand and modify the individual's behavior through collaborative goal setting and patient and family education before referring him for psychological services. See reference: Pedretti (ed): Matthews, MM, Foderaro, D, and O'Leary, S: Cardiac dysfunction.

65. (C) By learning to use a sliding board with car transfers Using a sliding board with all functional transfers is the primary way to educate a client with paraplegia to perform independent car transfers. Answers A and B, teaching a family member to assist and using public transportation, would not constitute an independent car transfer. Answer D, tenodesis, would not be implicated as a strategy to use with individuals with paraplegia. See reference: Pedretti (ed): Adler, C, and Tipton-Burton, M: Wheelchair assessment and transfers.

66. (B) "Scoot forward to the edge of the wheelchair." When the therapist has the individual scoot forward to the edge of the wheelchair, this helps the individual position the body over the feet and causes the weight to shift forward during a transfer. The individual is much easier to transfer when the weight is shifted forward. If the person attempts to stand up (answer A) from a regular seated position, and the weight is shifted back during a transfer, the individual may require more than one person to assist with the transfer or it may be a total lift by one or more in-

dividuals. Answer C, unfasten the wheelchair brakes, is incorrect because the wheelchair needs to be stabilized in a locked position before standing. Positioning the wheelchair facing the mat table (answer D) allows no room for the therapist to stand and assist with the pivot. See reference: Palmer and Toms: Body mechanics and guarding techniques.

67. (C) biomechanical. The biomechanical approach uses voluntary muscle control during performance of activities for people with deficits in strength, endurance, or range of motion. The biomechanical approach focuses on decreasing deficits in order to improve performance of daily activities. The neurophysiological approach (answer A) is applied to individuals with brain damage. Emphasis is on the nervous system and methods for eliciting desired responses. The neurodevelopmental approach (answer B) also focuses on the nervous system, but emphasizes eliciting responses in a developmental sequence. The rehabilitative approach (answer D) is to teach a person how to compensate for a deficit on either a temporary or permanent basis. See reference: Trombly (ed): Zemke, R: Remediating biomechanical and physiological impairments of motor performance.

68. (B) A call system for emergency and non-emergency use A call system for emergency and nonemergency use. A call system is necessary for a person with a high-level spinal cord injury to allow the caretaker to leave the room, but remains available to answer the person's call for assistance for daily needs or an emergency. This is frequently the first opportunity that a person with a spinal cord injury would have to control some part of his or her life, giving some feeling of independence or choice. An ECU does allow independence in operating appliances, lights, and so on through the use of switches or voice control but would not be a necessity for safety. A remote control power door opener that would allow a caretaker to enter would be useless if the person is unable to call for assistance. An electric page turner is useless without the ability to call for someone to position or replace reading material. See reference: Trombly (ed): Dow, PW, and Rees, NP: High-technology adaptations to overcome disability.

69. (D) has good UE range of motion but difficulty accessing small targets. A large keyboard would be best for someone who has good range of motion but difficulty accessing small targets. A person with limited range of motion but adequate fine coordination (answer A) would benefit from a smaller or contracted keyboard. If someone fatigues rapidly when reaching for the keys (answer B), having to reach further on a large keyboard would cause more fatigue. A large keyboard would be more difficult for a person using one hand (answer C), because the hand would have to move farther to complete typing, adding more work to the process. See reference:

Pedretti (ed): Cook, AM, and Hussey, SM: Electronic assistive technologies in OT practice.

70. (C) get the shirt all the way on, then line up the buttons and holes and begin buttoning from the bottom. It is easier to see the buttons and buttonholes at the bottom of the shirt than at the top (answer B); therefore, beginning to button from the bottom is more likely to result in success for the individual with motor or visual-perceptual deficits. Buttoning first (answer A) may result in ripping off the buttons as the shirt is pulled over the head. A buttonhook with a built-up handle (answer D) would be helpful for an individual with finger weakness or incoordination (e.g., quadriplegia), not hemiparesis. See reference: Pedretti (ed): Foti, D, Pedretti, LW, and Lillie, S: Activities of daily living.

71. (B) sip-and-puff switch. A sip-and-puff switch allows control through respiration: blowing air into and sucking air out of a straw positioned in front of the mouth activates the switch. This method would be particularly appropriate for a client with no functional movements. Answers A and C, joysticks and single digital switches, require mechanical activation through movement of some part of the body—hand, foot, head, chin. Answer D, mouth sticks, are usually used for direct access on keyboards or on ECU control panels. See reference: Neistadt and Crepeau (eds): Bain, BK: Assistive technology in OT.

72. (A) elevate the arm on pillows so it rests higher than the heart. Elevation, contrast baths, retrograde massage, pressure wraps, and active range of motion are effective methods for managing edema. When massaging an edematous extremity, stroking should be performed from the distal area to the proximal, not the reverse (answer B). Because active and PROM can both be beneficial to managing edema (answers C and D) instructing the patient to avoid range of motion activities would be incorrect. See reference: Pedretti (ed): Kasch, MC: Hand injuries.

73. (B) Explain to the patient and caregiver that one must be "homebound" in order to be eligible for home care services. In order to be eligible for home care services, the patient must be confined to home, a condition referred to as homebound. The patient need not be bedridden, but leaving the residence must require a considerable or taxing effort. Absences from the home are permitted but must be infrequent in nature, short in duration, or for the purpose of receiving medical treatment. Given that this patient is able to leave the home for a social visit and tolerate riding in a car for 30 minutes, he is not considered homebound. The OT practitioner would first inform and explain this criteria to the patient and caregiver (answer B). After this has been explained, the OT practitioner would communicate with the PT (answer D) and refer the patient for outpatient therapy (answer C). Simply providing a home

program and discharging the patient would not meet the patient's needs because he continues to required therapeutic intervention. See reference: Piersol and Ehrlich (eds): Zahoransky, M. The system and its players.

74. (D) a raised-bed garden. The individual with back pain must avoid activities that stress the lumbar spine such as "prolonged static postures with a flexed lumbar spine, repetitive bending with a flexed spine, and lifting and carrying when the normal lumbar curve is not maintained" (p. 723). A raised-bed garden would allow gardening without bending. A wheelbarrow with elongated handles (answer B) would be harder to control while pushing than a wheelbarrow with normal handles and would place undue stress on the low back. A 12-inch-high seat with tool holders could benefit an individual with low endurance, but working on the ground from that position would be very difficult for an individual with back pain. See reference: Pedretti (ed): Smithline, J: Low back pain.

75. (C) Provide lateral trunk support A lateral trunk support in the frontal plane stabilizes the side, helping to maintain correct alignment of the pelvis and trunk in the chair by counteracting the twisting effect of asymmetrical muscle tone. By providing upper extremity support, the lateral trunk support would also prevent improper loading onto an unstable shoulder joint. Using a reclining wheelchair (answer A) is incorrect because doing so would shift the client's weight to the posterior but would not prevent the lateral shift of the trunk. An arm trough (answer B) may help maintain a more centered position of the trunk, but the weight of the affected extremity would result in instability and improper alignment of the shoulder, which could lead to shoulder pain. A lateral pelvic support (answer D) would provide stabilization of the pelvis to prevent it from shifting sideways, but this support would be too low to prevent the trunk from moving laterally. See reference: Neistadt and Crepeau (eds): Dutton, R: Treatment of performance components.

76. (B) Sliding board transfer Sliding board transfers, or push-up-and-over transfer techniques, are the safest and most efficient technique when transferring to a tub seat. Answer A, stand pivot transfers, would only be effective with unilateral amputations or crutches and answer C, dependent lifting, would not address independent transfer training with the client; neither would answer D, not initiating transfers until the client is fit with prosthetics. See reference: Pedretti (ed): Adler, C, and Tipton-Burton, M: Wheelchair assessment and transfers.

77. (D) incoordination. A person who has tremors or poor coordination could limit much instability by stabilizing the limb proximally before working distally. Stabilization adds a secure base of support from which to work. Reduced vision, poor endurance, and limited fine movement would not require stabilization when writing, but they would require stronger contrast of guiding lines or ink on paper, more frequent rests, or built-up writing tools. See reference: Trombly (ed): Trombly, CA: Retraining basic and instrumental activities of daily living.

78. (B) use a guiding technique: place food in the resident's hand and bring it to the mouth. Use of a guiding technique is particularly effective because the person receives sensory cues that something is approaching the face ahead of time. This can facilitate opening of the mouth. Answer C, wiping food particles off a person's face, is not recommended until after the person swallows, as this can start a reflexive opening of the mouth and interfere with eating. Answer A, clearing food pocketed in the resident's cheeks, should be performed by the person themselves, not the therapist. Allowing the resident to select what food or beverage they prefer (answer D) would not have a particular effect on a resident who is tactilely defensive. See reference: Larson, Stevens-Ratchford, Pedretti, and Crabtree (eds): Foti, D: Evaluation and interventions for the performance area of self-maintenance.

79. (A) remedial treatment, such as rubbing or stroking the involved extremity. When sensation begins to return, it is appropriate to initiate remedial activities for sensory retraining. Stimulating the involved extremity by rubbing or stroking (to provide tactile input) or through weight-bearing activities (to provide proprioceptive input) are examples of remedial activities. Compensatory activities, which are essential for individuals with decreased or absent sensation, would have been part of the original treatment plan. Answers B, C, and D are all examples of compensatory strategies. See reference: Pedretti (ed): Evaluation of sensation and treatment of sensory dysfunction.

80. (D) observe for signs of pain, redness, and irritation, then discontinue use and report to therapist. Of the answers listed, the most important aspect of splint education is the need of monitoring splinted skin areas for presence of problems related to splint use, such as pain, redness, blisters or skin irritations, which can lead to injury. If such signs exist the next step is to discontinue use of the splint and report the problem to the therapist, who can then reevaluate the splint. Answer A, teaching the client to bend or modify the splint themselves would be inappropriate, could make the splint ineffective or cause injury. Poor cosmesis (answer B) would be an inadequate reason to discontinue splint use. Splint care instructions (answer C) are important to maintain the splint but are much less of a priority than informing the patient about precautions. See reference: Neistadt and Crepeau (eds): Wylett-Rendall, J.: Treatment of performance components.

81. (A) provide verbal cues, external aids such as calendars and family pictures, and opportunities to practice using the external aids. Verbal cues, external aids, and opportunities to practice using the external aids would be most appropriate for clients with deficits in orientation. Answer B, reducing distractions, and answer C, presenting information in short units, would be adaptive strategies to promote attention and information processing. Answer D, connecting new information to previously held knowledge and skills, is a technique to aid retrieval of information and improve memory. See reference: Unsworth (ed): Schwarzberg, S: Clinical reasoning with groups.

82. (B) Use heavy utensils, pots, and pans Heavy kitchen items increase stability for individuals with incoordination. Other suggestions include using prepared foods, nonskid mats, easy-open containers, serrated knives, and tongs. Built-up handles (answer A) are useful for individuals with limited grasp. A high stool (answer C) benefits those who fatigue easily. Placing the most commonly used items on shelves just above and below the counter (answer D) is a useful way to adapt the environment for individuals with limited reach. See reference: Pedretti (ed): Foti, D, and Pedretti, LW in Self-care/home management.

83. (A) soft to hard to rough. Hypersensitivity stimuli is graded by texture and force. Texture begins with soft, progresses to hard, and moves to rough. The force begins with touch, progresses to rub, and moves to tapping. The texture and force of the stimuli are graded together. Light, medium, and heavy do not specify what the texture and force of the stimuli would be during training. A person with hypersensitivity would be unable to tolerate training beginning with a rough texture. See reference: Trombly (ed): Bentzel, K: Remediating sensory impairment.

84. (A) Prevent loss of joint and skin mobility During the acute stage, when burn wounds are partial or full thickness in nature, maintenance of joint range of motion and skin mobility is the primary goal of intervention. Providing adaptive equipment (answer B) is typically performed during the surgical or postoperative stage, and compression and vascular garments (answer C) and the prevention of scarring (answer D) are goals most commonly implemented during the rehabilitation phase. See reference: Pedretti (ed): Jordan, CL, and Allely, RR: Burns and burn rehabilitation.

85. (A) Holding the hammer Holding the hammer is the only activity listed that requires gripping with the entire hand. Holding the stamping tools and needle (answers B and D) requires pinch patterns. Squeezing the sponge (answer C) offers less resistance than holding the hammer and would therefore be less effective for strengthening. See reference: Breines: Folkcraft.

86. (D) Weaving on a frame loom Use of and attention to the entire loom area is essential for weaving on a frame loom. The shuttle must slide across the entire width of the loom, which involves crossing the midline. It is possible to build a coil pot (answer A), to make macramé objects (answer B), and string beads for a necklace (answer C) without crossing the midline. See reference: Breines: Folkcraft.

87. (D) Eggs Eggs provide a uniform texture and density. Answers A, B, and C are all foods that are contraindicated in those with dysphagia diets because vegetable soup and salad (answers A and B) provide too many textures, and watermelon (answer C) because of the seeds. See reference: Pedretti (ed): Nelson, KL: Dysphagia: Evaluation and treatment.

88. (C) environmental modification. Environmental modification is the area of intervention that can best assist in maintaining safety and supporting function at home by providing the physical and sensory environments to compensate for deficits. Strength and endurance activities (answer A) will have no direct affect on safety in the home. Cognitive rehabilitation techniques (answer B) are not indicated for conditions with progressive cognitive deterioration. Use of assertiveness skills (answer D) would be inappropriate for dealing with the kinds of communication problems encountered with persons who have Alzheimer's. See reference: Pedretti (ed): Atachison, P, Pedretti, LW, McCormack, GL: Alzheimer's disease.

89. (B) flaccidity. Flaccidity, or hypotonicity, is often present immediately after a stroke and may later change to spasticity (answer D) or increased muscle tone. The flaccid extremity feels heavy and hangs limply at the individual's side. The weight of the arm may eventually pull the humerus out of the glenohumeral joint, resulting in subluxation (answer C). Answer A is inadequate because paralysis may be accompanied by either flaccidity or spasticity. See reference: Pedretti (ed): Undzis, MF, Zoltan, B, and Pedretti, LW: Evaluation of motor control.

90. (A) isometric muscle contractions. Isometric muscle contraction involves contracting the muscle without joint movement or a change in muscle length. Isotonic contractions (answer B) shorten the muscle length with accompanying joint movement. Progressive resistance (answer C) is a type of isotonic exercise that uses an increase in weight during consecutive exercise repetitions. A person who has a cast obstructing movement would be unable to perform either type of isotonic exercise. Passive movements (answer D) are performed by an outside force to the arm and involve joint motion but no muscle contraction. Passive movement could not be performed with a casted joint. See reference: Pedretti (ed): Pedretti, LW, and Wade, IE: Therapeutic modalities.

91. (B) figure-ground perception. Figure-ground perception is the ability to visually separate an object from the surrounding background. An example of this would be an individual's having the ability to find a button on a plaid shirt. A problem with spatial relations is seen in dressing when a person overestimates or underestimates the need for reaching when attempting to button buttons. The person is unable to judge the relationship between the object and the body. Body image is a mental picture of the person's body that includes how the person feels about the body. Visual closure is the ability to recognize an object even though only part of it is seen, for example, recognizing a partially covered button. See reference: Zoltan: Visual discrimination skills.

92. (A) work locks and latches on doors and windows. The ability to manipulate the locks and latches is a safety concern because the individual may be unable to open them to let family members into their home or close them to keep intruders from entering. Built-up handles (answer B), energy conservation techniques (answer C), and adaptations to clothing fasteners (answer D) are not safety issues. See reference: Trombly (ed): Feinberg, JR, and Trombly, CA: Arthritis.

93. (C) Minimizing scar hypertrophy through compression garments and proper skin care Minimizing scar hypertrophy through compression garments and proper skin care is imperative upon wound closure. Answer A, preventing scar formation via static splinting, is typically performed during the surgical or postoperative phase of treatment. Controlling edema (answer B) and promoting self-care skills (answer D) are not goals directly related to scar management and are commonly initiated during acute care intervention. See reference: Pedretti (ed): Jordan, CL, and Allely, RR: Burns and burn rehabilitation.

94. (A) "Client will purchase 10 items at the supermarket with supervision." Short-term goals must relate to the long-term goal being addressed. Since the long-term goal being addressed is independence in grocery shopping, the short-term goal must relate to grocery shopping. Answers B and C do not relate to grocery shopping. "Goals need to be written to show what the patient will accomplish, not what the therapist will do" (p. 94). Answer D is an appropriate treatment intervention but is written in a way that describes what the OT, not the client, will do. See reference: AOTA: Effective documentation for OT.: Writing goals.

95. (C) Ability to consistently follow hip precautions Many factors are considered when a short-term goal is reset. These factors may include items such as consistency of performance, cognitive or perceptual impairments, the amount of time required, and any change in attention or concentration. For the short-term goal to be changed, the individual needs to be able to demonstrate a consistency of performance in the use of hip precautions, because improved performance in the dressing has already been demonstrated. The amount of time needed or concentration have not been problems or they would have been part of the original goal. The ability to use the adaptive equipment appropriately has also been demonstrated. See reference: Trombly (ed): Trombly, CA: Planning, guiding, and documenting therapy.

96. (D) fracture to the distal radius. A fracture to the distal radius is most commonly referred to as a Colles' fracture. Colles' fractures are one of the most frequent injuries to the wrist. These fractures "may result in limitations in wrist flexion and extension, as well as pronation and supination resulting from the involvement of the radioulnar joint" (p. 669). Answers A, B, and C are not anatomically representative of a Colles' fracture. See reference: Pedretti (ed): Kasch, MC: Hand injuries.

97. (D) Obtain a narrower wheelchair because this one is too wide. The recommended wheelchair seat width is 2 inches wider than the widest point across the hips and thighs of the seated individual. If the seat is 2.5 inches wider than the patient (answer A), it is too wide, not too narrow. In addition, "wheelchairs should be as narrow as possible while allowing for comfort, ease of repositioning, and transfers" (p. 605). The narrower the wheelchair, the easier it is to maneuver. Because a narrower wheelchair would be better, padding the sides (answer C) is a less desirable option. The need to lose or gain weight (answer B) should be discussed first with a patient's physician. In this client's situation, losing weight would result in a worse wheelchair fit. See reference: Trombly (ed): Deitz, J, and Dudgeon, B: Wheelchair selection process.

98. (B) Implement a pureed diet and allow adequate time for eating As ALS progresses, speaking and swallowing become more difficult and a pureed diet becomes necessary. The individual runs the risk of aspiration or choking if meals are rushed. Adaptive equipment (answer A) is provided much earlier in the disease process. The independence achieved with adaptive equipment has a positive psychological effect on the individual who sees his or her independence slipping away. See reference: Pedretti (ed): Pedretti, LW, and McCormack, GL: Amyotrophic lateral sclerosis.

99. (B) hyperextension of the PIP joint and flexion of the DIP joint. Answer B is the only answer provided that describes a swan-neck deformity. The pattern of hyperextension of the PIP and DIP joints (answer A) may be seen in lower-motor-neuron palsies. Flexion of the PIP joint and hyperextension of the DIP joint (answer C) is descriptive of a boutonniere deformity. An individual who has overstretched the volar plates at the PIP and DIP joints would have

hyperextension of the MP joint and flexion of the DIP joint (answer D). See reference: Pedretti (ed): Hittle, JM, Pedretti, LW, and Kasch, MC: Rheumatoid arthritis.

100. (C) cumulative trauma disorders. Cumulative trauma disorders are viewed as a mechanism of injury for tendonitis, nerve compression syndromes, and myofascial pain because of the nature of repetitive strain and motion disorders. Answer A, osteoarthritis disorders, frequently present with stiffness, redness, and edema. Answer B, peripheral vascular disease, is unrelated to the diagnoses mentioned in the question and is more commonly associated with the vascularity of the client. A neuroma (answer D) is specifically related to an amputation, nerve injury or suture. See reference: Pedretti (ed): Kasch, MC: Hand injuries.

101. (B) below the MCP joints. The MCP joints are stabilized proximally, or below the MCP joints, to isolate the joint movement being measured and to eliminate any combined movements. Answers A, above the MCP joints, and C, at the wrist, would allow combined movements of the joints and would invalidate the individual joint measurements. Answer D, on top of the MCP joints, would block joint movement and make any individual joint measurements incorrect. See reference: Norkin and White.

102. (D) pressure marks or redness from the splint should disappear after 20 minutes Many types of splints may be made without the fingers flexed, or the thumb opposed and abducted: for example, an antispasticity ball splint or a dynamic splint for extension. Most splints are not worn at all times but are removed for activities such as self-care or exercise. A therapist issues a wearing schedule when a splint is fitted or given to a patient. All splints that are made or given to a patient are checked for correct fit by adjusting any areas that still have redness or pressure marks after the splint has been removed for 20 minutes. See reference: Trombly (ed): Linden, CA, and Trombly, CA: Orthoses: Kinds and purposes.

103. (B) pinch meter. A pinch meter is used to measure the strength of a three-jaw-chuck grasp pattern (also known as palmar pinch), as well as key (lateral) pinch and tip pinch. For each of these tests, the individual performs three trials, which the tester averages together; the result is compared to a standardized norm. An aesthesiometer (answer A) measures two-point discrimination. A dynamometer (answer C) measures grip strength, and a volumeter (answer D) measures edema in the hand. See reference: Trombly (ed): Trombly, CA: Evaluation of biomechanical and physiological aspects of motor performance.

104. (D) Airplane and burn hand splint Airplane and burn hand splints are typically seen in the treatment of patients with burn injuries, especially when the wounds involve the crossing of a joint. The burn hand splint prevents ligamentous stress at the interphalangeal joints while aiding in the reduction of edema, and the airplane splint maintains the shoulder in 90 degrees of abduction in attempts to prevent contracture development at the axillary region. Answer A is incorrect and is often contraindicated because of the nature of a resting splint's placing too much stress on the extensor tendon mechanism of the hand. Answers B and C are splints that are occasionally used in burn centers, (with the exception of the posterior neck splint, which is contraindicated; it is common to see anterior neck splints) but are primarily fabricated in settings not specific to burn care intervention. See reference: Neistadt and Crepeau (eds): Rivers, EA, and Jordan, CL: Skin system dysfunction: Burns.

105. (A) carpeting with low or looped pile. Carpeting with low pile would be the best choice for an elderly person who may be prone to falls because it provides the fewest tripping hazards and provides a sense of security during walking. Answer B, a wood floor, is a hard surface that can be slippery and hazardous for someone who may fall easily. Answer C, area rugs, would not be recommended because of the potential for tripping on the rug edges. Answer D, carpeting with deep pile and padding may be comfortable and provide cushioning if the person does fall, but can add resistance or "drag" when walking and present an additional tripping hazard. See reference: Larson, Stevens-Ratchford, Pedretti, and Crabtree (eds): Christenson, MA: Environmental design, modification and adaptation.

106. (D) strength. Exerting enough pressure to twist off the lid requires strength. He demonstrates adequate range of motion (answer A) when he grasps the knife. He demonstrates adequate coordination (answer B) by spreading peanut butter on the bread and accurately positioning the lid onto the jar opening. He demonstrates adequate endurance (answer C) by standing during the entire activity of making a peanut butter sandwich. See reference: AOTA: Uniform Terminology for OT, third edition.

107. (A) clearly direct a caregiver in preferred head position, food portion size, and choice of food to eat. An individual with C3 quadriplegia lacks the strength necessary to use an MAS or any cuff device (answers B, C, and D). It is important for this individual to be able to instruct a caregiver how to assist with feeding in a manner that is pleasant and enjoyable. See reference: Christiansen (ed): Garber, SL, Gregorio, TL, Pumphrey, N, and Lathem, P: Self-care strategies for persons with spinal cord injuries.

108. (B) dressing apraxia. To some extent, dressing apraxia is a result of impaired awareness of the affected side and the relation of body parts to the clothing, as well as difficulty with assembly of the clothing onto the body. Difficulty with spatial relations (answer A) is a problem with awareness of the relationship of one's self to another object. A person with anosognosia (answer C) is unaware of any deficits. Figure-ground discrimination (answer D) is the ability to distinguish an object from its background. See reference: Trombly (ed): Quintana, LA: Evaluation of perception and cognition.

109. (C) have the individual visualize the task first and then provide general statements such as "Let's get ready." Answer C is correct because visualizing a task and its movement sequences helps the individual with motor apraxia by giving a visual model to refer to during the activity. Using general comments such as "Let's get ready" rather than specific step-by-step directions is more effective because individuals with motor apraxia have difficulty imitating or initiating motor tasks on command, though they understand the concept of the task. Answer A, step-by-step commands, would add to the confusion for an individual with motor apraxia but would be helpful for the individual with ideational apraxia who may not understand the concept of the task but may be able to perform individual steps of the task on command. Removing visual distractions and enhancing the visual environment, as in answer C, is useful for individuals with visual perceptual deficits rather than motor apraxia. Answer D, having the individual move slowly and touch objects during the task, is a method aimed at improving spatial relations' perception. See reference: Gillen and Burkardt (eds): Rubio, KB: Treatment of neurobehavioral deficits.

110. (B) Use a walker Ambulatory aids may be used to substitute for lost motion, reduce weight bearing on the lower extremities, or widen the base of support to increase stability. An individual with a balance deficit requires a wider base of support, which is provided by walkers and quad canes. A standard cane (answer A) is effective for reducing weight bearing, and does not provide as much stability as a walker or quad cane. This individual is ambulatory; therefore, working on meal preparation from a wheelchair (answer C) in a home without kitchen modifications would create an unnecessary hardship. See reference: Dutton: Rehabilitation postulates regarding intervention.

111. (D) Ice application, immobilization, and splinting Ice, immobilization, and splinting are all interventions that are considered to be appropriate adjunct activities to be used during the acute stages of tennis elbow. Answers A, B, and C, are all contraindicated because of their potential to increase edema, pain, and immobility. See reference: Cailliet: Elbow pain.

112. (C) fair minus (3-). The definition of fair minus (3-) is that the part moves through incomplete range of motion (< 50%) against gravity or through complete range of motion with gravity eliminated against slight resistance. A grade of good (4), answer A, indicates strength on the manual muscle test and ability to move through full range of motion against gravity and to take moderate resistance. A fair grade (3), answer B, would be the ability to move through the full range of motion and against gravity but not take any additional resistance. A grade of poor plus (2+), answer D, would move through full range of motion with gravity eliminated and take minimal resistance before suddenly relaxing. See reference: Trombly (ed): Trombly, CA: Evaluation of biomechanical and physiological aspects of motor performance.

113. (C) take the individual's vital signs at rest. First, vital signs should be taken at rest. The individual should then perform an activity while being monitored by the OT practitioner for any signs or symptoms (answer B). The third step is to take vital signs again immediately after completion of the activity (answer A). The final step is to retake vital signs after the individual has rested for 5 minutes (answer D). This process provides the OT practitioner with baseline information about the individual's endurance level. See reference: Dutton: Introduction to biomechanical frame of reference.

114. (B) perform the evaluation over several sessions. Upper extremity evaluation is lengthy and can be fatiguing, and fatigue should be avoided with individuals with Guillain-Barré syndrome. In addition, results may be invalid if the individual is fatigued and not performing at the highest level possible. Strength, range of motion, and sensory testing (answers A, C, and D) are all important when evaluating an individual with Guillain-Barré syndrome, but must be administered using a method that will yield valid results. See reference: Pedretti (ed): McCormack, GL, and Pedretti, LW, in Motor unit dysfunction.

115. (C) dysphagia. Dysphagia is the inability to swallow. Answer A, deglutition, is the term used to describe the normal process of consuming liquids and solids. Answer B, dysmetria, "is the inability to estimate how much motion is required to reach a desired target" (p. 160). Answer D, dysarthria, is best described as slurred speech secondary to cerebral lesions. See reference: Pedretti (ed): Nelson, KL: Dysphagia: Evaluation and treatment.

116. (C) the client is receiving nasal tube feedings. Nasal tube feedings (or nasal gavage) is a process of feeding that is introduced through a tube that enters the nasal passage and leads to the stomach. Answers A, thin liquid feedings; B, stage I foods only; and C, pureed foods only, are all considered to be oral feedings. See reference: Pedretti (ed): Nelson, KL: Dysphagia: Evaluation and treatment.

117. (A) using effective communication skills. Clarifying expectations, honestly defining needs, and providing tactful and constructive feedback are communication skills that promote understanding. Successful communication with the patient's children will most likely help them deal with their fears and concerns, increase their understanding of their father's condition, and elicit greater cooperation. Although time management techniques, deep breathing, and laughter (answers B, C, and D) are all useful and valid stress reduction techniques, they do not address the issue at hand, which is communication between the father and his children. See reference: Neistadt and Crepeau (eds): Giles, GM, and Neistadt, ME, in Treatment for psychosocial components: stress management.

118. (D) washing windows. Washing windows is a repetitive activity that involves resisted, elevated upper extremity activity. Rests can be taken as needed. Vacuuming, peeling potatoes, and polishing furniture (answers A, B and C) do not provide adequate resistance to achieve upper extremity strengthening. See reference: Dutton: Introduction to biomechanical frames of reference.

119. (C) swimming in a cool water pool. Swimming is an excellent activity for promoting physical fitness, and the cool water pool (temperature under 84 degrees) will prevent the overheating that is contraindicated for individuals with MS. Jogging and volleyball (answers A and D) are both likely to result in overheating, and volleyball would probably fatigue weak hand muscles. Painting (answer B) is a lightweight activity that would probably appeal to an artist, but would do very little to promote physical fitness. See reference: Pedretti (ed): Hietpas, J, Hooks, ML, Atchison, P, et al, in Degenerative diseases of the central nervous system.

120. (D) "Family will demonstrate independence in current positioning and feeding techniques." Goals should be functional, measurable, and objective. In addition, short-term goals must relate to the long-term goal being addressed. This answer meets those criteria. Answer A does not provide measurable criteria, nor does it directly relate to the long-term goal of family training. Answer B, while measurable, does not relate to the long-term goal. Answer C describes the long-term goal of family independence in the feeding program. See reference: AOTA: Effective documentation for OT.: Moorhead, P, and Kannenberg, K: Writing functional goals.

121. (D) Touch The senses included in the somatosensory system are touch, movement, pain, and temperature. The auditory, olfactory, visual gustatory, and vestibular systems are special systems that directly give input into the brain. The somatosensory system has receptors located throughout the body (muscles, tendons, ligaments, joints, skin, and so forth). In the brain, receptors are located in the thalamus, cortex, and brain stem. Receptors also exist in certain tracts of the spinal cord. See reference: Trombly (ed): Woodson, AM: Stroke.

122. (B) Two A person in stage two of Brunnstrom's levels of recovery demonstrates weak, associated movements, usually in a flexor synergy; there may be little or no finger flexion. A person in stage one, flaccidity (answer A), has no movement or spasticity on the affected side of the body. In stage three (answer C), all movements occur in synergy, spasticity is present and mass grasp is present in the affected hand. In stage four (answer D), spasticity begins to decrease, there is some deviation from synergistic patterns, and lateral prehension and partial finger extension may be present in the hand. See reference: Pedretti (ed): Pedretti, LW: Movement therapy: The Brunnstrom approach to treatment of hemiplegia.

123. (D) Playing balloon volleyball An activity such as balloon volleyball may be graded for improving strength by adding resistance to the arm in the form of weights. Endurance may be improved by adding more repetitions of the movement. Raising the height of the net can increase the range of motion required. Blowing up and tying balloons (answer A) and painting faces on balloons (answer B) are primarily fine motor activities. An individual who throws darts at balloons (answer C) would be able to increase the resistance needed for shoulder strengthening by adding weight to the arms or using balloons with thicker rubber. However, there would not be an appropriate method to increase the number of repetitions necessary for improving endurance because the repeated noise would be annoying. See reference: Pedretti (ed): Pedretti, LW, and Wade, IE: Therapeutic modalities.

124. (A) training to inspect for pressure sores on bony prominences and affected areas. Visual inspection of an area is important to prevent pressure sores, which may develop because there are no sensory cues to alert a person to the skin breakdown. It is recommended that an individual with absent sensation not trim his or her own nails (answer B) because of safety issues. Another person may be able to assist by trimming the nails or the individual could file his or her own nails; however, the second option is often difficult and time consuming. Extra padding on a splint (answer C) would cause increased pressure and redness to an area, which would lead to skin breakdown. Hypersensitivity training (answer D) is performed with exaggerated sensation, not absent sensation. See reference: Trombly (ed): Bentzel, K: Remediating sensory impairment.

125. (C) Provide transfer tub bench and install grab bars The best adaptation to achieve access to the tub would be providing the client with a transfer tub bench, which is recommended for individuals who cannot step over the edge of the tub, and bathroom grab bars to provide stability during the move into the tub. Answer A, repositioning the light switch would help to enhance visual cues and safety. Providing long-handled adaptive devices (answer B) would enhance bathing performance, if the person had difficulty with reaching the legs and feet. Answer D, nonskid decals and mats are also a safety measure to prevent slipping and falling. See reference: Pedretti (ed): Smith, P: Americans with Disabilities Act: Accommodating persons with disabilities.

126. (A) using the strongest joint, avoiding positions of deformity, and ensuring correct patterns of movement. The significance of using these principles for individuals with preexisting joint conditions and adverse musculoskeletal changes may help to restore function as well as prevent further impairments. Answers B, C, and D involve common muscle relaxation and stress management techniques not related to joint protection techniques. See reference: Trombly (ed): Bear-Lehman, J: Orthopaedic conditions.

127. (D) present important principles in small units that are spaced at a slower than normal pace. According to learning principles for older adults, learning will be more effective if the information is presented in small units at a slower pace. Answer A is incorrect because learning will be impeded if information is presented too quickly and in large chunks. Answer B is incorrect because presentations that are highly organized will enhance retention of information more than loosely structured presentations. Attempts to persuade clients on points which may not be in agreement of the older adult's preconceived ideas, values, or habits may also impede learning (answer C), where a more collaborative approach may result in better learning of concepts. See reference: Larson, Stevens-Ratchford, Pedretti, and Crabtree (eds): Stevens-Ratchford, RG: OT services within the rehabilitation health care system.

128. (B) Reposition the person in the wheelchair to allow optimal range of motion. When a person in a wheelchair who uses an augmentative communication device suddenly begins making errors, it is necessary to FIRST check the position of the individual. Improper positioning could result in the wheelchair's interfering with access or with range of motion needed to use the communication device. A person may eventually need to be referred to a physician for a physical examination (answer A); however, it is best for the therapist to first problem solve and seek a solution if the person's medical status has not changed. The person's communication abilities would not be reassessed (answer C) until the person has been optimally positioned in the wheelchair. A communication device would only need to be replaced (answer D) if there were a mechanical problem within the system causing the errors that could not be fixed. See reference: Angelo and Lane (eds): Taylor, SJ, and Kreutz, D: Powered and manual wheelchair mobility.

129. (C) 10 degrees of head flexion from the midline. When an individual's neck is kept at 10 degrees of flexion past midline, this closes the passage to the lungs, but allows food to easily pass down the esophagus. Answers A and B both involve extension of the neck, which should be avoided as this opens the passageways to the lungs and may cause choking or aspiration. Answer D, extreme flexion of the head, narrows the passageway to the stomach and causes a feeling of food sticking in the throat. See reference: Pedretti (ed): Nelson, KL: Dysphagia: Evaluation and treatment.

130. (B) Avoid internal rotation and adduction of the involved hip Following hip arthroplasty, positions such as flexion of the hip past a prescribed range (usually 60 to 90 degrees), internal rotation, and adduction can result in dislocation of the hip. Therefore, this answer is the priority. OT practitioners instruct patients in hip precautions and provide them with adaptive equipment so they can safely perform self-care, work, and leisure activities. Answers C and D may help an individual comply more easily with hip precautions. Sitting during LE dressing (answer A) is also recommended. See reference: Pedretti (ed): Morawski, D, Pitbladdo, K, Bianchi, EM, Lieberman, SL, Novic, JP, and Bobrove, H: Hip fractures and total hip replacement.

131. (B) weight bearing through the upper extremity in sitting or standing. Weight bearing is the most effective way of normalizing tone, according to the NDT treatment approach for adult hemiplegia. Placing a weighted cuff on the extremity (answer A) would have the effect of increasing muscle tone, making reaching more difficult. Answer C, using only the unaffected upper extremity would accomplish the reaching task, but would not normalize muscle tone in the affected upper extremity. Answer D, "forced use" is a treatment concept used to encourage functional motor return in hemiplegic upper extremities, but is not a method designed to normalize muscle tone, nor is it a specific technique of the NDT treatment approach. See reference: Pedretti (ed): Davis, JZ: Neurodevelopmental treatment of adult hemiplegia: The Bobath approach.

132. (B) a hook provides better prehensile function and allows greater visibility of objects. The fact that a hook TD provides better prehensile function and allows greater visibility of objects would be the most important consideration for a person whose primary concern is functioning as a carpenter. Answers A, C, and D are incorrect, because though they can be important considerations for some people with UE amputations, they are not as relevant to this person's goals. See reference: Pedretti (ed): Rock, LM, and Atkins, DJ: Upper extremity amputations and prosthetics.

133. (C) Toothbrush with built-up handle An individual with C7-8 quadriplegia has the hand strength to hold a toothbrush with a built-up handle. An alternate method can be to position the toothbrush between the fingers. An individual with a C5 injury may require an MAS for brushing teeth (answer A). Other individuals with injuries at the C5-6 level may be able to use a universal cuff (answer B) or a wrist support with a utensil holder (answer D) to hold the toothbrush. See reference: Christiansen (ed): Garber, SL, Gregorio, TL, Pumphrey, N, and Lathem, P. Self-care strategies for persons with spinal cord injuries.

134. (C) attending a rehabilitation program in a skilled nursing or extended care facility. The most appropriate recommendation for this person is to receive rehabilitation in a skilled nursing or extended care facility because the patient requires rehabilitation services provided at a lower level of intensity but has the goal of returning home. An intensive inpatient rehabilitation program (answer A) requires a person to tolerate 3 hours minimum per day, which would be unlikely for this patient. Answer B, extending the patient's stay in the acute care hospital, is not possible because the length of stay is usually determined by third-party payers, and patients are discharged once medically stable. Answer D, seek nursing home placement, is incorrect because this person has the potential to become sufficiently independent to return home. See reference: Neistadt and Crepeau (eds): Freda, M: Facility-based practice settings.

135. (B) Increase the number of towels from 10 to 20 Endurance is improved by increasing the number of repetitions so the muscle has to work over a longer period of time. Placing towels on a higher shelf (answer A) would help to increase range of motion. Placing towels on a lower shelf (answer C) decreases the difficulty of the activity and does not lengthen the period of time needed to improve endurance by providing more repetitions. The arm could be strengthened by adding a 1-pound weight (answer D), but that would not increase the repetitions needed to improve endurance. See reference: Pedretti (ed): Pedretti, LW, and Wade, IE: Therapeutic modalities.

136. (D) Aesthesiometer People with sensory loss in the hand often drop things because they are not receiving adequate sensory input. An aesthesiometer measures two-point discrimination with a moveable point attached to a ruler that has a stationary point at one end. The dynamometer (answer B) and pinch meter (answer C) are both used to measure strength. An individual with a loss of strength would drop heavy, not lightweight items. A goniometer (answer A) is a tool with two arms used to measure movement at a joint. One arm is held stationary while the other arm moves around an axis of 360 degrees. See reference: Pedretti (ed): Kasch, MC: Hand injuries.

137. (B) activity adaptation. Modifying how directions are provided is one way to adapt activities. Activity analysis (answer A) is the process of identifying the aspects, steps, and materials used in performing the activity. Grading activities (answer C) is a gradual progression of steps toward a goal. Clinical reasoning (answer D) is the problem-solving process that practitioners use in thinking about a client's treatment. See reference: Early: Analyzing, adapting, and grading activities.

138. (C) Implement compensatory strategies to manage the environment Interventions directed toward improvement are typically unrealistic when working with individuals diagnosed with cognitive disorders. These disorders are characterized by deteriorating courses. A social skills emphasis (answer A) is more appropriate for individuals with schizophrenia. Habit restructuring (answer B) is more appropriate for those with substance use disorders. Role resumption (answer D) is more appropriate for those with mood disorders. See reference: Early: Understanding psychiatric diagnosis: the DSM-IV.

139. (B) emotional lability. Emotional lability is the rapid shifting of moods. Emotional lability may be one of the symptoms observed in individuals experiencing mania (answer A). Paranoia (answer C) describes enduring beliefs about being harmed. Denial (answer D) is not acknowledging the presence of information. See reference: Early: Responding to symptoms and behaviors.

140. (A) Controlled stimulation with meaningful sensory cues An environment that provides controlled stimulation with visual, tactile, and auditory cues that are meaningful to the resident is preferable because it will best facilitate correct perception of the environment. Difficulty in perceiving or misunderstanding environmental cues can lead to behavioral problems or agitation. Environments that are too stimulating (answer B) or too unstimulating (answer C) can increase confusion. Answer D is incorrect because while dementia units should have a homelike atmosphere, and residents should have familiar objects near them to maintain links with memories, the more important consideration in overall environmental design is to incorporate the special environmental adaptations that will enhance function. See reference: Larson, Stevens-Ratchford, Pedretti, and Crabtree (eds): Christenson, MA: Environmental design, modification, and adaptation.

141. (B) teaching the person to use a diary or log. Compensation techniques are used to work around a deficit area by using alternative methods to accomplish the same task. Teaching the use of a diary or log is an example of an external memory aid which provides cues to compensate for memory deficits. Answers A and C are incorrect because they are examples of internal memory strategies (retracing and rehearsal) which rely on mental effort by the person. Answer D, use of a memory training computer program, is a technique for remediation of memory skills and, therefore, not an example of a compensation method. See reference: Trombly (ed): Quintana, LE: Remediating cognitive impairments.

142. (D) Assess the individual's topographical orientation skills. In order to plan an appropriate intervention, the individual's community mobility skills must first be assessed. Constantly getting lost is a strong indicator that the individual may be impaired in the area of topographical orientation. Learning to take the bus and obtaining a library card (answers A and C) are important steps toward independent library use but should occur after evaluation has been completed. Individuals may enjoy using a library whether they can read or not, so the ability to read is not essential to this goal and does not need to be evaluated (answer B). See reference: Early: Activities of daily living.

143. (C) Hallucinations The symptoms of schizophrenia are generally classified as either negative or positive. Negative symptoms tend to persist after the positive, or acute, symptoms are treated with medications. Negative symptoms greatly impact an individual's level of functioning. Answers A, B, and D are all negative symptoms. See reference: Early: Understanding psychiatric diagnosis: The DSM-IV.

144. (D) the measurability of activity performance. The potential to measure an activity's results is central to a behavioral frame of reference. Answer A is linked to developmental frames of reference, answer B is linked to psychoanalytic frames of reference, and answer C is linked to sensory integrative frames of reference. See reference: Neistadt and Crepeau (eds): Crepeau, EB and Neistadt, ME: Activity analysis: A way of thinking about occupational performance.

145. (C) applying grout to a tile trivet and waiting for it to dry. Activities provide a variety of opportunities for therapeutic gains. The process of grouting a tile trivet involves covering the individual's tile design with the grout mixture and is a messy step. The individual then sees that the tile pattern is emphasized with the addition of the grout. Waiting for the grout to dry requires an individual to delay gratification. See reference: Neistadt and Crepeau (eds): Crepeau: Activity analysis, a way of thinking about occupational performance.

146. (B) remote memory. The ability to recall events from one's distant past is remote memory and is commonly assessed through verbal interviews and informal testing, such as this question about an individual's recall of childhood events. Retention (answer A) is determined by giving the individual information and asking about the same information a few minutes later. Orientation (answer C) is determined by asking about the current time and date. Recent memory (answer D) is determined by asking about meals eaten that day. See reference: Neistadt and Crepeau (eds): Golisz, KM, and Toglia, JP: Evaluation of perception and cognition.

147. (D) Ask the employer to provide an isolated cubical as the work space An isolated cubical is a reasonable accommodation for an individual who is highly distractible. The Americans with Disabilities Act (ADA) requires employers to provide reasonable accommodations for individuals with documented disabilities that will enable them to work despite the disability. A job coach (answer A) is more appropriate for an individual who needs frequent cueing or assistance to perform the job. Frequent breaks (answer B) are a reasonable accommodation for individuals with anxiety who need to manage stress. Although explaining the problem of distractibility to the employer (answer C) may provide useful information and open the lines of communication with the employer, it does not offer a solution. See reference: Early: Work, homemaking and childcare.

148. (D) Arrange for the patient to attend a discharge group to discuss these concerns. The OTR can structure a discharge-planning group to encourage patients to share similar concerns regarding adjustment after hospitalization. The group can provide support and encouragement for fellow patients as well as opportunities for brainstorming and problem-solving issues related to the return to community living. Answers A and B do not provide opportunities for the patient to gain the insight and perspective of other patients who may share similar concerns. Suggesting that the patient lie (answer C) is not ethical. See reference: Early: Psychosocial skills and psychological components.

149. (A) provide each patient with an individual project and have him or her choose a tile color for the project. The activity should begin with the most basic level of decision making. Each of the other choices provide increasingly more challenging decision making abilities. Choosing from an assortment of projects (answer B) requires higher level decision making ability than selecting a color. Answer C requires not only decisions on design, color, and size, but also involves decision making among group members. Answer D involves decision making on two separate aspects, pattern and colors, resulting in a higher level of complexity than answer A. See reference: Early: Analyzing, adapting, and grading activities.

150. (C) Alcoholics Anonymous (AA). Self-help groups focus on personal growth in which leadership comes from the membership. AA is an example of such a group. MADD is an example of an advocacy group that focuses on changing the legal system. Group therapy involves leadership and expertise from outside of the membership itself. Al-Anon is a combination of support group and self-help group for

family members of the alcoholics. See reference: Posthuma: Self-help groups.

151. (C) memory impairment. Cognitive abilities such as memory are most often the first to be affected in individuals with Alzheimer's disease. Receptive and expressive aphasia (answer A), personality changes, and loss of independence in ADL (answer D) appear in the middle stage of the disease. Incontinence (answer B), the inability to recognize family members, and the inability to walk are evident in the late stage of Alzheimer's disease. See reference: Ryan (ed): Practice Issues in OT: Brown, I, and Epstein, CF: The elderly with Alzheimer's disease.

152. (D) select appropriate evaluation procedures. OT evaluation begins with the initial interview and chart review, which guide the OT in deciding on a frame of reference and the identification specific evaluation procedures or assessments. Assessments are then performed (answer C) to gather information to identify problem areas and plan treatment. After the assessments are complete, the OT uses clinical reasoning skills to analyze data (answer A) and to identify the person's strengths and weaknesses. The treatment plan (answer B) is developed after the individual's problems have been identified and evaluation data have been analyzed. Finally, specific interventions are selected. See reference: Pedretti (ed): Pedretti, LW: OT evaluation and assessment of physical dysfunction.

153. (C) Digging a garden with a shovel Activities that include bilateral use of tonic muscles against resistance, such as digging a garden, playing volleyball, or playing tug of war, can help to normalize tone in this population. Dancing with rapid alternating movements (answer A) may heighten arousal. Playing Twister (answer B) may facilitate balance and promote interpersonal skills. Rocking in a rocking chair (answer D) may reduce the level of arousal. See reference: Bruce and Borg: Movement-centered frame of reference.

154. (C) baking cookies using a recipe. This is a well-delineated meal preparation activity that provides structure with a specific sequence of tasks. Setting a table or preparing a shopping list (answers A and D) do not necessarily require sequencing of tasks. Planning a meal (answer B) involves a great deal of organizational ability and would not be an appropriate choice for an initial activity to address goals relating to sequencing tasks. See reference: Early: Responding to symptoms and behaviors.

155. (B) Go out for lunch to fast-food restaurant A key principle in intervention for effective transition includes using natural environments and cues and increasing community-based instruction as the student gets older. Classroom-based activities (answers A, C, and D) are not as effective in promoting development of the community member role as activities that actually take place in the community. See reference: Case-Smith (ed): Spencer, K: Transition services: From school to adult life.

156. (A) "It sounds as if you're not sure whether you are ready to be discharged." Paraphrasing is repeating what someone has said in your own words. Chitchat (answer B) is a conversational response unrelated to what the individual said. Confrontation (answer D) is a response that requires the individual to acknowledge difficult or painful issues. Proposing a solution (answer C) does not help the individual improve his or her decision-making skills or sense of competence. See reference: Denton: Effective communication.

157. (B) Socialization, task performance, daily living skills, and time management Evaluation of children who have psychosocial problems is centered on behavioral, affective or interpersonal areas, with visual motor and motor assessment following when screening suggests the need. But specific emphases in evaluation vary according to the age of the client with psychosocial disorders. Answer A reflects primary evaluation areas for toddlers and preschoolers. Answer C is more consistent with adult populations. Answer D reflects evaluation priorities for children with neurological, rather than psychosocial, dysfunction. See reference: Neistadt and Crepeau (eds): Florey, LL: Psychosocial dysfunction in childhood and adolescence.

158. (C) use simple and highly structured activities. Projective media, isolation, and discussing delusions are all contraindicated for people with schizophrenia. Projective activities (answer A) are most useful for encouraging expression of feelings. It may be appropriate to separate individuals (answer B) who are violent or unable to tolerate the presence of others nearby. Discussing delusions (answer D) is undesirable because it is likely to reinforce them. See reference: Early: Responding to symptoms and behaviors.

159. (B) a class about job-seeking strategies. The OT practitioner's remediation of identified deficits can be organized into three general approaches in psychosocial settings: enhancing the individual's skills and performance, assisting the individual in adjusting his or her perspective on skills and performance, and altering the environment. Teaching and training methods predominate the skill and performance remediation approach. Answer A is more consistent with object relations approaches; answer C is consistent with cognitive disabilities; and answer D is consistent with occupational behavior and human occupation approaches. See reference: Zoltan: Executive functions.

160. (D) Encourage group members to share similar experiences and reactions with each other Answer D is a strategy designed to develop cohe-

siveness among members. Many people have reported that recognizing one's similarities with other people is a very valuable experience. Answers A and C are designed to impart information. Answer B is an example of catharsis, which may not be helpful to all members; moreover, the OT practitioner must be aware of and understand the precautions necessary for the use of catharsis. See reference: Early: Group concepts and techniques.

161. (D) The staff may need to monitor water temperature and the amount of soap being used. This individual is functioning within the level 4 range of Allen's Cognitive Levels. Because this individual can recognize whether items are clean or dirty, cueing to place dirty items in the hamper (answer A) is not necessary. However, independent use of the washer and dryer (answer C) and problem solving (answer B) are more appropriate for individuals functioning at level 5, in which the individual demonstrates flexibility in response to change. See reference: Allen, Earhardt, and Blue: Analysis of activities.

162. (C) initiation. Initiation, or the ability to begin a task, affects a person's spontaneity in performing activities and how much he or she is able to perform. An individual with initiation problems may be able to plan or carry out activities but may be unable to begin until prompted by another person. Problems with attention (answer A), concentration (answer B), or apraxia (answer D) are evidenced as the incomplete or incorrect completion of an activity. See reference: Zoltan: Executive functions.

163. (C) needs assessment. Needs assessment is the necessary first step of gathering data about the population, treatment needs, and resources available. Program planning (answer A) involves establishing goals and objectives based on the results of the needs assessment. Program implementation (answer B) occurs following program planning and involves coordination, assessment, and intervention selection. Program evaluation (answer D) occurs after implementation and involves systematic review and analysis of the program based on achievement of program goals. See reference: Cottrell (ed): Grossman, J, and Bortone, J: Program development.

164. (B) "This program will help you to learn about the skills you have that are needed on MOST jobs and about your potential for work." Prevocational evaluation programs are designed to assess work skills that the client possesses, to identify their potential for work, and to help participants acquire skills by practicing skills that are important in the work environment. Vocational evaluation programs identify the actual interests and skills for specific types of work, such as assembly line work (answer A). Work role maintenance programs are for individuals who are employed but whose involvement in treatment has temporarily interrupted their employment (answer C). Developing job search skills (answer D) is needed for clients who have job skills but who have difficulty finding employment. See reference: Early: Treatment settings.

165. (C) provide a summary of observations of the patient's behavior, including what the patient said and did during the interview. An observation summary should present a concise and accurate picture of what happened so that the OTR can understand almost as well as if she were present during the interview. It is a summary and should not include extensive descriptions (answer A) or interpretations of the interview (answer D). A treatment plan (answer B) should be developed collaboratively with the OTR. See reference: Early: Data collection and evaluation.

166. (C) tardive dyskinesia. Long-term use of antipsychotic medications can lead to tardive dyskinesia in approximately 15% of individuals. Because the behavioral side effects described in this question can seriously impact the individual's daily living skill performance as well as his or her self-concept, OTs are responsible for knowing these side effects. Tremors, muscular weakness, and "rigid gait" are behaviors of parkinsonian syndrome, sometimes seen as side effects of antipsychotic medications (answer A). Overdose symptoms (answer B) vary according to the specific antipsychotic medication ingested. Lithium toxicity (answer D) is linked to antimanic medications. See reference: Early: Psychotropic medications and other biological treatments.

167. (A) baking brownies. A correctly sequenced progression of difficulty in meal preparation is access a prepared meal; prepare a cold meal; prepare a hot beverage, soup, or prepared dish; prepare a hot one-dish meal; and prepare a hot multidish meal. Making a fresh fruit salad (answer D) is a less challenging activity because no cooking is involved. Although both involve heating an item, preparing toast (answer C) is more simple than heating soup because opening a plastic bag is a less complex task than opening a can. Baking brownies (answer A) is slightly more complex because of the progression from stove top to oven and the addition of several ingredients that need to be mixed. Therefore, this would be the appropriate upgrade. Making an apple pie (answer B) requires a higher level of task performance and complexity than brownies and would be an appropriate task after the individual demonstrates competence in the less complex task of baking brownies. See reference: Neistadt and Crepeau (eds): Rogers, JC, and Holm, MB: Evaluation of activities of daily living (ADL) and home management.

168. (A) specific measurable statements with time frames. Goals can be either short term (i.e., in the immediate future) or long term (i.e., over an extended period). The purpose of a goal is to provide a specific statement that is measurable and indicates what is to be accomplished. Patients and significant others play vital roles in working with the therapist to establish goals that are meaningful and realistic. Time frames (answer B) may be only a part of a measurable goal or objective. Specific measurements of the patient's skill and performance (answer C) are parts of the assessment information that assists the therapist in establishing appropriate goals and objectives for treatment. Activities to be completed that correspond with the goals (answer D) are part of the objective and treatment plan. See reference: AOTA: The OT Manager: Acquaviva, JD: Documentation of OT services.

169. (A) begin with activities that have obvious solutions and high probabilities of success and then gradually increase the complexity. This strategy is effective in developing problem-solving skills. Gross and fine motor activities (answer B) can heighten awareness of self- and develop coordination. Increasing the time spent on the activity (answer D) helps development of attention span. Structuring the number and kinds of choices (answer C) is a method for developing decision-making skills. See reference: Early: Analyzing, adapting, and grading activities.

170. (C) simply stated, concrete verbal instructions. Answer C is correct because the individual is most likely able to understand simple concrete verbal instructions and abstract information may be very difficult to understand. Answer B is incorrect because an individual with an injury to the right nondominant cerebral hemisphere will have difficulty understanding facial expressions and body gestures as a result of difficulty processing visuospatial information. The individual will often have neglect to the left side of the visual field so answers A, presenting written information on the left side, and answer D, pictures of instructions on the left side, are incorrect as the individual is able to see to the right, but not to the left side. See reference: Pedretti (ed): Pedretti, LW, Smith, JA, and Pendleton, HM: Cerebral vascular accident.

171. (A) discharge recommendations. The COTA would contribute to the process of making discharge recommendations (answer A), but this section of the discharge evaluation is to be completed by the OTR. Answers B, C, and D may be completed independently by the COTA because these areas reflect factual data at the time of discharge. This information may include discharge disposition and data on the patient's current status. See reference: AOTA: OT roles.

172. (A) Punctuality, accepting directions from a supervisor, and interacting with coworkers Psychosocial components include time management, social conduct, interpersonal skills, and self-control. Punctuality and accepting feedback are examples of prevocational skills within these psychosocial performance components and are important prevocational skills. Memory, decision making, attention to task, and sequencing (answer B) are considered to be cognitive components. Standing tolerance, endurance, and eye–hand coordination (answer C) are categorized as sensorimotor components. Grooming and adhering to safety precautions (answer D) are work performance areas and are not psychosocial performance components. See reference: AOTA: Uniform Terminology for OT, third edition.

173. (A) reminiscence group. In a reminiscence group, the focus is on providing social opportunities for sharing life stories and feelings, expressing pride in past life experiences, and gaining support for past life difficulties, all of which would enhance self-esteem and help the resident to achieve acceptance of past and present life. See reference: Hellen: Appendix 9-10, Activity therapy care conference report form information: therapeutic value.

174. (B) Aerobic exercise Gross motor activities, involving either aerobic exercise or stretching and relaxation, can help to reduce the physical symptoms associated with anxiety. Although line dancing (answer C) involves all of the elements of gross motor activities, it requires the individual to follow specific steps and movements, which could cause the patient to become more anxious. Copper tooling and woodworking kits (answers A and D) are primarily fine motor activities. See reference: Early: Responding to symptoms and behaviors.

175. (B) to offer even-tempered acceptance, reflecting back what is heard without agreeing the situation is hopeless. A cheerful approach (answer A) can be perceived as denying the importance of the person's feelings. Silence (answer C) may also be perceived as unaccepting. Answer D is incorrect because the therapist needs to provide the structure; initiating and maintaining discussions is often difficult for depressed individuals. See reference: Early: Responding to symptoms and behaviors.

176. (B) insecurity. Feelings of insecurity are often covered up by projecting difficulties onto other objects (the collage) or other people. Hopelessness (answer C) involves negative statements about oneself or about changing. A comment or action which demonstrates the inability to choose between tasks typically reflects indecision, (answer D). Passivity (answer A) is often only "heard" through nonverbal communication. See reference: Posthuma: Observations and analysis.

177. (A) When the COTA consistently obtains the same results as the OTR The term "service competency" indicates an interrater reliability between two OT professionals. Service competency is determined by skill level, not by years of experience

(answer D). Passing the NBCOT examination (answer B) establishes entry-level competence, not service competence in a particular area. OT practitioners have a professional responsibility to maintain competence, and continuing education (answer C) is one method for maintaining competence and promoting lifelong learning. See reference: Neistadt and Crepeau (eds): Sands, M: Practitioners' perspectives on the OT and OT assistant partnership.

178. (D) senior COTA will evaluate, guide, and teach the staff COTAs. A supervisor has administrative, evaluative, and teaching roles. COTAs always require at least a general level of supervision, never minimal (answer A). Under general supervision, contact is made monthly. Minimal supervision is provided on an as-needed basis. It is possible that this may be less than once a month. Taking a supervisory position does not always result in a decreased caseload (answer B). If the role of COTAs in a department is to be redefined, all OT staff should participate in the process (answer C). See reference: Early: Supervision.

179. (C) once a month. The description of general supervision given by the AOTA includes a minimum of monthly direct contact with supervision available as needed by phone or other forms of communication. Answer A describes close supervision with direct contact occurring daily. Answer B refers to routine supervision or direct contact occurring a minimum of every week. Answer D is minimal supervision, which occurs on an as-needed basis. See reference: AOTA: Guide for supervision of OT personnel in the delivery of OT services.

180. (C) Notify NBCOT of the situation and reassign the patient to a different therapist. According to the Code of Ethics, therapists are responsible for maintaining relationships that "do not exploit the recipient of services sexually, physically, emotionally, financially, socially or in any other manner." The patient–therapist relationship is compromised when the therapist enters into a social or intimate relationship with a patient. Every therapist is responsible to report "any breaches of the Code of Ethics to the appropriate authority," whether they are a supervisor or not. Because the issue is practice related, the NBCOT is the appropriate authority. It is then the responsibility of the NBCOT to determine if and what type of disciplinary action should be taken. Maintaining a relationship with a patient (answer A) is unacceptable. The Code of Ethics does not require the supervisor to take a disciplinary action, such as terminating or reassigning the employee (answers B and D), but the facility might. See reference: AOTA: OT code of ethics.

181. (B) at or above the minimal entry level of competence. The AOTA statement "Purpose and value of OT fieldwork education" states that "Upon completion of Level II fieldwork education, the student is expected to function at or above the minimum entry level of competence" (p 845). In answer A, the student would not be performing at a passing level. Answers C and D are levels far above where a successful fieldwork student would be expected to be. See reference: AOTA: Purpose and value of OT fieldwork education.

182. (A) partial hospitalization. Partial hospitalization is appropriate for individuals who are experiencing acute psychiatric symptoms and who have a place or family to stay with at night. Except for overnight care, partial hospitalization offers most of the structure, staffing, and services available on an inpatient unit. Home health care (answer C) is an option for individuals who are medically unable to attend outpatient treatment because of significant medical or immobility issues. Day care (answer B) is long-term care that provides structured daily activities and medications to maintain current levels of functioning. Community mental health centers (answer D) provide a wide range of individual and outpatient services that address a variety of individual goals. See reference: Neistadt and Crepeau (eds): Treatment settings.

183. (D) wear gloves, a gown, a mask, and goggles. Answer D is the action that is consistent with universal precaution guidelines for working with an individual when there is a risk of coming in contact with body fluids such as sputum from coughing. Answers A, B, and C would not provide adequate protection against exposure to an infectious agent. See reference: Neistadt and Crepeau (eds): Pizzi, M, and Burkhardt, A: OT for adults with immunological diseases.

184. (B) have at least 1 year of experience as a certified OT practitioner. An individual who passes the NBCOT examination becomes a certified OT practitioner. In order to be a primary supervisor for a level-II OT student, the individual must be a registered OT with at least 1 year of experience. To supervisor level-II OTA students, the individual must be a certified OT practitioner with at least 1 year of experience. There is no minimum experience requirement for supervising level-I students. Although it may help to develop supervisory skills to work with a level-I student before taking a level-II student (answer D), there is no such requirement. See reference: AOTA: Standards for an accredited educational program for the OT.

185. (A) levels of self-care skills attained by clients with head trauma at discharge. The process of program evaluation includes reviewing the outcomes of providing services. Evaluating the levels of self-care skills attained by clients with head trauma on standardized tests would provide data about the effectiveness of therapy in achieving goals and would be an example of area of program evaluation. Answers B, C, and D are incorrect because they focus on evaluating departmental operations, rather than results achieved through the provision of care. See reference: Neistadt and Crepeau (eds): Perinchief, JM: Management of OT services.

186. (D) A patient with the diagnosis of a CVA and left neglect caught his left arm in the wheel of the wheelchair, resulting in a cut and bruise. An incident report should be completed whenever a situation occurs that is harmful to the patient or practitioner. This includes but is not limited to falls, burns, cuts, and contact with hazardous materials. See reference: AOTA: OT roles.

187. (C) Both OTRs and COTAs should have liability insurance. Liability insurance protects OT practitioners from financial damage should they be sued for negligence or misconduct. Most facilities maintain coverage for licensed professionals, but the level of coverage may not be sufficient to cover the amount sought for by the claimant. Therefore, OT practitioners may chose to insure themselves at a higher level. See reference: Ryan (ed): Practice Issues in OT: Jones, RA: Service operations.

188. (B) No, it violates the OT Code of Ethics. Despite the level of training she has achieved, according to the code it is still necessary for the COTA to demonstrate service competency in order to administer PAMs "Physical agent modalities may be used by OT practitioners when used as an adjunct to or in preparation for purposeful activity by a practitioner who has demonstrated service competency" (p. 1075). Service competency in this area includes the theoretical background and technical skills for the safe and effective use of the modality. Although study and practice are necessary to establish service competency, they are not by themselves sufficient; an OTR must determine that the COTA is competent before she can administer PAMs (answers A and C). Having an OTR on duty in the facility (answer D) does not make it acceptable for a COTA to administer a modality if the COTA has not demonstrated service competency. See reference: AOTA: Registered OTs and certified OT assistants and modalities.

189. (D) Yes, if the state law does not require a physician referral. AOTA does not require individuals to have a physician referral or prescription (answers A and B) in order to receive OT services, whether group or individual (answer C). However, OT practitioners must be aware of and adhere to the requirements of local, state and federal laws; government agencies; third-party payers; and facilities. Because the individual is going to pay for the services herself, the third-party payer policy is not an issue. In private practice, the OTR/COTA team may establish their own facility policies and can accept self-referrals if they so choose. Therefore, as long as state law does not require a physician referral or prescription, the individual can be accepted into the stress management group. See reference: AOTA: Statement of OT referral.

190. (D) "The patient has been provided with a lumbar support and a written copy of the home program." The plan section of a discharge summary contains the patient's discharge disposition (e.g., to a nursing home or to outpatient therapy), recommendations for additional therapy or actions on the part of the patient (e.g., outpatient therapy, home health, or performing a home program), equipment needs or equipment provided to the patient, and plans for discharge. Answer A is a subjective report. Answer B is an example of a statement that belongs in the objective section of a discharge summary. Answer C belongs in the assessment section. See reference: AOTA: Effective documentation for OT.

191. (C) Obtain a physician's plan of care identifying services to be provided Within the home care setting, the therapist must have a physician's order, which identifies the services that are to be provided. After the OT's assessment, identification of deficits as well as short- and long-term goals (answers A and B) can be established. The individual's history of the current illness (answer D) is contained within the initial assessment. See reference: Piersol and Ehrlich (eds): Zahoransky, M: The system and its players.

192. (D) Help place food on the spoon for a patient practicing the use of a universal cuff in the patient's room at lunchtime, while the OT supervisor runs a lunch group in the dining room An aide may be delegated client-related tasks when (1) the outcome of the task being delegated is predictable; (2) the situation is stable and will not require judgment or adaptation; (3) the client has previously demonstrated the ability to perform the task; (4) the aide has demonstrated competence in the specific task; (5) the aide has been instructed in how to carry out the task with the specific client; (6) the aide knows the relevant precautions; and (7) continuous supervision is provided. When these conditions are met, answers A, B, and C are all acceptable. While answer C may meet the other criteria, continuous supervision is absent, since the supervising OT is in the dining room. See reference: AOTA: Guidelines for the Use of Aides in OT practice.

193. (A) Treatments from the OT plan provided by an OT practitioner Based on the OT Code of Ethics regarding competence, OT may only be done by "those individuals holding appropriate credentials for providing services." These credentials are certification from NBCOT and, when appropriate, state licensure as an OT or OT assistant. Therefore, answers B, C, and D are incorrect because recreational, music, and art therapists do not hold these credentials. See reference: AOTA: OT code of ethics.

194. (C) a numbers table to select the popula-

tion. Numbers tables are used to select members of a population at random. An example is an OT department's choosing to study the charts of patients who had rehabilitation services to identify the typical OT charges that these patients are most likely to incur. For example, within 1 year, the OT department treated more than 170 individuals with the diagnosis of CVA. Instead of reviewing all of the cases, the department may choose to review 10% of the cases and use a numbers table to identify which charts should be reviewed. Answers A and B represent studies of an entire population. Answer D is an example of a sample population. See reference: Neistadt and Crepeau (eds): Deitz, JC: Research: Discovering knowledge through systematic investigation.

195. (D) Transdisciplinary In the transdisciplinary method of teamwork, one member provides the direct intervention and other team members function in collaborative consultant roles. This allows the family to interact with one service provider rather than several. Answer A is incorrect because a unidisciplinary team is not really a team; as the term implies, there is only one member. Answer B is not correct because the multidisciplinary team uses several disciplines, but they may not work in a collaborative manner. Answer C is also incorrect because in the interdisciplinary team, although it has group consensus regarding program planning, the members carry out their programs in their own environments. See reference: Case-Smith (ed): Stephens, LC, and Tauber, SK: Early intervention.

196. (B) The COTA updates the OTR on the progress a patient has made in the past week, and both provide information to update the goals. A collaborative relationship between an OTR and a COTA supports sharing of information and the use of each professional's skills. In this type of relationship, communication is two way, and both individuals work as a team to the benefit of the patient. Answers A and D demonstrate one-way communication in which the OTR tells the COTA what to do. In answer C, the OTR takes information from the progress note but does not get input or recommendations from the COTA for the patient's discharge summary. See reference: AOTA: OT roles.

197. (C) Supervision of noncertified personnel Under the supervision of an OTR, COTAs often participate in orienting, training, and evaluating the performance of unlicensed or noncertified personnel. Quality-assurance programs (answer A) should be established by team members and not independently. COTAs may supervise other COTAs (under the supervision of an OTR), but supervision of OTRs must be carried out by OTRs (answer B). Management responsibilities such as marketing (answer D) are also within the scope of practice of the OTR. See reference: AOTA: OT roles.

198. (D) use brochures, posters, videotapes,

and films available from the AOTA to enhance the presentation. The emphasis of this question is that it is every OT practitioner's responsibility to promote the profession. Simple, daily public relations activities occur each time an OT practitioner (whether it is a COTA or an OTR) describes the services to be provided to patients and families. More complex public relations may include developing a plan to promote community awareness regarding the profession. A public relations program is designed to increase the public's awareness about the role and importance of OT services. See reference: Ryan (ed): Practice Issues in OT: Jones, RA: Service operations.

199. (D) Label each item with the individuals' names. Cosmetics should never be shared. Federal regulations prohibit the sharing cosmetics if there is any likelihood of the cosmetics coming in contact with bodily fluids. This likelihood would be high in a geropsychiatric population. See reference: Early: Safety techniques.

200. (D) federal, state and local regulations, and third-party payers. "To provide OT services, the type of referral required (e.g. whether a physician's referral is necessary) is determined by federal, state, and local regulations and the policies of third-party payers. AOTA does not dictate whether a physician's referral is required" (p. 125). Answers A, B, and C are incorrect because professional organizations do not control referral policies. See reference: Sabonis-Chafee and Hussey: Overview of the OT process.

SIMULATION EXAMINATION 5

> **Directions:** Circle the correct answer to the following questions. When you have completed this examination, check your answers against the answer key that follows. As you will see, an explanation is given for each answer along with a reference for further study. The book author is listed as well as the chapter author. See the bibliography for complete references.

Randomized Questions

1. **A person with a long history of Parkinson's disease is experiencing considerable fatigue during the day. The OT practitioner's MOST appropriate response to help the person maintain his or her level of function is to teach the person how to:**
   A. "work through" the fatigue.
   B. perform desired activities in a simplified manner, to conserve energy.
   C. perform additional exercises to increase energy level.
   D. eliminate activities and reduce activity level as much as possible.

2. **An OT practitioner realizes that an adult worker with a developmental disability is having difficulty learning an assembly sequence. The practitioner decides to use backward chaining. Backward chaining can BEST be implemented by:**
   A. encouraging the individual to reverse the packaging sequence.
   B. having the worker put only the last piece into the game package.
   C. putting only the pencil or the pad into the game box.
   D. having the therapist demonstrate and repeat the correct sequence before each of the worker's attempts.

3. **The OT practitioner is treating a person with mild carpal tunnel syndrome. The MOST important instruction for the therapist to give the patient is to avoid:**
   A. extension.
   B. flexion.
   C. ulnar deviation.
   D. radial deviation.

4. **An individual with mental illness wants to travel to the library independently but keeps getting lost. Which of the following actions should the OT practitioner take FIRST?**
   A. Take the individual to the library and obtain a library card.
   B. Assess the individual's ability to read.
   C. Identify the bus that goes to the library and obtain a bus schedule.
   D. Assess the individual's topographical orientation skills.

5. **While observing a client who has just been admitted to the rehabilitation unit after a right cerebrovascular accident (CVA) with left hemiplegia, the OT practitioner notices that the patient's right arm lays limply by the patient's side. In documenting this observation, the OT will MOST likely use the term:**
   A. paralysis.
   B. flaccidity.
   C. subluxation.
   D. spasticity.

6. **An OT practitioner is working in a outpatient upper extremity and hand clinic. The practitioner's case load consists of clients who have tendonitis, nerve compression syndromes, and myofascial pain. The OT practitioner can assume that these diagnoses are MOST commonly associated with:**
   A. osteoarthritis conditions.
   B. peripheral vascular diseases.

C. cumulative trauma disorders.

D. neuroma-related conditions.

7. **An OT practitioner positions an infant in the supine position and places attractive toys overhead to provide an opportunity to work against gravity. This position is MOST effective for developing which ability?**

A. Shoulder flexion and protraction

B. Shoulder extension and retraction

C. Development of head control

D. Development of trunk control

8. **The OT practitioner is observing dressing skills in an individual with chronic obstructive pulmonary disease (COPD). While putting on his shirt, the individual becomes short of breath and stops to rest before finishing with the shirt and going on to his trousers. The OTR would recognize this as a deficit in:**

A. postural control.

B. muscle tone.

C. strength.

D. endurance.

9. **The OT is developing a treatment plan to promote developmental acquisition for an infant in the neonatal intensive care unit (NICU). Which of the following actions will have the most PERMANENT impact?**

A. Modify the environment to protect the infant from additional stressful stimuli

B. Recommend early intervention referral to assess infant upon discharge home

C. Complete the neurobehavioral assessment and identify interventions emphasizing developmental skill acquisition

D. Create a comfortable foundation for fostering parent skills through parent-therapist collaboration

10. **The therapist needs to identify an activity that will address psychosocial goals by (1) allowing the individual to experience success using a messy process and (2) requiring the individual to delay gratification. The activity process that is the BEST for providing this experience is:**

A. working in a group of three other individuals.

B. selecting the design pattern for a tile trivet.

C. applying grout to a tile trivet and waiting for it to dry.

D. encouraging the individual to clean off the table at the end of the group session.

11. **A preteen with a history of traumatic brain injury (TBI) is relearning to prepare simple foods but has been having difficulties with sequencing so the OT practitioner has provided the patient with a chart of steps to follow. The child has just learned to prepare his favorite sandwich without "losing his place" in the process but continues to need occasional verbal reminders to look at the chart and to ensure safety. At this point, the child's MOST recent level of independence would be documented as:**

A. independent.

B. independent with setup.

C. supervision.

D. minimal assist.

12. **A computer programmer arrives at an OT clinic complaining of pain while on the job. Which of the following are MOST likely to be considered work-related injuries specifically linked to the age of technology?**

A. Systemic diseases

B. Edema and paresthesias

C. Burns and electrocution

D. Carpal tunnel and chronic cervical tension

13. **A second grade child has a diagnosis of muscular dystrophy. The child operates a manual wheelchair, but his mobility is slow because of muscle weakness. The OT should consider a powered wheelchair when the:**

A. child starts junior high school and will be expected to switch classrooms several times daily.

B. child's speed over long distances becomes less than that of a walking person.

C. child's home can be made accessible for a power wheelchair.

D. child becomes unable to propel a manual wheelchair.

14. **Which of the following is the MOST appropriate goal to address when working with clients diagnosed with cognitive disorders?**

A. Improve their social skills in relating to others

B. Create new habits of time use

C. Implement compensatory strategies to manage the environment

D. Facilitate resumption of previous life roles

15. **An individual was unable to achieve the goal "the client will initiate two requests to other group members for sharing materials within a 1-week period." The BEST revised goal is:**
    A. "The client will initiate two requests to other group members for sharing group materials within a 2-week period."
    B. "The client will initiate one request to one other group member for sharing or using group materials within a 1-week period."
    C. "The client will initiate two requests to each of the five group members for sharing one group tool within 2 weeks."
    D. "The client will say hello to the group leader at the start of each group session."

16. **An OT practitioner is treating a client who demonstrates pain, progressive weakness of the thumb, atrophy of the thenar muscles and numbness and tingling in the thumb, index, long, and half of the ring fingers. The client is not experiencing proximal upper extremity limitations so the practitioner will MOST likely suspect problems with which of the following?**
    A. Ulnar nerve
    B. Median nerve
    C. Radial nerve
    D. Brachial plexus

17. **An OT practitioner treats most clients under the behavioral frame of reference. The activity feature that is MOST consistent with a behavioral frame of reference is:**
    A. the level of skill required is appropriate for the generally expected skills for that age.
    B. the symbolic potential of the activity.
    C. the combined activity demands of sensations, perceptions, and motor skills.
    D. the measurability of activity performance.

18. **An OT practitioner is assessing the range of motion of an individual who demonstrates internal rotation of the shoulder to 70 degrees. The practitioner would MOST likely document the patient's active range of motion as:**
    A. within normal limits.
    B. within functional limits (WFL).
    C. hypermobility that requires further treatment.

D. limited mobility that requires further treatment.

19. **After assessing a client who had recently lost his spouse in a house fire, the psychiatrist classifies the client as having an anxiety disorder caused by the occurrence of a major life event. Which of the following BEST represents this disorder?**
    A. Cyclothymic disorder
    B. Dysthymia
    C. Schizophrenia
    D. Post-traumatic stress disorder (PTSD)

20. **Which aspects of psychosocial performance are MOST important to emphasize in developing a client's work potential in a prevocational program?**
    A. Punctuality, accepting directions from a supervisor, and interacting with coworkers
    B. Memory, sequencing of the work tasks, attending to work tasks, and making decisions
    C. Standing tolerance, eye–hand coordination, and endurance
    D. Maintaining personal cleanliness and adhering to safety precautions

21. **An OT practitioner is working with a client in a work program setting. What is the FIRST step to achieving the program objective of preventing reinjury within a work program?**
    A. Performing a prework screening
    B. Learning proper body mechanics
    C. Participating in work hardening
    D. Engaging in vocational counseling

22. **The goal of an arts and crafts group for chronically mentally ill individuals is to improve their decision-making abilities. The MOST appropriate approach to initiating a mosaic tile activity would be to:**
    A. provide each patient with an individual project and have him or her choose a tile color for the project.
    B. have the patients choose from a variety of projects.
    C. have the patients decide on a design, size, shape, and colors for a group mosaics project.
    D. have each patient decide on a pattern and two tile colors to use in the his or her mosaic project.

23. In order for an individual sitting in a wheelchair to achieve maximal pelvic stability, the seat belt should be positioned:

A. inferior to the ischial tuberosity.
B. superior to the iliac crest.
C. inferior to the anterior superior iliac spine.
D. superior to the posterior superior iliac spine.

24. A young client who is diagnosed with depression tells an OT practitioner about feelings associated with being alone and afraid. A chart review reveals that the individual leads a very isolated lifestyle. The BEST way for the practitioner to respond is to:

A. reassure the client that they can be friends.
B. tell the client, "I know how you feel."
C. encourage the client to socialize more often.
D. use active listening techniques.

25. In a home program to promote beginning symbolic play for a child with developmental delay, the OT practitioner would MOST likely recommend playing with:

A. busy box, nesting toys, and blocks.
B. board games.
C. craft kits.
D. doll house and dress-up clothes.

26. "The patient arrived without her walker 3 out of 3 days this week." The MOST appropriate section of a SOAP note for the OT practitioner to place this statement is the:

A. subjective.
B. objective.
C. assessment.
D. plan.

27. When providing OT for children who have been diagnosed with a terminal illness, the PRIMARY focus for OT intervention would be:

A. educational activities.
B. play and self-care activities.
C. socialization activities.
D. motor activities.

28. An adult with schizophrenia walks with a shuffling gait and hunched posture. Using a movement-centered frame of reference, which of the following activities would MOST effectively contribute to normalization of this individual's posture?

A. Dancing with rapid alternating movements
B. Playing the game Twister
C. Digging a garden with a shovel
D. Rocking in a rocking chair

29. When ordering a wheelchair for an individual with multiple sclerosis (MS), the MOST important consideration is the adaptability of the wheelchair in anticipation of:

A. gradual gains in strength.
B. growth of the individual
C. further decline.
D. improved wheelchair mobility.

30. An OT practitioner requests that an OT student treat a client with a condition involving the upper extremity. The OTR suggests the use of contrast baths, retrograde massage, and pressure wraps. The OT student can consider these interventions as PRIMARY techniques to address:

A. heterotopic ossification.
B. edema.
C. wound healing.
D. scar management.

31. An OT practitioner observes a 5-year-old child with Down syndrome who has low muscle tone sitting on the floor exclusively using a "W" sitting position. This observation MOST likely indicates that the child is:

A. developing abnormally.
B. using a noncompensatory position to achieve stability.
C. demonstrating typical development for a child with Down syndrome.
D. using a position normal for a younger child, not for a 5-year-old child.

32. An individual with a history of substance abuse lives in a group home. The residential manager has asked the OT practitioner to work with the individual to develop house cleaning skills. Which of the following interventions is most appropriate when a COGNITIVE approach is desired?

A. Reward the individual with a snack bar token when chores have been successfully completed
B. Praise the individual when chores have been successfully completed

C. Post a schedule of each individual's chore responsibilities in a highly visible location

D. Conduct a group discussion about responsibilities people have when living in a group home

33. **An auto mechanic is currently in a work-hardening program after being in a car accident that left him with numerous upper and lower extremity impairments. The ultimate goal for this individual is to return to full employment as an auto mechanic. Which of the following BEST represents a work-hardening activity for this individual?**

A. Lifting weights

B. Working on a mock car engine

C. Visiting the work site garage

D. Preparing a light lunch for mealtime

34. **The OT practitioner has fitted a 6-year-old child for an adapted seat for use in the home for mealtime and other table-top activities. Which of the following instructions is MOST appropriate to convey to the parents?**

A. Adapt the seat as needed

B. Bring the seat in for each weekly therapy session in order to adjust it according to the child's growth

C. Bring the seat in for reevaluation within 6 months

D. Keep the seat until the end of the IEP

35. **An OTR observes an individual having difficulty trying to find white socks on a bed with white sheets. The MOST appropriate performance component for the OT to address is:**

A. figure-ground discrimination.

B. unilateral neglect.

C. position in space.

D. cognitive mapping.

36. **An OTR has asked a COTA to identify how a patient spends his leisure time, which leisure activities he especially enjoys, and which others he has participated in that he would be interested in renewing. The MOST appropriate tool for the COTA to use is:**

A. an evaluation of living skills

B. an interest checklist.

C. an activity configuration.

D. a self-care evaluation.

37. **An OT practitioner is preparing for the discharge of a preadolescent child with limited strength and endurance. Which of the following home adaptations is MOST important to recommend?**

A. Mount lever handles on doors and faucets

B. Remove all throw rugs

C. Install nonskid pads on steps

D. Mount a table-top easel for written home work

38. **During a stress management group, an individual recently diagnosed with MS complains that his teenage children are resistive to helping with chores that were previously his responsibility, such as mowing the lawn and taking out the trash. The stress management technique that would MOST successfully address this concern is:**

A. using effective communication skills.

B. applying time management techniques.

C. deep breathing.

D. laughter.

39. **An OT practitioner is developing transition activities for a group of 16-year-old students diagnosed as trainable mentally retarded. Which of the following activities would be BEST for addressing goals related to transition?**

A. Role-play ordering food in the classroom

B. Go out for lunch to a fast-food restaurant

C. Order a take-out lunch by phone

D. Select lunch items from a picture menu in the classroom

40. **A client that the OT practitioner is working with uses a wheelchair and requires minimal assistance with all transfers and basic ADL. The client is expected to remain at this functional level. Which of the following would be the MOST appropriate community living option for this client at discharge?**

A. A cradle-to-grave home

B. A transitional living center

C. An adult day program

D. A clustered independent living arrangement

41. **Which of the following instructions should the OT practitioner follow when administering standardized tests to young children?**

A. Test in a stimulating environment

B. Follow test manual directions

C. Always administer tests in a single session

D. Carry on a conversation with the child

42. An OT practitioner providing home-based care to an individual with acquired immunodeficiency syndrome (AIDS) learns from his caregiver that he has become too weak to turn himself in bed. What is the MOST important modification to the treatment plan for the OT practitioner to recommend?

A. To begin a strengthening program

B. To begin a bed-mobility program

C. To teach the caregiver how to lift and turn the client safely

D. To provide an environmental control unit (ECU) to the client

43. The treatment goal for a 4-year-old child with hypotonia is to improve grasp. Which of the following activities would be BEST for preparing the child's hand for grasp activities?

A. Dropping blocks into a pail

B. Placing pegs on a pegboard

C. Weight-bearing on hands

D. Holding and eating a cookie

44. When providing adaptive equipment to an individual with arthritis, the OT practitioner would explain that the PRIMARY purpose of using this equipment is to:

A. decrease joint stress and pain.

B. correct deformity.

C. simplify work.

D. decrease independence.

45. An individual alternately exhibits laughing and crying throughout a treatment session. This behavior should be documented as:

A. mania.

B. emotional lability.

C. paranoia.

D. denial.

46. When administering an evaluation of upper extremity function to a newly admitted patient with Guillain-Barré syndrome, it is MOST important to:

A. test proximal muscle strength first.

B. perform the evaluation over several sessions.

C. include sensory testing.

D. evaluate range of motion.

47. An OT practitioner is working with an individual who demonstrates the inability to begin a task or activity. The practitioner documents that the client MOST likely has problems with:

A. attention.

B. concentration.

C. initiation.

D. apraxia.

48. A child with poor anticipatory postural control demonstrates inadequate playground skills, losing her balance when trying to anticipate movement. Which of the following activities will BEST promote the development of these skills?

A. Ballet

B. Soccer

C. Basketball

D. Ping-pong

49. When leading groups, OT practitioners should demonstrate consistency from day to day. Inconsistent behavior would MOST likely result in:

A. overdependence of group members.

B. group members' knowing what to expect from the group leader.

C. anxiety and confusion among group members.

D. group members' receiving too much praise.

50. An individual with lower extremity paralysis uses a standard manual wheelchair and is ready to be discharged to home. During the home evaluation, the OT practitioner notes that the entrance to the bathroom is 32 inches wide and the toilet is 15 inches high. Which of the following recommendations will MOST facilitate use of the bathroom for this individual?

A. Widen the doorway

B. Raise the toilet

C. Widen the doorway and raise the toilet

D. Widen the doorway and lower the toilet

51. An OT practitioner has planned to assess group interpersonal skills in an activity-based group of seven individuals. Shortly before the group is to begin, the therapist is asked to add two newly admitted clients to the group. Which of the following actions would yield the MOST efficient and effective result?

A. Ask one or two of the original seven members to wait until later and include the two new clients in the group

B. Add the two new clients and then divide the members into two groups

C. Interview the two new clients separately and continue with the original evaluation group of seven

D. Proceed with the group as planned, adding both new clients to the original seven

52. An OT practitioner is making a home visit to an elderly client who lives alone. The client exhibits severe hand weakness. When addressing safety in the home, the OTR should be MOST concerned with the client's ability to:

A. work locks and latches on doors and windows.

B. use built-up utensils while eating.

C. use energy conservation techniques.

D. manipulate fasteners on clothing.

53. An 8-year-old boy is being treated in OT for social withdrawal and depression. At the time of discharge, the BEST recreational activity for the OT practitioner to recommend for the child is:

A. swimming lessons.

B. Boy Scouts.

C. computer games.

D. piano lessons.

54. The home health OT practitioner is seeing a client in the middle stages of Alzheimer's disease. The family is very concerned that the client's memory loss is now interfering with performance of daily activities, even familiar self-care activities. The MOST relevant OT intervention at this point would be:

A. memory retraining activities for the client.

B. ADL retraining program for the client.

C. instructing caregivers in task breakdown.

D. leisure activity planning.

55. The OT practitioner is making recommendations to a community living site for a 13-year-old child who has mental retardation. Which of the following statements most accurately describes the functional ability of this child who is in the moderate (trainable) range of intellectual ability?

A. The client requires nursing care for basic survival skills.

B. The client can usually handle routine daily functions.

C. The client requires supervision to accomplish most tasks.

D. The client is able to learn academic skills at the third to seventh grade level.

56. An OT practitioner in an acute care hospital is using the SOAP note format to document information about an individual with dementia. Which statement is the BEST example of subjective information?

A. The therapist will establish a daily self-feeding routine using verbal and physical cues to encourage the individual to open containers on the lunch tray.

B. The individual has been able to identify closed liquid-beverage containers on the meal tray for four of six presentations.

C. The individual is able to identify and drink liquids presented in cups without lids but leaves beverages in closed containers untouched.

D. The individual asks for more beverages during meals, but appears surprised when the therapist indicates beverages in closed containers are on the meal tray.

57. OTs working in the area of early intervention have frequent contact with a child's parents. Which of the following statements BEST describes how parents should be involved in the OT program?

A. Parents should not be present during OT sessions.

B. Parents should be trained as substitute therapists.

C. Parents should be considered as part of a collaborative partnership with therapists.

D. Only one parent needs to be present when the OT program is discussed.

58. An OT practitioner is planning a meal preparation activity for an adult client with attentional and organizational deficits secondary to alcohol abuse. The treatment goals address the client's difficulties in properly sequencing tasks. The MOST appropriate activity to use FIRST is:

A. setting the table.

B. planning an entire meal.

C. baking cookies using a recipe.

D. preparing a shopping list.

59. An OT practitioner is working with a client who complains of pain while completing kitchen cleaning tasks. Which of

the following positions would be **MOST** effective in alleviating low back pain when the patient is loading the dishwasher?

A. Place dishes next to dishwasher and load from a standing position
B. Wash dishes in the sink
C. Place dishes next to dishwasher and load from the front of the dishwasher
D. Place dishes near the dishwasher, bend down on one or both knees, and load

60. **The OT practitioner is selecting activities for an 8-year-old child with Duchenne's muscular dystrophy. Which of the following developmental issues is MOST important to consider when identifying activities for this child?**

A. Establishment of basic trust
B. Freedom to use his initiative
C. Development of self-identity
D. Reinforcement of competence

61. **Each morning, an OT practitioner performs ADL training with a teenage client who has quadriplegia. On the first day, the practitioner works with the client, arranging the shirt on the lap. When the client masters that particular skill, they work on sliding both arms into the sleeves and pushing the shirt up past the elbows. When this skill is mastered, they will work on gathering the shirt up at the collar and pulling it on over the head. This technique is BEST known as:**

A. repetition.
B. cueing.
C. rehearsal.
D. chaining.

62. **When preparing a home program with the goal of independent toileting for a young child with postural instability, the MOST important adaptation the OT practitioner can recommend is:**

A. replacing zippers and buttons with Velcro closures.
B. mounting a safety rail next to the toilet.
C. introducing toilet paper tongs.
D. placing a colorful "target" in the toilet bowl.

63. **An elderly man was admitted to the hospital after a car accident. He sustained a right pelvic fracture and verbalizes extreme pain with ambulation. The orthopedic doctor has recommended that the patient perform "toe touch only" weight**

bearing on his right foot for 6 to 8 weeks. The OT should instruct the patient to use a walker when performing which of the following activities?

A. Transferring on and off a commode seat
B. Working on bed mobility
C. Performing self-feeding
D. Working on distal lower extremity dressing

64. **A preschooler has poor visual tracking skills, which affect her performance on tasks requiring eye–hand coordination. Which of the following activities is most appropriate for the OT practitioner to recommend to the child's parents in order to promote beginning visual tracking skills during summer vacation?**

A. Tossing and catching a water balloon
B. Catching and bursting soap bubbles
C. Throwing and catching a beach ball
D. Playing softball

65. **An OT manager is preparing the outpatient OT staff for a visit from an accrediting agency. The accrediting agency that surveys inpatient and comprehensive outpatient rehabilitation programs is BEST represented by which of the following:**

A. AOTA.
B. JCAHO.
C. CARF.
D. NBCOT.

66. **An individual has sustained a large, full-thickness burn to both upper extremities while running a fireworks display. The client is in the acute care phase of treatment. Which of the following BEST represents an acute care rehabilitation goal?**

A. Prevent loss of joint and skin mobility
B. Provide adaptive equipment
C. Provide compression and vascular support garments
D. Prevent scar hypertrophy through scar management techniques

67. **The OT is working with a patient on an acute care floor when the patient's IV equipment disengages, splashing the therapist in the eye with the medication and IV "backwash" fluid. The therapist's FIRST response should be to:**

A. rub the eye and continue treatment.
B. rinse the eye with an eye wash or water immediately.

C. write an incident report.

D. cover the eye with a bandage and contact the immediate supervisor.

68. During an interview, the OT practitioner decides to respond to an individual by paraphrasing. The PRIMARY reason for this type of response is to:

A. refocus or redirect the individual's comments.

B. show acceptance and understanding to the individual.

C. force the individual to make a choice.

D. encourage an individual to give additional information.

69. An OT manager is attempting to find a way to have financial success in the department while ensuring patient satisfaction. Which of the following is MOST likely to be implemented to assess patient flow, develop critical pathways, and cut costs?

A. Quality improvement

B. Peer review teams

C. Cost accounting

D. Interdisciplinary care improvement teams

70. In establishing a wellness program for older adults, the OT practitioner is MOST likely to incorporate activities that:

A. improve weakness following a CVA.

B. increase physical activity and fitness.

C. improve social skills for depressed elders.

D. increase independent performance of transfers.

71. In an acute mental health facility, an individual refuses to participate in OT activities, and the therapist notes the refusal in the subjective section of a documentation note. Which form of refusal would MOST likely reflect acute depression?

A. "I had an argument with another group member and I'm too angry."

B. "I don't want to participate because I don't know how to do the activity."

C. "I'm just too tired."

D. "I'm waiting for my visitors to come."

72. An OT manager in a large department is trying to determine which staff will be able to supervise level-II fieldwork students in the upcoming months. OT practitioners may only be selected to be primary student supervisors if they:

A. are certified OT practitioners with at least 6 months of experience.

B. have at least 1 year of experience as a certified OT practitioner.

C. are certified by the NBCOT.

D. have supervised a level-I student before the level-II student.

73. An OT practitioner is educating a client with a cumulative trauma disorder about common work-related risk factors. The OTR explains to the client that many of the PRIMARY risk factors are:

A. repetition, high force, and awkward joint postures.

B. progressive resistive exercise, joint mobilization, and weight bearing.

C. inflammation, swelling, and pain.

D. fatigue, muscle cramps, and paresthesias.

74. The OT practitioner is leading a grooming group for female clients in a psychosocial treatment setting. Which of the following options BEST complies with universal precautions?

A. Use disposable cotton swabs and have clients bring their own cosmetics

B. Use disposable gloves when combing client's hair

C. Wash and dry makeup brushes between uses

D. Avoid bringing cosmetics in glass containers to the group

75. In preparing a patient with a unilateral below-knee amputation for discharge from a rehabilitation facility, the MOST important adaptive equipment for the OT to recommend is:

A. lightweight cooking utensils.

B. a tub bench and toilet rails.

C. long-handled dressing devices.

D. a reacher.

76. In screening a child who has been referred to OT, the PRIMARY goal of the OT is to:

A. obtain necessary information for an OT consultation with teachers or parents.

B. test a wide variety of developmental behaviors.

C. establish an information base for the OT treatment plan.

D. determine the need for further evaluation.

77. While practicing wheelchair-to-tub transfers an individual's external cathe-

ter is dislodged and urine spills onto the floor. The therapist notes that the urine appears to have blood in it. Which one of the following responses is the MOST appropriate?

A. An exposure has not occurred; clean up the area with paper towels and resume treatment as quickly as possible.

B. An exposure has occurred; close off the area until it can be disinfected and resume treatment as quickly as possible.

C. An exposure has occurred; clean up the spill with towels, place towels in the dirty laundry bin, and resume treatment as quickly as possible.

D. An exposure has occurred; put on gloves, clean up the spill with paper towels, put the soiled paper towels in a plastic bag, seal the bag, disinfect the area, and finish the patient's session with whatever time is still left.

78. Which individual would benefit the MOST from using a wrist-driven flexor hinge splint during a prehension activity?

A. A client with a C1 injury
B. A client with a C3 injury
C. A client with a C6 injury
D. A client with a T1 injury

79. A child with limited upper extremity range of motion is being readied for discharge. The MOST important home adaptation for the OT practitioner to recommend concerning use of the toilet is:

A. installation of safety bars next to the toilet seat.
B. mounting of a wide-base toilet seat.
C. placement of a skidproof stepping stool next to the toilet.
D. installation of a bidet with a spray wash and air-drying mechanism.

80. A hospital-based multidisciplinary team meets bimonthly to monitor their services in regard to the creation of an environment that meets or exceeds consumer needs. This model is MOST appropriately called:

A. total quality management.
B. cost accounting.
C. employee empowerment.
D. horizontal structuring.

81. An individual with depression is ready to return to the job held before taking a leave of absence. Which of the following

is the FIRST action the OT practitioner should take?

A. Perform a job analysis.
B. Request reasonable accommodation.
C. Emphasize activities that promote a sense of self-efficacy.
D. Encourage the individual to participate in a weekly support group.

82. A school-age child with fine motor difficulties is ready for discharge from outpatient OT services. Which of the following is the MOST important information to focus on?

A. The child's interests and hobbies
B. The child's writing, dressing, and self-feeding skills
C. The child's academic achievement
D. The availability of the child's parents for follow-up services

83. A child is observed grabbing toys from others, becoming easily frustrated, and is unable to sit still. This behavior MOST likely indicates:

A. attention-deficit hyperactivity disorder (ADHD).
B. mood disorder; manic episode.
C. conduct disorder.
D. anxiety disorder.

84. An OT practitioner is working with an individual with impaired memory. When the client is unable to follow verbal instructions, the practitioner changes the approach to demonstration. This is an example of:

A. activity analysis.
B. activity adaptation.
C. grading the activity.
D. clinical reasoning.

85. A client that the OT practitioner is treating brings an order from his physician requesting treatment for epicondylitis. Which of the following adjunct activities should be used to treat the ACUTE symptoms of tennis elbow?

A. Passive range of motion (PROM), weight bearing, and mobilization
B. Resistive exercises, heat application, and work simulation
C. Heat application, PROM, and strengthening
D. Ice application, immobilization, and splinting

86. **An individual with strong dependency needs is able to lace a leather wallet only with consistent verbal cueing. Which is the BEST way to grade this activity in order to decrease dependency?**
    A. Provide written instructions on lacing techniques and ask the individual to continue on her own
    B. Ask the individual to try some lacing with distant supervision and praise her for what she has been able to do
    C. Ask the individual to take the lacing to her room and continue without the OT's assistance
    D. Tell the individual to complete a small amount of lacing while the OT assists another patient in the same room

87. **After administering an interest checklist, the therapist documents that the individual has identified a few solitary leisure interests and no interests involving social interaction. Based on this information, what is the BEST activity to use in the next session of a leisure counseling group?**
    A. A leisure inventory assessment
    B. An activity exploring leisure opportunities and problems
    C. A magazine picture collage
    D. A calendar of community leisure activities for the first week after discharge

88. **An OT practitioner is instructing a person with arthritis how to maintain range of motion while performing household activities. Which of the following activities MOST effectively accomplishes this?**
    A. Use short strokes with the vacuum cleaner
    B. Keep elbow flexed when ironing
    C. Keep lightweight objects on low shelves
    D. Use dust mitt to keep fingers fully extended

89. **Using the Model of Human Occupation as a frame of reference, evaluation of an individual should focus PRIMARILY on which of the following?**
    A. Identification of problem behaviors that need to be extinguished
    B. Clarification of thoughts, feelings, and experiences that influence behavior
    C. Cognitive function, including assets and limitations
    D. The effect of personal traits and the environment on role performance

90. **A child has difficulty controlling food in her mouth when swallowing. In helping the parents to plan snacks, the OT practitioner would be MOST likely to recommend:**
    A. chicken noodle soup.
    B. peanut butter.
    C. carrot sticks.
    D. applesauce.

91. **An OTR is working on sitting balance with an individual with C6 quadriplegia. The BEST position for the individual's hands to be in when using them for support is to have the fingers:**
    A. extended and adducted.
    B. flexed at all joints.
    C. extended and abducted.
    D. adducted and flexed only at the MCP joints.

92. **When working with a child who exhibits tactile defensiveness, which of the following areas should be evaluated FIRST?**
    A. Reading skills
    B. Dressing habits
    C. Social skills
    D. Leisure interests

93. **An individual who works as a nurse reports difficulty squeezing the bulb of the sphygmomanometer when taking blood pressures and difficulty opening pill bottles. Which of the following instruments would be MOST appropriate for assessing this individual?**
    A. Goniometer
    B. Aesthesiometer
    C. Volumeter
    D. Dynamometer

94. **An OT practitioner working in a sheltered workshop with adult clients with developmental disabilities is preparing for a group of clients functioning at Allen's Cognitive Level 4. Which of the following is the BEST method for introducing an assembly activity?**
    A. Provide repetitive, one-step activities
    B. Demonstrate a three-step assembly process
    C. Provide project samples for clients to duplicate
    D. Provide written directions for the individuals to follow

95. **An individual with MS reports extreme frustration because her house is so dir-**

ty. When she does attempt to clean it, she is too exhausted to do anything else afterward. She does not think she can afford to pay someone else to clean. Which of the following strategies is MOST appropriate for this individual?

A. Convince the individual to hire a house cleaner

B. Prescribe activities that will increase strength

C. Use the largest joint available for the task

D. Alternate tasks that require standing with those that can be performed sitting

96. An individual with the goal of increasing attention span is frequently observed watching the person next to her instead of performing her assigned task. This behavior MOST likely indicates:

A. memory deficits.

B. spatial operations.

C. generalization of learning.

D. distractibility.

97. When instructing the parents of a toddler in the use and care of a hand splint, the OT practitioner should put MOST emphasis on:

A. checking for irritation and pressure problems.

B. avoiding excessive heat exposure.

C. cleansing the splint regularly.

D. adhering strictly to the wearing schedule.

98. An OT practitioner is evaluating a client who is unable to name or demonstrate the use of common household objects. The practitioner documents this as:

A. apraxia.

B. stereognosis.

C. visual agnosia.

D. alexia.

99. While in the hospital, a 48-year-old roofing contractor experienced extrapyramidal syndrome after being placed on neuroleptic medications. The patient is to continue taking the medication after discharge from the hospital. It is MOST important to advise the patient to:

A. keep time in the sun as brief as possible.

B. avoid use of power tools and sharp instruments.

C. get up slowly from a standing, sitting, or lying position.

D. be aware of the dehydrating effects of caffeinated drinks and alcohol.

100. An OT wishes to assess the results of a life-skills training program provided to individuals at a shelter for abused women. Which of the following methods would be BEST for obtaining this information?

A. Final evaluation of each client involved

B. Client satisfaction survey

C. Program evaluation

D. Utilization review

101. During a routine transfer, a patient's legs buckle, causing him and the OT practitioner to fall to the floor. The most appropriate way for the OT practitioner to document this accident is in a(n):

A. incident report.

B. daily progress note.

C. letter to the department head.

D. verbal report to the department head.

102. An individual with hand weakness has difficulty holding a fork. Using a biomechanical frame of reference, which of the following interventions would be MOST appropriate?

A. Elicit functional grasp using reflex inhibiting postures

B. Stimulate the hand flexors to promote a functional grasp

C. Repeatedly squeeze with the hand against increasing amounts of resistance

D. Build up utensil handles

103. An OTR performing a motor skills evaluation observes that a child is awkward at many gross motor tasks, particularly those which require relating the body to objects in space. Though able to skip rope in the regular forward pattern of movement, the child is unable to skip rope backwards, even after several attempts. This information would lead the therapist to be particularly observant for additional signs of:

A. delayed reflex integration.

B. inadequate bilateral integration.

C. developmental dyspraxia.

D. general incoordination.

104. A supervising OT asks an experienced COTA to complete a portion of an assessment. The portion that is MOST appropriate for the COTA to complete independently would be:

A. collecting chart review information.

B. analyzing and interpreting assessment information.

C. establishing the treatment goals.

D. establishing the treatment plan.

105. An OT practitioner is treating a client who developed a severe PIP joint contractures in the third digit, 2 months after a burn injury. Which of the following static splinting techniques would BEST address the needs of this individual?

A. Plaster cylindrical splint

B. Dynamic outrigger splint

C. Blocking splint

D. PIP-DIP splint

106. In administering an assessment of fingertip pinch strength, the OT practitioner would instruct the individual being tested to place the fingers in which position?

A. Thumb against the tip of the index finger

B. Thumb against the side of the index finger

C. Thumb against the tips of the index and middle fingers

D. Thumb against the tips of all the fingers

107. A COTA frequently administers the Allen Cognitive Level Test and then discusses it with the supervising OTR. Which of the following MOST accurately describes the OTR's role during these discussions?

A. Determine the COTA's service competency

B. Collect data on the patient's performance

C. Interpret the results based on data collected by the COTA

D. Develop the treatment plan

108. A method that an OT practitioner can use to document total finger flexion without recording the measurement in degrees would be to:

A. measure the passive flexion at each joint and total the numbers.

B. measure the distance from the fingertip to the distal palmar crease with the hand in a fist.

C. measure the active flexion at each joint and total the measurements.

D. measure the distance between the tip of the thumb and the tip of the fourth finger.

109. While preparing for his first presentation at a professional conference, an OT realizes he does not have the name of the author of an article containing critical information he planned on photocopying and distributing. Which of the following is the MOST appropriate action for the OT to take?

A. Distribute the handout and apologize for not having the author's name.

B. Show the handout with an overhead projector and apologize for not having the author's name.

C. Use the handout only as a resource while developing the presentation.

D. Refrain from using the handout in any way.

110. An OTR is preparing to do a parachute activity as part of a sensory integration program and several of the patients in the group are taking antipsychotic medications. The OTR should be alert for which possible side effect that could occur as a result of this activity?

A. Postural hypotension

B. Photosensitivity

C. Excessive thirst

D. Blurred vision

111. When there is not a referral for OT services, it is MOST important for the COTA involved in the provision of services to know that:

A. the OTR is operating outside the scope of practice and regulating agencies should be notified.

B. the OTR must assume responsibility for all OT services delivered.

C. a written letter of consent must be received from the patient or a significant other.

D. the COTA should seek a referral from the patient's family physician.

112. An OTR is working as a consultant to a health care facility to assist the facility in achieving compliance with the Americans with Disability Act (ADA), Title III. The PRIMARY focus of the OT's efforts would be to make recommendations about:

A. improving accessibility in building access, building interiors, and rest rooms.

B. modifying equipment, providing assistive aids, and training in adaptive methods so a disabled person can perform a particular job.

C. providing education to persons who hire personnel concerning nondiscriminatory behaviors and procedures regarding persons with disabilities.

D. assistive technology systems to facilitate job performance of disabled employees.

113. An OT practitioner working for the school system has identified a general need to enhance the fine coordination skills of the elementary school students to facilitate better writing skills. The BEST population-based intervention would be to:

A. screen students for writing problems and provide in-depth assessment of those identified.

B. provide remedial activities for those students identified having fine coordination deficits.

C. recommend activities develop fine coordination that teachers can incorporate into classroom programming.

D. recommend additional OT staff to provide direct services for students.

114. An artist recently diagnosed with MS is interested in pursuing a leisure activity that will promote physical fitness. Because the individual's symptoms are limited to mild UE numbness and slight weakness in the dominant hand at this point, the BEST activity to recommend is:

A. volleyball.

B. painting with the dominant hand.

C. swimming in a cool water pool.

D. jogging on a track or treadmill.

115. An entry-level OT practitioner wants to know the extent of her liability when providing occupational therapy. Which of the following answers is MOST accurate?

A. Only OTRs need to have liability insurance.

B. Only COTAs need to have liability insurance.

C. Both OTRs and COTAs should have liability insurance.

D. Neither OTR or the COTA need to have liability insurance.

116. In establishing long-term goals for an individual with T4 paraplegia in a rehabilitation setting, the OT practitioner would MOST likely predict that the patient will attain what level of independence with bathing, dressing, and transfers?

A. Complete independence with self-care and transfers

B. Independence with self-care and minimal assistance with transfers

C. Minimal assistance with self-care and moderate assistance with transfers

D. Dependence with both self-care and transfers

117. An OT practitioner is planning to use remedial strategies to prepare individuals treated in a psychosocial setting for job hunting. The activity MOST consistent with this approach is:

A. reviewing an interest checklist.

B. holding a class about job-seeking strategies.

C. modifying the work environment to reduce stress.

D. using an expressive group magazine collage using pictures of different types of jobs.

118. An OT practitioner is performing sensation testing on an individual with hemiplegia. The therapist should FIRST:

A. apply the stimuli distally to proximally.

B. test the involved area then the uninvolved area.

C. present test stimuli in an organized pattern to improve reliability during retesting.

D. apply the stimuli to the uninvolved area proximally to distally in a random pattern.

119. When developing play activities for a child with acute juvenile rheumatoid arthritis, which of the following precautions should the OT practitioner follow?

A. Avoid light touch

B. Avoid rapid vestibular stimulation

C. Avoid resistive materials

D. Avoid elevated temperatures

120. An OT practitioner is assessing hand function in a man with arthritis by observing him as he makes a peanut butter sandwich. The individual is unable to remove the lid from a 28-ounce peanut butter jar but is able stand at the counter, spread peanut butter on the bread with a knife, and replace the lid when he has finished making the sandwich. These observations would MOST accurately reflect deficit in the performance component:

A. range of motion.

B. coordination.

C. endurance.

D. strength.

121. Adults with mental retardation can be offered a variety of work alternatives. Which of the following MOST likely involves simple assembly or sorting and packaging tasks with supervision and subcontracted piecework?

A. An adult activity center
B. Supervised employment
C. Job coaching
D. A sheltered workshop

122. **Upon completion of a level-II fieldwork placement on a rehabilitation unit, a student is functioning slightly below minimal entry-level competence. The supervising fieldwork educator should:**

A. fail the student.
B. pass the student with the requirement that the student not practice in a rehabilitation setting.
C. pass the student and recommend additional training or volunteer work in a rehabilitation setting.
D. pass the student.

123. **While observing a newly referred child in the playground, the OT practitioner suspects that the child has dyspraxia. The MOST relevant assessment to determine the child's level of performance will be one which determines the child's ability to:**

A. print or write.
B. read.
C. calculate mathematics.
D. plan new motor tasks.

124. **The OT practitioner is evaluating two-point discrimination in an individual with a median nerve injury. The MOST appropriate procedure is to:**

A. apply the stimuli beginning at an area distal to the lesion progressing proximally.
B. test the involved area first, then the uninvolved area.
C. present test stimuli in an organized pattern to improve reliability during retesting.
D. allow the individual unlimited time to respond.

125. **An OT practitioner has been hired to develop a community-based program for patients with chronic mental illness. The FIRST step in the process which the practitioner must complete is:**

A. program planning.
B. program implementation.
C. needs assessment.
D. program evaluation.

126. **In planning a therapeutic dressing program for a first grade child who is mentally retarded, the therapist's FIRST consideration should be the need for:**

A. adaptive equipment.
B. adaptive clothing.
C. proper positioning.
D. adapted teaching techniques.

127. **As part of an initial evaluation of an individual with carpal tunnel syndrome, the OTR evaluates light touch sensation using a cotton ball. After wearing a wrist splint for 2 weeks the patient returns for a reevaluation, which the COTA performs. At this time, the MOST appropriate method for reevaluation of light touch is to use:**

A. a cotton ball.
B. an aesthesiometer.
C. Semmes-Weinstein monofilaments.
D. a pin or straightened paper clip.

128. **On the way to lunch, an OT practitioner is stopped by a patient's spouse and questioned for 15 minutes about the patient's progress. What is the MOST appropriate action for the OT practitioner to take when determining how the patient will be treated and charged for the scheduled one hour treatment session?**

A. Charge the patient for an additional 15 minutes of treatment for the time spent with family member.
B. Reduce the patient's therapy to 45 minutes and charge for 1 hour of treatment to cover the time spent with the family member.
C. Reduce the patient's therapy to 45 minutes and charge patient for 45 minutes of treatment.
D. Treat the patient as scheduled and charge for the 1 hour of direct time spent with the patient.

129. **An OT practitioner is instructing an individual with left hemiplegia how to remove a t-shirt. The correct sequence is:**

A. (1) remove shirt from unaffected arm; (2) remove shirt from affected arm; (3) gather shirt up at the back of the neck; and (4) pull gathered back fabric off over head.
B. (1) remove shirt from affected arm; (2) remove shirt from unaffected arm; (3) gather shirt up at the back of the neck; and (4) pull gathered back fabric off over head.
C. (1) gather shirt up at the back of the neck; (2) pull gathered back fabric off over head;

(3) remove shirt from affected arm; and (4) remove shirt from unaffected arm.

D. (1) gather shirt up at the back of the neck; (2) pull gathered back fabric off over head; (3) remove shirt from unaffected arm; and (4) remove shirt from affected arm.

130. The supervisor of OT is off work and in a local establishment listening to a band with her friends. She observes one of the therapists she supervises at another table being intimate with a gentleman she is currently treating on an outpatient basis. Which of the following actions should the supervisor take in order to be consistent with the OT Code of Ethics?

A. Indicate to the therapist that she may maintain the relationship as long as it does not impair the patient's treatment

B. Notify the state licensure board and terminate the employee

C. Notify NBCOT of the situation and reassign the patient to a different therapist

D. Discipline the employee and refer the patient to another outpatient center

131. An OT practitioner is using a sensory integration approach with a group of regressed individuals with limited attention spans. Most group members can tolerate a group situation for no more than a half-hour. Which of the following activities would be BEST for beginning the session?

A. Go around the circle and ask each patient to introduce himself/herself

B. Pass around a scent box and ask each patient to smell the contents

C. Ask each patient to select a favorite poem and read it

D. Discuss the lunch menu and healthy eating habits

132. Staff members in a group home report to the OT practitioner that several of the men repeatedly try to touch female clients and staff and often make sexual gestures and comments. Which of the following environmental modifications would be MOST likely to reduce this behavior?

A. Provide a relatively active and stimulating environment with opportunities for these individuals to engage in real-life activities

B. Stand to the side of these individuals instead of face to face during interactions with them

C. Avoid having these individuals in close proximity to others to reduce opportunities for physical contact

D. Advise these individuals in a calm, nonjudgmental manner about the behavior you expect

133. A hospital's public relations department plans to take some pictures of the OT staff working with patients. Before proceeding, which of the following MUST be obtained?

A. The correct spelling of the patients' names for the photograph caption

B. The patients' written consents to take the photographs and use them for publicity

C. The department head's written consent to take the photographs and use them for hospital purposes

D. The correct spelling of the patients' diagnoses and names for the photographs' captions

134. An OT practitioner is planning to demonstrate and then involve a group of individuals in practicing "broken record" behaviors. Which of the following interventions BEST encompasses the broken record technique?

A. Music therapy activities

B. Self-awareness activities

C. Assertiveness training

D. Psychodrama approaches

135. An OTR/COTA team need to report discharge information and document the information in the patients' chart. At what level does the COTA participate in making discharge recommendations?

A. An entry-level COTA may perform the task independently.

B. An intermediate-level COTA may perform the task independently.

C. A COTA contributes to the process but does not complete the task independently.

D. A COTA cannot perform the task.

136. A woman experienced repeated sexual abuse by her father as a child and now describes her father's abusive actions as being caused by his stress of being fired from a job because of new management. The defense mechanism she is MOST likely to be using is:

A. identification.

B. projection.

C. denial.

D. rationalization.

137. Many COTAs are employed in long-term care facilities and perform many functions. The function which the OTR MUST perform in this setting is:

A. activity programming, environmental adaptations, and caregiver and staff education.

B. ADL training, and running feeding and leisure activity groups.

C. interpreting results of assessments for the purposes of treatment planning.

D. positioning, providing adaptive devices, and instructing in use of splints.

138. An OT manager is developing a proposal for OT services in the NICU. Using the developmental support care approach as the basis for services, how would the OT BEST describe OT's scope of practice in the NICU?

A. Modifying the environment to protect the infant from overstimulation and inappropriate stimuli

B. Providing PROM, positioning and handling, fabrication of splints, and referral to early intervention

C. Educating parents and hospital staff

D. Implementing motor and behavioral skill acquisition through developmental milestone positioning

139. Which of the following would be the BEST cup for the OT practitioner to recommend using when working with an individual who tends to drink too quickly?

A. A vacuum feeding cup

B. A "nosey cup" (cut out for the nose)

C. A mug with two handles

D. A cup with a large drinking spout

140. The OT practitioner is attempting to better understand a particular phenomenon by conducting a small research study. Initially, the OTR identifies a potential research question. The NEXT step in the process would be to:

A. state the purpose.

B. design the research.

C. complete a review of the literature.

D. establish boundaries for the study.

141. An OT practitioner is evaluating a young cabinetmaker who complains of sensory changes over the dorsal thumb and proximal phalanx of the index, long, and half of the ring finger. The practitioner will MOST likely suspect involvement of the:

A. ulnar nerve.

B. median nerve.

C. radial nerve.

D. brachial plexus.

142. An OT practitioner is requested to evaluate and make recommendations to a job site that is in search of ergonomic adaptations. An example of this type of adaptation might be:

A. introducing relaxation seminars for employees to decrease stress while on the job.

B. treating corporate clients for cumulative trauma disorders.

C. initiating a smoking cessation program.

D. suggesting furniture and accessories that promote better positioning at work.

143. OT services in a long-term care facility are provided by two OTRs and one COTA through a contract agency. When the absence of one of the OTRs creates a staffing shortage, the administration instructs the present OTR to perform evaluations only and instructs the COTA, a new graduate, to perform all treatment planning and implementation until they are full staffed again. No time is designated for supervision. What is the MOST appropriate way for the OT staff to respond?

A. Follow the administrator's instructions.

B. Express concern to the administrator about inadequate supervision and then follow administrator's instructions.

C. Express concern in writing to contract agency and then carry out the administrator's instructions.

D. Explain to the administrator this is not an appropriate solution and then develop an alternate solution.

144. An OT practitioner is fabricating a dynamic splint for a butcher who sustained a low-level radial nerve injury while slicing lunchmeat at the deli where he works. The OTR explains to the client that a dorsal dynamic splint for this type of nerve injury should:

A. provide wrist extension, MCP flexion, and thumb flexion.

B. prevent wrist extension, MCP extension, and thumb extension.

C. prevent wrist extension, MCP flexion, and thumb flexion.

D. provide wrist extension, MCP extension, and thumb extension.

145. On completion of an evaluation of a child with CP, the OT has identified the primary objective of inhibition of flexor spasticity in the hand. The activity that would be **MOST** appropriate in meeting this objective would be:

A. building a block tower.

B. active release of blocks into a container.

C. traction on the finger flexors.

D. weight-bearing over a small bolster in prone.

146. An OT practitioner is working with an individual who is about to be discharged from OT after rehabilitation for a hand injury. The client has not been able to work for 3 months and is still unable to perform the job requirements as a sales manager in a clothing store. Which of the following recommendations should the OT practitioner recommend concerning OT services?

A. The client should continue to perform a home program at time of discharge.

B. The client should receive home health OT.

C. The client should enroll in a work-hardening program.

D. The client should discontinue OT services at the time of discharge.

147. A 78-year-old individual who is ambulating with a walker in the home informs the OT practitioner that improving balance is a major concern. Although the patient took showers in the past, now his fear of falling limits him to sponge baths. The OT practitioner tells the individual that it is wise to avoid situations in which the risk of falling is high. Which of the following should the OT practitioner advise the individual to do **NEXT**?

A. Try the bathtub instead of the shower

B. Purchase a shower chair

C. Describe how using a shower chair improves safety

D. Explain that therapy will improve his balance

148. In selecting a standardized test to use with a child, an **OT** practitioner can assume that the test:

A. is valid.

B. has normative data.

C. has a standard format.

D. is reliable.

149. A young client who will be using a wheelchair after discharge from the rehabilitation facility is going home. In determining accessibility of the interior home environment, the **FIRST** area of evaluation the OT will be concerned with is:

A. location of telephones and appliances.

B. arrangement of furniture in bedrooms.

C. steps, width of doorways, and threshold heights.

D. presence of clutter in the environment.

150. An OT providing services to a community mental health program has been asked to examine the effectiveness of the OT groups that have been provided over the past 6 months. Which of the following procedures should be used to accomplish this goal?

A. Quality assurance

B. Peer review

C. Utilization review

D. Program evaluation

151. The **MOST** effective method of compensation for both unilateral neglect and absence of sensation in an upper extremity with good motor control is to:

A. avoid the use of sharp tools or scissors and to avoid extreme water temperatures.

B. wear noisy bracelets on the wrist or ankle as a reminder to visually scan toward the affected side.

C. use an electric shaver.

D. wear elbow pads on the affected side.

152. The benefits that a correct sitting position has in relation to hand function is explained to the parents of a child with **CP**. The child currently uses compensatory movements because of the inability to sit independently. Which aspect of therapeutic positioning should the OTR stress?

A. Stabilizing the trunk

B. Placing weight on the arms

C. Stabilizing the pelvis, hips, and legs

D. Stabilizing the head and neck

153. An individual complains of perspiration which is causing his resting hand splint to be uncomfortable. The **BEST** action for the **OT** practitioner to take is to:

A. recommend putting talcum powder in the splint.

B. line the splint with moleskin.

C. fabricate a new resting hand splint with perforated material.

D. provide a stockinet for the individual to wear inside the splint.

154. An OT practitioner is administering a standardized test to a young client who suddenly becomes uncooperative and complains that the test is "too hard." The MOST appropriate response for the OT practitioner would be to:

A. switch to easier items to improve the child's self-esteem.

B. terminate the session and schedule another session for the remainder of the test.

C. follow administration instructions and note changes in behavior.

D. adapt the remaining test items to ensure success.

155. An OT practitioner is assessing hand sensation in an older adult with diabetic neuropathies who frequently complains of hand pain. It appears that the client would benefit from a desensitization program. The OT informs the client that hypersensitivity training is typically graded from:

A. soft to hard to rough.

B. tap to rub to touch.

C. light to medium to heavy.

D. rough to hard to soft.

156. A child with motor delays is being evaluated to determine how he performs self-care activities. Which evaluation procedure is MOST likely to provide relevant information about self-care function?

A. Standardized tests of motor development

B. Review of the medical record

C. Developmental screening test

D. Home observation and parent interview

157. A client with hemiplegia and her spouse are working on toilet transfer training activities with the OT practitioner. The BEST way for the OT practitioner to teach the couple to perform transfers will be:

A. only to the unaffected side of the client's body.

B. only to the affected side of the client's body.

C. to both sides of the client's body.

D. only to the side of the body from which the client will be approaching the toilet.

158. A COTA and OTR have effectively worked together for the past 5 years. Which of the following BEST describes the supervisory process between a COTA and a supervising OTR at this level?

A. A mutual process

B. A evaluative process

C. A counseling process

D. A learning process

159. An OT practitioner working in a sheltered workshop with individuals with mental retardation must be aware of how the agency that provides services to the developmentally disabled population is accredited. Which of the following is responsible for accrediting these workshops?

A. JCAHO

B. CARF

C. AC MRDD

D. NLN/APHA

160. A child displays poor postural stability because of low muscle tone. To promote beginning antigravity control, the FIRST activity that should be performed is:

A. pull-to-sit, leaning back against therapy ball.

B. prone scooter obstacle course.

C. hippity-hop races.

D. batting a balloon while the child is suspended in net.

161. An individual with poor writing skills needs to produce large amounts of legible material upon returning to work. The MOST appropriate method of compensation the OT could recommend would involve having the person:

A. learn to type.

B. practice fine motor coordination exercises.

C. practice letter or shape formations.

D. strengthen the finger flexors and extensors.

162. An adolescent with mental retardation is planning to enter a supported employment program in the community after leaving school. Which area of intervention would the OT practitioner be MOST likely to focus on?

A. Developing the student's leisure interests and play skills

B. Developing the student's vocational interests, social skills, and community mobility skills

C. Facilitating development of the student's gross motor skills

D. Facilitating development of the student's fine motor skills

163. A 4-month-old infant being seen for an OT assessment shows a strong preference for the left hand when reaching for a rattle at midline. Considering the development of dominance in normal children, the OT practitioner should conclude that:

A. further observation and evaluation of right-sided dysfunction is indicated.

B. development of hand dominance is proceeding in a typical manner.

C. hand dominance will not develop until age 1 year.

D. unilaterality precedes bilaterality in typical development.

164. A research question has been identified and a literature review completed by an OT practitioner. The NEXT step for the OT researcher is to:

A. refine the question and develop the background.

B. decide on methodology.

C. establish boundaries for the study.

D. collect and analyze data.

165. A 1-year-old child is working on increasing neck flexor strength. At this time, the child can maintain head alignment when tilted backward from an upright supported sitting position, to a 45-degree incline, but loses control when tilted further back. The NEXT important step in the intervention is to work on head and neck alignment:

A. in a sidelying position while batting a toy.

B. in a prone position while watching a peek-a-boo game.

C. by tilting backwards up to 60 degrees while rocking.

D. in a supine position, while watching an overhead mobile.

166. The OT practitioner is instructing a patient who has had a myocardial infarction (MI) in energy conservation techniques. The BEST example of limiting the amount of work needed for a task is:

A. using a side-loading washer.

B. wearing permanent-press clothing.

C. using an extended-handle dustpan.

D. using good body mechanics.

167. An individual with underreactive sensory processing has been referred to OT. Based on a sensory integration frame of reference, activities for this individual should have which of the following facilitory characteristics?

A. Arrhythmic and unexpected

B. Arrhythmic and slow

C. Sustained and slow

D. Unexpected and rhythmic

168. An OT practitioner is instructing a client with a total hip replacement how to perform a passenger side car transfer. Which of the following BEST represents the initial steps of this transfer?

A. Stand the body parallel to the car, hold onto a stable section of the car, lift and place the left leg into the car, and slowly sit and follow with opposite leg

B. Back up the body to the passenger seat, hold onto a stable section of the car, extend the involved leg, and slowly sit in the car

C. Back up the body to the passenger seat, hold onto a stable section of the car, flex both legs simultaneously, and slowly sit in the car

D. Back up the body to the passenger seat, hold onto a stable section of the car, flex the involved leg, and slowly sit in the car

169. An OT practitioner is working on functional mobility skills with a child who has a pes varus deformity of the foot. The OT can BEST document this as a(n):

A. enlarged great toe.

B. club foot.

C. pronated foot.

D. unstable heel.

170. A home health OT is working with an individual who is ambulatory but demonstrates poor balance. The individual has a walker, a standard cane and a wheelchair at home, but financial constraints have prevented any home modifications. Which of the following ambulatory methods would be MOST appropriate for use during meal preparation training?

A. Use a standard cane

B. Use a walker

C. Use a wheelchair

D. Hold on to counters and walls

171. The husband of an individual who is being treated for bipolar disorder describes his frustration with the ups and downs

of his wife's condition. Which of the following is the BEST support group to recommend to this husband?

A. Al-Anon
B. Family therapy
C. National Alliance for the Mentally Ill
D. Recovery, Inc.

172. An OT practitioner is working with a client diagnosed with a mild sprain. The client cradles her hand and appears to be hypersensitive to light touch. The individual also presents with edema, pain, shiny skin, and excessive dryness of the extremity. Based on this, the OTR assumes that the client is MOST likely suffering from:

A. neuromas.
B. reflex sympathetic dystrophy.
C. carpal tunnel syndrome.
D. desensitization.

173. The OT is working with an individual in a psychosocial partial hospitalization program who is having difficulty making decisions. The therapist has suggested a baking activity but the client as unsure if she wants to do this activity. The therapist's response that would BEST facilitate decision making is:

A. "I think baking would be a helpful activity to try. Baking something you like offers you several choices and decisions. You wanted to bake cookies today, didn't you?"
B. I think baking would be a helpful activity to try. Baking something you like offers you several choices and decisions. Why do you want to bake?
C. I think baking would be a helpful activity to try. Baking something you like offers you several choices and decisions. These choices and decisions can help you feel more positive about making other decisions. You can choose a cake mix or a cookie mix. Which would you like?
D. I think baking would be a helpful activity to try. Baking something you like offers you several choices and decisions. These choices and decisions can help you feel more positive about making other decisions. Do you want to bake cookies?

174. A toddler diagnosed with developmental delays does not finger-feed when presented with food in the clinic. The BEST way to obtain further information about his feeding skills is to:

A. interview his parents to determine his favorite foods.
B. observe him in his home during feeding time.
C. review his chart for food allergies.
D. repeat the observation in a quiet area (in order to minimize distractions).

175. An OT practitioner is transferring a client with hemiplegia from a wheelchair to an elevated mat. The client is able to place both feet on the floor and move the buttocks to the edge of the wheelchair. The therapist then places one hand on the client's right anterior pelvis and the other hand on the client's left shoulder. The client is set up so the transfer can be performed toward the client's stronger side. The client then pushes to a standing position and pivots with the therapist's guidance. This is MOST likely an example of a(n):

A. independent transfer from wheelchair to mat.
B. assisted stand pivot transfer.
C. pneumatic lift transfer.
D. dependent stand pivot transfer.

176. The OT treatment goal for a child with athetoid CP is self-feeding. Which of the following adaptations would BEST solve the problem of food sliding off the plate when the child attempts to pick it up with a spoon?

A. Swivel spoon
B. Nonslip mat
C. Mobile arm support
D. Scoop dish

177. The OT practitioner is treating a patient with a standard above-elbow amputation who is experiencing hypersensitivity of the residual limb. The OT would most likely perform which of the following interventions in the preprosthetic phase of treatment?

A. Activities to strengthen the residual limb
B. Activities to increase the range of motion of the residual limb
C. Activities which provide tapping, application of textures, and weight bearing to the residual limb
D. Activities for practicing putting on and taking off the UE prosthesis

178. An OT practitioner is attempting to decide which type of group to institute

within an acute psychiatric setting. The supervising OT suggests the directive group treatment approach because it is MOST appropriate in acute care mental health for individuals with:

A. substance abuse problems.

B. eating disorders.

C. adjustment disorders.

D. disorganized psychosis.

179. An OT practitioner is working on a feeding program for an individual with amyotrophic lateral sclerosis (ALS) who is in the late stages of the disease process. Which of the following is the MOST appropriate intervention for this individual?

A. Provide a rocker knife, plate guard, and nonskid mat

B. Implement a pureed diet and allow adequate time for eating

C. Emphasize upper extremity strengthening

D. Minimize the use of adaptive equipment

180. An OT practitioner is assessing a client who has schizophrenia and appears to be experiencing acute symptoms of the disease. Which of the following is considered to be an acute or positive symptom of schizophrenia that the OT might document in her assessment?

A. Flat affect

B. A lack of pleasure

C. Hallucinations

D. Withdrawal from others

181. When working with clients who experience low back pain, it is important to practice functional techniques such as lifting and carrying. Which of the following BEST represents a correct lifting method?

A. Keep both knees straight, flex the back, and keep object an arm's distance away from the body

B. Bend both knees, keep the back straight, and bring object close to the body when lifting

C. Keep both knees and back straight and bring object close to the body when lifting

D. Bend one knee while keeping the other leg straight and keep the object an arm's length away from the body

182. An individual tells the OT practitioner, "I don't know about going home tomorrow. I wanted to be discharged yesterday and the doctor suggested I stay in the hospital another day." Which of the following responses MOST accurately reflects an active listening approach?

A. "It sounds as if you're not sure whether you are ready to be discharged."

B. "You know, your doctor is a very intelligent person."

C. "How about calling your doctor when you get home if you feel a panic attack coming on."

D. "You've been doing extremely well; what are you afraid of?"

183. A young individual with MS is about to be discharged to home. The client is independent in bathtub transfers using a grab bar. The MOST important self-care recommendation the OT practitioner can make regarding bathing is to:

A. use cool water.

B. use moderately heated water.

C. take showers and avoid bathing.

D. bathe at the sink with a basin.

184. A therapist is working with an individual who was admitted to an inpatient psychiatric program for major depression. This individual is also diagnosed with stage 4 AIDS. The BEST general focus of treatment at this point would be to:

A. restore and maintain functional performance of self-chosen occupations that enhance competent performance of valued occupational roles.

B. increase physical endurance and maintain desired self-care tasks.

C. facilitate resolution of current and anticipated losses through the grieving process.

D. restore and maintain functional performance of the individual's primary work role.

185. An individual with ALS swims three times a week to maximize strength and endurance. Initially able to swim for only 10 minutes, the individual is now able to swim 20 minutes without becoming fatigued. The NEXT step is:

A. continue the program of swimming 20 minutes three times a week.

B. decrease swimming frequency to two times a week.

C. increase swimming time to 25 minutes or to tolerance.

D. provide adaptive equipment that will enable the individual to swim using less energy.

186. An OTR is performing an UE functional assessment on an elderly client with rheumatoid arthritis. The OTR is MOST likely to determine that the client has limited internal rotation if the client is unable to touch the:

A. back of the neck.

B. top of the head.

C. lower back.

D. opposite shoulder.

187. A patient who has had a TBI is beginning OT. The OTR practitioner needs to assess whether this person can transfer learning from one activity to another in order to plan treatment appropriately. The MOST appropriate way for an OT to observe this learning ability would be to:

A. describe situations that might be unsafe and ask the patient how he would respond.

B. give the patient a simple jigsaw puzzle to solve.

C. have the patient get dressed in a certain way, then change the task at the next session.

D. give the patient simple calculations to perform.

188. The OT observes that a child moves from a completely prone position to a prone-on-elbow position. In reporting the child's progress, the OTR documents that the child is gaining control in the midline position through the development of:

A. primitive reflexes.

B. prehensile reactions.

C. righting reactions.

D. equilibrium reactions.

189. The BEST method for handling a child who exhibits tactile defensiveness is to:

A. tickle him during play times.

B. play loud music when undressing him.

C. lightly stroke his arms and legs during baths.

D. hold him firmly when picking him up.

190. An individual demonstrates the ability to pick up a penny from a flat surface. This represents which of the following prehension patterns?

A. Lateral

B. Palmar

C. Tip

D. Three-jaw chuck

191. An older adult with diabetes is working on a macramé project as a way of increasing standing tolerance. The MOST relevant safety factor for the OT practitioner to take into consideration is the:

A. length of the cords she will start with.

B. thickness of the cords she will be using.

C. texture of the cords she will be using.

D. type of surface she will be standing on.

192. An OT practitioner who is leading a stress management group explains to the members that stressors can be MOST accurately described as the:

A. process by which individuals adjust to daily stressful events within their environments.

B. body's reactions to threat, often described as "fight or flight."

C. precipitating conditions and events that elicit stress reactions.

D. process of "fit" between the individual and his or her environment.

193. An OT practitioner is teaching a client who recently sustained an above-elbow amputation how to dress with one hand. Teaching a client to perform a familiar activity or skill is called the:

A. problem-solving method.

B. retraining method.

C. altered task method.

D. compensation method.

194. A school-age child has Duchenne muscular dystrophy. Although he is able to use a manual chair for distances between classes, he is tired on arrival. What would be the BEST recommendation the OTR could make for wheelchair use at school?

A. Retain the manual chair to build up strength

B. Change to an ultralight sports model because it requires less strength

C. Change to a power wheelchair to reduce effort

D. Encourage walking with a walker to alternate mobility methods

195. An OT practitioner is helping a family plan a wheelchair ramp to the front door of their home. What is the minimum amount of space needed in front of the door to allow easy access by wheelchair?

A. 3 feet by 5 feet

B. 4 feet by 4 feet

C. 4.5 feet by 3 feet

D. 5 feet by 5 feet

196. The spouse of a patient with a progressive disease has come into the OT department to learn how to help the spouse perform functional activities at home. The FIRST focus of caregiver education for this person should be:

A. methods for motivating the patient to perform ADL.

B. how to analyze activities to solve problems.

C. instruction in how to provide cues to the patient.

D. instruction in how to perform the activities safely.

197. Direct OT services are being discontinued for a student with attention deficit disorder, but consultation will be provided to help the child adjust to the new classroom. Which of the following recommendations is MOST appropriate?

A. Use dim lighting and reduce glare by turning down lights

B. Remove all posters and visual aids to reduce visual distractions

C. Provide a screen to reduce peripheral visual stimuli

D. Restructure classroom activities into a series of short-term tasks

198. The BEST way to instruct an individual with hemiparesis to button a shirt is to:

A. button all the buttons before putting the shirt on.

B. get the shirt all the way on, then line up the buttons and holes and begin buttoning from the top.

C. get the shirt all the way on, then line up the buttons and holes and begin buttoning from the bottom.

D. use a buttonhook with a built-up handle.

199. An OT practitioner is speaking with parents who believe that their child with CP could benefit from OT consultation at school. In order for a school-aged child to receive OT services within a school system, which of the following forms must be completed FIRST?

A. UB-82

B. FIM

C. IEP

D. HCFA-1500

200. An OT practitioner is performing an environmental assessment to determine accessibility for a client who will be returning home. The FIRST step in this process is to:

A. identify the barriers to movement and function in the home environment.

B. identify and analyze the tasks and occupations that the client will be performing in the home.

C. identify the aspects of the environment which support movement and function in the home.

D. determine the social environment of the client.

ANSWERS FOR SIMULATION EXAMINATION 5

1. (B) perform desired activities in a simplified manner, to conserve energy. One method used to extend a person's occupational performance as Parkinson's disease progresses is to introduce task simplification. This allows conservation of energy which can then be expended on desired activities. In a person with long-standing Parkinson's disease, encouragement to "work through" fatigue (answer A) and to perform additional exercises (answer C) would further deplete available energy. Recommendations to decrease activity level as much as possible (answer D) would also be detrimental to maintaining occupational performance levels. See reference: Neistadt and Crepeau (eds): Pulaski, KH: Adult neurological dysfunction.

2. (B) having the worker put only the last piece into the game package. Working backwards from the last (successful) step of a sequence is known as "backward chaining." Answer A represents the opposite of backward chaining. Answer C is more descriptive of shaping behaviors, and answer D is more descriptive of modeling behaviors. See reference: Pedretti (ed): Pedretti, LW, and Umphred, DA: Motor learning and teaching activities in occupational therapy.

3. (B) flexion. Flexion at the wrist, especially while grasping or pinching, should be avoided. Repetitive flexion and extension movements also cause compression of the median nerve. Answers A, extension, C, ulnar deviation, and D, radial deviation, do not cause inflammation to the area surrounding the median nerve by repetitive compression or a static hold to that area of the wrist. See reference: Hunter, Schneider, Mackin, and Bell (eds): Baxter-Petralia, P: Therapist's management of carpal tunnel syndrome.

4. (D) Assess the individual's topographical orientation skills. In order to plan an appropriate intervention, the individual's community mobility skills must first be assessed. Constantly getting lost is a strong indicator that the individual may be impaired in the area of topographical orientation. Learning to take the bus and obtaining a library card (answers A and C) are important steps toward independent library use but should occur after evaluation has been completed. Individuals may enjoy using a library whether they can read or not, so the ability to read is not essential to this goal and does not need to be evaluated (answer B). See reference: Early: Activities of daily living.

5. (B) flaccidity. Flaccidity, or hypotonicity, is often present immediately after a stroke and may later change to spasticity (answer D) or increased muscle tone. The flaccid extremity feels heavy and hangs limply at the individual's side. The weight of the arm may eventually pull the humerus out of the glenohumeral joint, resulting in subluxation (answer C). Answer A is inadequate because paralysis may be accompanied by either flaccidity or spasticity. See reference: Pedretti (ed): Undzis, MF, Zoltan, B, and Pedretti, LW: Evaluation of motor control.

6. (C) cumulative trauma disorders Cumulative trauma disorders are viewed as a mechanism of injury for tendonitis, nerve compression syndromes, and myofascial pain because of the nature of repetitive strain and motion disorders. Answer A, osteoarthritis disorders, frequently present with stiffness, redness, and edema. Answer B, peripheral vascular disease, is unrelated to the diagnoses mentioned in the question and is more commonly associated with the vascularity of the client. A neuroma (answer D) is specifically related to an amputation, nerve injury or suture. See reference: Pedretti (ed): Kasch, MC: Hand injuries.

7. (A) Shoulder flexion and protraction Answer A is correct because the infant changes from extensor influences on posture to development of flexion in the supine position. This requires the ability to flex and protract the shoulders against gravity in order to reach forward and upward to grasp toys. Answer B is not correct because shoulder extension and retraction would not be encouraged during supine activities when the toys are placed overhead. Answers C and D are not correct because most activities of looking and reaching can be accomplished without using head or trunk control against gravity in the supine position. See reference: Kramer and Hinojosa (eds): Colangelo, CA: Biomechanical frame of reference.

8. (D) endurance. A deficit in endurance is demonstrated by the person's inability to sustain cardiac, pulmonary, and musculoskeletal exertion for the duration of the activity. Answer A, a deficit in postural control, would be correct if the client had been unable to maintain his balance while putting on the shirt. A deficit in muscle tone (answer B) would have been evident if the client had demonstrated spasticity while putting on the shirt. Inability to push his arms through the resistance created by the shirt sleeve would demonstrate a deficit in strength (answer C). See reference: AOTA: Uniform Terminology for Occupational Therapy, third edition.: .

9. (D) Create a comfortable foundation for fostering parent skills through parent-therapist collaboration All four answers describe possible ways for an OT to impact an infant's developmental outcome. However, the most permanent action would capitalize upon developing family-centered mutual collaboration. With this approach, communication is the key to creating a relationship that will foster parental skill development and expertise. This then provides the parents with effective tools to best nurture and care for their infant at any time and in any environment, and has a permanent impact on the developmental outcome for the infant. See reference: Case-Smith (ed): Hunter, JG: Neonatal Intensive Care Unit.

10. (C) applying grout to a tile trivet and waiting for it to dry. Activities provide a variety of opportunities for therapeutic gains. The process of grouting a tile trivet involves covering the individual's tile design with the grout mixture and is a messy step. The individual then sees that the tile pattern is emphasized with the addition of the grout. Waiting for the grout to dry requires an individual to delay gratification. See reference: Neistadt and Crepeau (eds): Crepeau: Activity analysis, a way of thinking about occupational performance.

11. (C) supervision. At this level, the child performs the task on his or her own but cannot be safely left alone, or the child may need verbal cueing or physical prompts for 1 to 24% of task. At the independent level (answer A) the child performs the complete task, including the set-up. At the independent-with-setup level (answer B) the child performs the task after someone sets it up. Minimal assist (answer D) signifies that the child performs 50 to 75% of the task independently, but needs physical assistance or other cueing for the remainder of the task. See reference: Case-Smith (ed): Shepherd, J: Self-care and adaptations for independent living.

12. (D) Carpal tunnel and chronic cervical tension Carpal tunnel syndrome and chronic cervical tension are just some of the work-related occurrences secondary to the arrival of visual display terminals and specialized technology that require repetition and unusual body positioning. Answers A and C are injuries typically not associated with repetitive motion or cumulative trauma disorders. Answer B, edema and paresthesias, are typical symptoms (not injuries) of repetitive motion and cumulative trauma disorders. See reference: Neistadt and Crepeau (eds): Fenton, S, and Gagnon, P: Treatment of work and productive activities: Functional restoration, an industrial approach.

13. (B) child's speed over long distances becomes less than that of a walking person. This child should be considered for a power wheelchair when the current means of locomotion proves less efficient and slower than locomotion by walking. Because the child will be experiencing progressive muscle weakness, energy conservation is of primary importance. Answers A and C address valid environmental considerations to be made after determining the general need for a powered chair. Waiting until the child becomes unable to propel the wheelchair (answer D) would make the transition more difficult and prevent the child from getting around independently in the meantime. See reference: Case-Smith (ed): Wright-Ott, C, and Egilson, S: Mobility.

14. (C) Implement compensatory strategies to manage the environment. Interventions directed toward improvement are typically unrealistic when working with individuals diagnosed with cognitive disorders. These disorders are characterized by deteriorating courses. A social skills emphasis (answer A) is more appropriate for individuals with schizophrenia. Habit restructuring (answer B) is more appropriate for those with substance use disorders. Role resumption (answer D) is more appropriate for those with mood disorders. See reference: Early: Understanding psychiatric diagnosis: the DSM-IV.

15. (B) "The client will initiate one request to one other group member for sharing or using group materials within a 1-week period." Reducing the number of requests and the variety or number of individuals the client is expected to interact with is the best way to simplify the initial goal. Extending the amount of time to accomplish the goal (answer A) does not make the goal easier to achieve. Increasing the number of individuals (answer C), and subsequently the number of requests, to five also makes the goal more difficult to achieve. Changing interactions to the group leader (answer D) moves the goal away from the original problem area of peer social conversation to authority conversations. See reference: Early: Analyzing, adapting, and grading activities.

16. (B) Median nerve The median nerve passes through the carpal tunnel at the wrist. Impingement in this region causes sensory changes in the thumb, index finger, long and half of the ring finger. Prolonged impingement in the carpal tunnel results in atrophy of the thenar eminence and weakness of the opponens pollicis. Injury to the radial nerve in the wrist area causes sensory damage only. Damage to the ulnar nerve at the wrist causes decreased grip strength and complete or partial loss of sensation over half of the fourth digit (ring finger) and all of the

fifth digit (little finger) plus the proximal hypothenar region. A brachial plexus injury may result in damage to any or all of the UE peripheral nerves. This may cause motor and/or sensory impairments. See reference: Pedretti (ed): Kasch, MC: Hand injuries.

17. (D) the measurability of activity performance. The potential to measure an activity's results is central to a behavioral frame of reference. Answer A is linked to developmental frames of reference, answer B is linked to psychoanalytic frames of reference, and answer C is linked to sensory integrative frames of reference. See reference: Neistadt and Crepeau (eds): Crepeau, EB and Neistadt, ME: Activity analysis: A way of thinking about occupational performance.

18. (A) within normal limits. The normal range of motion for internal rotation is 70 degrees. Rotation can be assessed with the humerus adducted against the trunk or with the shoulder abducted at 90 degrees. If the humeral movements for internal or external rotation are observed during the performance of activities and found to be adequate for the performance of any functional activities, the range of motion may be noted as WFL. The OT practitioner may choose not to perform a formal joint measurement if the joint is WFL, even though the end of the range may be lacking a few degrees, because the loss of movement may not be significant to the individual. Hypermobility at a joint is motion past the average range of motion, which at the shoulder would be past 70 degrees of internal rotation. If hypermobility is a deformity caused by an unstable joint as might occur after a surgical repair or a disease process, then splinting or another form of stabilization or immobilization can be used to correct the problem. If the practitioner observes hypermobility during range of motion, he or she should compare the range of motion to that on the individual's opposite side in order to assess normal range. A limitation of internal rotation at the shoulder would be less than 70 degrees of motion. If a limitation is apparent, the rehabilitation team may choose not to treat it unless it interferes with the function of the upper extremity. See reference: Trombly (ed): Trombly, CA: Evaluation of biomechanical and physiological aspects of motor performance.

19. (D) Post-traumatic stress disorder (PTSD) PTSD is an anxiety disorder that follows a traumatic event in a person's life. Answers A and B are mood disorders, and answer C is a psychotic disorder. See reference: Neistadt and Crepeau (eds): Giles, GM, and Neistadt, ME: Treatment for psychosocial components: Stress management.

20. (A) Punctuality, accepting directions from a supervisor, and interacting with coworkers Psychosocial components include time management, social conduct, interpersonal skills, and self-control. Punctuality and accepting feedback are examples of prevocational skills within these psychosocial performance components and are important prevocational skills. Memory, decision making, attention to task, and sequencing (answer B) are considered to be cognitive components. Standing tolerance, endurance, and eye–hand coordination (answer C) are categorized as sensorimotor components. Grooming and adhering to safety precautions (answer D) are work performance areas and are not psychosocial performance components. See reference: AOTA: Uniform Terminology for Occupational Therapy, third edition.

21. (B) Learning proper body mechanics Learning proper body mechanics (along with achieving a good fitness level) is one of the first steps to reducing the risk of reinjury in a work program. Answer C, work hardening, is appropriate to implement after the physical demands of the job specific task are achieved. Answer D, engaging in vocational counseling, is appropriate after it is determined that a client cannot return to the same job or employer. Answer A, a prework screening, is typically completed by the practitioner before the employer offers the new employee a job. See reference: Neistadt and Crepeau (eds): Fenton, S, and Gagnon, P: Treatment of work and productive activities: Functional restoration, an industrial approach.

22. (A) provide each patient with an individual project and have him or her choose a tile color for the project. The activity should begin with the most basic level of decision making. Each of the other choices provide increasingly more challenging decision making abilities. Choosing from an assortment of projects (answer B) requires higher level decision making ability than selecting a color. Answer C requires not only decisions on design, color, and size, but also involves decision making among group members. Answer D involves decision making on two separate aspects, pattern and colors, resulting in a higher level of complexity than answer A. See reference: Early: Analyzing, adapting, and grading activities.

23. (C) inferior to the anterior superior iliac spine. A seat belt placed across the lap inferior to the anterior superior iliac spine prevents the hips from being extended into a posterior pelvic tilt. If the seat belt is placed at an angle inferior to the ischial tuberosity (answer A), it would go across the thighs and allow a posterior pelvic tilt. A seat belt placed superior to the iliac crest or the posterior superior iliac spine (answers B and D, respectively) would be too high, allowing hip extension with posterior pelvic tilt to occur below the seat belt. See reference: Trombly (ed): Deitz, J, and Dudgeon, B: Wheelchair selection process.

24. (D) use active listening techniques. Active listening (answer D) is an effective listening response that enables the patient to know that his or her message has been communicated. Behaviors listed in answers A, B, and C can be counterproductive to developing a therapeutic relationship. Answers A and B may be perceived as enhancing a friendship, rather than a therapeutic relationship, and answer C may be considered inappropriate for someone who does not have adequate social skills. See reference: Ryan (ed): The Certified Occupational Therapy Assistant: Blechert, TF, and Kari, N: Interpersonal communication skills and applied group dynamics.

25. (D) doll house and dress-up clothes. To encourage symbolic play, the child should be exposed to toys offering imaginative, open-ended play opportunities, encouraging formulation of ideas and feelings. Answers A, B, and C are not only representative of the younger (answer A) or older child (answers B and C), but they also offer more defined, closed-ended play opportunities with predictable results. See reference: Case-Smith (ed): Morrison, CD, Metzger, P: Play.

26. (B) objective. Measured results based on an individual's performance are included in the objective section. The subjective portion (answer A) of the SOAP note contains information provided by the patient or family. Analysis of the measurements is recorded in the assessment area (answer C) of the SOAP note. Plans for future sessions are included in the plan section (answer D). See reference: Sabonis-Chafee and Hussey: Treatment planning and implementation.

27. (B) play and self-care activities. "When providing occupational therapy care for children with terminal illness, the underlying principle is to add quality to their remaining days. There are two performance areas that occupational therapists should address in children with terminal illness: (1) play activities and (2) activities of daily living" (p. 838). Educational activities (answer A) would not address the primary principle of adding quality of life. Play activities help the child to focus interest and express feelings and may incorporate socialization and motor activities (answers C and D), but neither of these types of activities alone would be the primary focus. Self-care activities allow the child to maintain independence and purposefulness. See reference: Case-Smith (ed): Barnstorff, MJ: The dying child.

28. (C) Digging a garden with a shovel Activities that include bilateral use of tonic muscles against resistance, such as digging a garden, playing volleyball, or playing tug of war, can help to normalize tone in this population. Dancing with rapid alternating movements (answer A) may heighten arousal. Playing Twister (answer B) may facilitate balance and promote interpersonal skills. Rocking in a rocking chair (answer D) may reduce the level of arousal. See reference: Bruce and Borg: Movement-centered frame of reference.

29. (C) further decline. Because MS is a degenerative disease, it is likely that the individual receiving a wheelchair will eventually decline further in functional performance. Improved wheelchair mobility and gains in strength (answers A and D) are not characteristic of progressive degenerative diseases. When ordering a wheelchair for a pediatric or adolescent client, it is important to anticipate growth of the individual (answer B). See reference: Neistadt and Crepeau (eds): Pulaski, KH, in Adult neurological dysfunction.

30. (B) edema. Contrast baths cause vasodilation and vasoconstriction, which facilitate a pumping out of the edema. Retrograde massage assists with the facilitation of blood and lymph movement. Pressure wraps (coban) are applied distal to proximal to address edema issues. Answers C and D, wound healing and scar management, may be contraindicated for these techniques because of possible inadequate wound closure and the potential for skin breakdown. Answer A, heterotopic ossification, is typically treated with gentle active range of motion within the pain free range and is often treated surgically. See reference: Pedretti (ed): Kasch, MC: Hand injuries.

31. (C) demonstrating typical development for a child with Down syndrome. Answer C is correct because exclusive "W" sitting is commonly seen in children with low muscle tone. The child is compensating for an inability to achieve stability in a variety of positions that require dynamic postural control, depending on skeletal rather than neuromuscular structures for stability. Answers A and D are not correct because exclusive "W" sitting would be considered both normal and age appropriate for a 5-year-old child with Down syndrome. Answer B is not correct because exclusive "W" sitting is considered to be a compensatory position. See reference: Kramer and Hinojosa (eds): Schoen, SA, and Anderson, J: Neurodevelopmental treatment frame of reference.

32. (D) Conduct a group discussion about responsibilities people have when living in a group home A cognitive approach is most appropriate with individuals "who must learn to do situational problem solving…when the individual has deficits in attention span, memory, or other cognitive abilities…or when the skills being learned need to be generalized." Discussion that heightens awareness in an attempt to modify behavior is one example of a cognitive intervention. Rewards and praise (answers A and B) are used when a behavioral approach is desired. Posting a schedule (answer C) is an example of an environmental adaptation that may facilitate compliance with chores but does not represent a cognitive approach. See reference: Christiansen (ed): Self-care strategies in intervention for psychosocial conditions.

33. (B) Working on a mock car engine Working on a mock car engine provides a work simulation that would be required by the client's job. This activity would also assist with increasing his endurance, strength, and productivity. Answer A, lifting weights, is not a work-hardening goal when performed in isolation of a simulated work task. Answer C, visiting the work site, would not be a work hardening activity but rather part of the onsite analysis that is typically completed by the practitioner and vocational retraining counselor. Answer D, meal preparation, is not considered to be a demand required by this particular vocation. See reference: Pedretti (ed): Kasch, MC: Hand injuries.

34. (C) Bring the seat in for reevaluation within 6 months Fit and function of seating and mobility should be reassessed within 6 months to account for the child's growth as well as any changes in posture. Parents should not make unsupervised adaptations (answer A) because improper positioning could harm the child. Weekly adjustment (answer B) is usually not necessary, and transporting the seat every week would be an unnecessary inconvenience to the parents. The end of the IEP (answer D) may be more than 6 months away and too long to wait. See reference: Case-Smith (ed): Wright-Ott, C, and Egilson, S: Mobility.

35. (A) figure-ground discrimination. Figure-ground discrimination is the ability to distinguish an object from the background. A person with impaired figure-ground discrimination would have difficulty finding the sock despite its position on the bed. Other deficits that may be demonstrated by the person would be an inability to see the sock on one side of the bed (unilateral neglect), to find it in relation to the bed (position in space), and to know how to get back to the bed to look for the sock (cognitive mapping). See reference: Trombly (ed): Quintana, LA: Evaluation of perception and cognition.

36. (B) an interest checklist. An interest checklist is frequently used to initiate discussion of how a patient usually spends his leisure time and to identify areas of specific interest. Although the evaluation of living skills and the self-care evaluations (answers A and D) address the use of leisure time, they are used primarily to assess skills in personal care, safety and health, money management, transportation, use of the telephone, and work. An activity configuration (answer C) is used to assess the patient's use of time and his feelings about all of the activities he performs in a typical day or week. See reference: Early: Data gathering and evaluation.

37. (A) Mount lever handles on doors and faucets For children with reduced strength and endurance, using less complex movements and less force results in energy conservation. Lever handles require less energy than knob handles on doors, faucets, and appliances. Answers B and C are environmental adaptations recommended to minimize the danger of slipping and falling for children with incoordination or postural instability. Answer D is contraindicated because work at a vertical surface against gravity requires more energy than movement in a horizontal plane. See reference: Case-Smith (ed): Dudgeon, BJ: Pediatric rehabilitation.

38. (A) using effective communication skills.
Clarifying expectations, honestly defining needs, and providing tactful and constructive feedback are communication skills that promote understanding. Successful communication with the patient's children will most likely help them deal with their fears and concerns, increase their understanding of their father's condition, and elicit greater cooperation. Although time management techniques, deep breathing, and laughter (answers B, C, and D) are all useful and valid stress reduction techniques, they do not address the issue at hand, which is communication between the father and his children. See reference: Neistadt and Crepeau (eds): Giles, GM, and Neistadt, ME, in Treatment for psychosocial components: stress management.

39. (B) Go out for lunch to a fast-food restaurant A key principle in intervention for effective transition includes using natural environments and cues and increasing community-based instruction as the student gets older. Classroom-based activities (answers A, C, and D) are not as effective in promoting development of the community member role as activities that actually take place in the community. See reference: Case-Smith (ed): Spencer, K: Transition services: From school to adult life.

40. (D) A clustered independent living arrangement These are usually composed of "apartment clusters or other types of housing in close proximity to each other, in which groups of residents with disabilities share services such as attendants and transportation" (p. 362). Cradle-to-grave homes (answer A) are houses designed and built with accessibility in mind. If a resident of a cradle-to-grave home begins to use a wheelchair later in life, the home will already be wheelchair accessible. Transitional living centers (answer B) "provide temporary living arrangements for individuals who are in a transitional phase between hospital or institution and independent community living" (p. 362). Adult day programs (answer C) are rehabilitation-oriented day programs for clients who live in the community; they are not residential. See reference: Trombly (ed): Law, M, Stewart, D, and Strong, S: Achieving access to home, community, and workplace.

41. (B) Follow test manual directions When administering a standardized test, directions from the test manual should be followed closely to ensure reliability of test results. The test environment should be free of visual or auditory distractions or the child may have difficulty concentrating; therefore, answer A, "test in a stimulating environment" is incorrect.

Answer C is incorrect because there are times when "...a child's fatigue, behavior, or time constraints" make it impossible to give the complete test in one session, and "most tests provide guidelines about how the test can be administered in two sessions" (p. 239). Answer D is wrong because, although the overall success of an evaluation can depend on the OT practitioner's ability to establish a rapport with the child and the family, too much conversation with the child may be distracting and prevent optimal performance. See reference: Case-Smith (ed): Richardson, PK: Use of standardized tests in pediatric practice.

42. (C) To teach the caregiver how to lift and turn the client safely Individuals unable to move themselves and those with sensory loss are susceptible to the development of decubiti. Skin damage results from pressure on the skin over a prolonged period of time. The skin over bony prominences is particularly prone to the development of decubitus ulcers. Frequent position changes are essential for these individuals to prevent skin breakdown and the risk of serious infection. If the patient were already involved in a strengthening program (answer A), it may be appropriate to change it to a maintenance program at this point. A bed-mobility program (answer B) and an ECU (answer D) would be appropriate if the individual has potential in these areas, but instructing the caregiver in how to reposition the patient is the highest-priority modification. See reference: Trombly (ed): Bentzel, K: Remediating sensory impairment.

43. (C) Weight-bearing on hands This is the only activity that will facilitate hand function in the preparation phase. Weight-bearing on the hands gives deep pressure to the surface of the hand and facilitates wrist and arm extension, as well as shoulder cocontraction, to prepare the arm for reach and stabilization of the hand for grasping. The other answers all provide different types of grasp activities that could be used as therapy. See reference: Case-Smith (ed): Exner, CE: Development of hand skills.

44. (A) decrease joint stress and pain. It is very important to preserve joint integrity in individuals with arthritis by using adaptive equipment to avoid or reduce the wear and tear stresses on fragile joints. Adaptive equipment would not correct deformities (answer B) because deformities are only corrected by surgery or with orthotic devices that reposition the joints in correct alignment. Adaptive equipment allows activities to be completed but would not simplify work by eliminating steps to an activity (answer C). Another reason adaptive equipment is used is to increase (not decrease) independence (answer D). See reference: Pedretti (ed): Hittle, JM, Pedretti, LW, and Kasch, MC: Rheumatoid arthritis.

45. (B) emotional lability. Emotional lability is the rapid shifting of moods. Emotional lability may be one of the symptoms observed in individuals experiencing mania (answer A). Paranoia (answer C) describes enduring beliefs about being harmed. Denial (answer D) is not acknowledging the presence of information. See reference: Early: Responding to symptoms and behaviors.

46. (B) perform the evaluation over several sessions. Upper extremity evaluation is lengthy and can be fatiguing, and fatigue should be avoided with individuals with Guillain-Barré syndrome. In addition, results may be invalid if the individual is fatigued and not performing at the highest level possible. Strength, range of motion, and sensory testing (answers A, C, and D) are all important when evaluating an individual with Guillain-Barré syndrome, but must be administered using a method that will yield valid results. See reference: Pedretti (ed): McCormack, GL, and Pedretti, LW, in Motor unit dysfunction.

47. (C) initiation. Initiation, or the ability to begin a task, affects a person's spontaneity in performing activities and how much he or she is able to perform. An individual with initiation problems may be able to plan or carry out activities but may be unable to begin until prompted by another person. Problems with attention (answer A), concentration (answer B), or apraxia (answer D) are evidenced as the incomplete or incorrect completion of an activity. See reference: Zoltan: Executive functions.

48. (A) Ballet To promote the development of anticipatory control, movement should be slow, predictable, and controlled from a stable base. Participation in a dance class would involve controlled movement from a stable base. Answers B, C, and D are activities that feature faster-moving objects whose speed and direction of movement cannot be controlled by the player and require quick reactions to unpredictable stimuli. See reference: Case-Smith (ed): Nichols, DS: The development of postural control.

49. (C) anxiety and confusion among group members. It is important for group leaders to demonstrate consistency by showing the same degree of respect, interest, and authority toward every group member. Overdependence (answer A) would be a result of the group leader's not giving group members enough autonomy. Group members know what to expect from the group leader (answer B) when the group leader demonstrates consistent behavior. Too much (answer D), too little, or inappropriate praise are aspects of nurturing behavior, which support growth and development of group members. See reference: Early: Group concepts and techniques.

50. (B) Raise the toilet The minimum doorway width that allows a standard wheelchair to pass through easily is 32 inches. A standard toilet is 15 inches, which is 3 inches lower than the standard

wheelchair seat. Raising the toilet 18 inches would make transfers easier for this individual. See reference: Neistadt and Crepeau (eds): Holm, MB, Rogers, JC, and Stone, RG: Person-task-environment intervention: a decision-making guide.

51. (B) Add the two new clients and then divide the members into two groups It is generally not cost-effective to run groups of less than three individuals, and it is not effective to have more than eight in a group. Maintaining an appropriate group size enables the OT practitioner to adequately observe the interpersonal skills of the members. Using interviews or groups with three or fewer members (answer C) will provide dyadic interaction information but not information about group interpersonal skills. Asking those originally asked to wait (answer A) is countertherapeutic to those individuals. A group of nine (answer D) would be too large to be effective. See reference: Cole: Writing a group treatment protocol.

52. (A) work locks and latches on doors and windows. The ability to manipulate the locks and latches is a safety concern because the individual may be unable to open them to let family members into their home or close them to keep intruders from entering. Built-up handles (answer B), energy conservation techniques (answer C), and adaptations to clothing fasteners (answer D) are not safety issues. See reference: Trombly (ed): Feinberg, JR, and Trombly, CA: Arthritis.

53. (B) Boy Scouts. While answers A, C, and D describe activities that may help build his sense of competence, only participation in Boy Scouts includes the necessary interaction with peers. Noncompetitive activities, a uniform to signify belonging, predictable routines, and exposure to role models are all elements of the Boy Scouts that can help him develop social competence. See reference: Case-Smith (ed): Cronin, AF: Psychosocial and emotional domains.

54. (C) instructing caregivers in task breakdown. Instructing the caregivers in task breakdown, or breaking down tasks into simple steps and then providing step-by-step instructions, will allow the client to perform activities as capabilities decline. At this stage of the disease, memory retraining (answer A) and ADL retraining (answer B) will probably not be effective. Leisure activities (answer D) structured to meet the needs of the client with Alzheimer's disease could be helpful but will not address the primary problem of performance of self-care activities. See reference: Pedretti (ed): Atchison, P, Pedretti, LW, McCormack, GL: Alzheimer's disease.

55. (B) The client can usually handle routine daily functions. Answer B is correct because it describes the skills of an individual with moderate or trainable mental retardation. This child would most likely be able to complete ADL, live in a group home setting, and do unskilled work in a sheltered workshop. Answer A describes a child with profound mental retardation, answer C describes a child with severe mental retardation, and answer D describes a child who is mildly mentally retarded and educable. See reference: Case-Smith (ed): Rogers, SL, Gordon, CY, Schanzenbacher, KE, and Case-Smith, J: Common diagnosis in pediatric occupational therapy.

56. (D) The individual asks for more beverages during meals, but appears surprised when the therapist indicates beverages in closed containers are on the meal tray. The subjective portion of the SOAP note should contain information that is gained through a chart review, or communication with the patient, his or her family, or staff. This information is not measurable and therefore is considered subjective. Answer A would be in the program plan. Answers B and C would be in the objective portion because they are either measurable or based on specific observations. See reference: Trombly (ed): Trombly, CA: Planning, guiding, and documenting therapy.

57. (C) Parents should be considered as part of a collaborative partnership with therapists. "The first interactions of the therapist with a family open the door to establishing a partnership" in which "the family and therapist collaborate using agreed upon roles to obtain agreed upon goals for the child". (p.117). Parents should be encouraged to observe their child in therapy so that they may better understand the program and their child's problems; therefore answer A is incorrect. Answer B is incorrect because although some parents may carry out therapy programs at home, "the goal is not for parents to become quasiprofessionals" (p. 117). It is also recommended that both parents be present when an OT program is discussed (answer D is incorrect), so that one does not become dependent on the other for information and communication. See reference: Case-Smith (ed): Humphry, R, and Case-Smith, J: Working with families.

58. (C) baking cookies using a recipe. This is a well-delineated meal preparation activity that provides structure with a specific sequence of tasks. Setting a table or preparing a shopping list (answers A and D) do not necessarily require sequencing of tasks. Planning a meal (answer B) involves a great deal of organizational ability and would not be an appropriate choice for an initial activity to address goals relating to sequencing tasks. See reference: Early: Responding to symptoms and behaviors.

59. (D) Place dishes near the dishwasher, bend down on one or both knees, and load. Bending down on one or both knees increases balance while reducing the need to bend at the waist. Answer A, loading from a standing position, is the traditional method of loading a dishwasher, and it increases

bending at the waist. Answer B, washing the dishes in the sink, does not address the most effective way to alleviate back pain when actually loading the dishwasher. Answer C, standing in front of the dishwasher and loading, is similar to answer A in that trunk rotation and flexion are required to effectively perform the activity. See reference: Pedretti (ed): Smithline, J: Low back pain.

60. (D) Reinforcement of competence According to Erikson, an 8-year-old is usually at the stage of industry versus inferiority, during which he or she develops a sense of competency. For a client who is expected to lose motor function gradually, a treatment plan that will provide him with an ongoing sense of competence (possibly in other areas) is especially relevant. Answers A, B, and C describe other developmental issues identified by Erikson that are typically achieved at other ages: basic trust (answer A) in infancy, initiative (answer B) during the toddler years, and self-identity (answer C) during adolescence. See reference: Case-Smith (ed): Law, M, Missiuna, C, Pollock, N, and Stewart, D: Foundations of occupational therapy practice with children.

61. (D) chaining. Teaching a task one step at a time, gradually adding more steps as steps are mastered, is called chaining. Chaining is frequently used when teaching a multistep task because it is easier to learn one step at a time than it is to learn a complete activity. Repetition and rehearsal (answers A and C) involve repeating the whole activity repetitively until the activity is learned. Cueing (answer B) uses an external source to remind a person of the next step or part of that step. See reference: Zoltan: Executive functions.

62. (B) mounting a safety rail next to the toilet. In order to sit independently on the toilet and relax sufficiently to control muscles needed for elimination, the child has to feel posturally secure. Safety rails next to the toilet, low toilets that allow the child to put both feet on the ground, and reducer rings to decrease the size of a toilet seat all help to provide maximal stability for the child with unstable posture. Answers A, C, and D describe adaptations used for other deficits. Replacing zippers and buttons with Velcro closures (answer A) is helpful for a child with reduced strength or fine motor coordination. Introducing toilet paper tongs (answer C) helps increase reach in a child with limited range of motion. Placing a colorful target (answer D) helps boys aim into the bowl, a difficulty associated with perceptual or cognitive limitations. See reference: Case-Smith (ed): Shepherd, J: Self care and adaptations for independent living.

63. (A) Transferring on and off a commode seat The patient will most likely utilize a walker to transfer on and off a commode seat. In this case, the assistive device (the walker) will permit the patient to adhere to the mandated toe touch precautions, while providing balance, decreasing pain and encouraging safe transfers. Answer B, bed mobility, does not indicate the need for a walker. In this case, the patient may benefit from the use of a trapeze attached to the bed to increase the use of both upper extremities while performing bed mobility. Answer C, self-feeding, can be performed in bed, or at the patient's bedside prior to performing a kitchen/meal preparation task which would include the use of an assistive device. While answer D, distal lower extremity dressing, can be performed in bed with devices such as a long-handled shoehorn, sock aid, dressing stick, elastic shoelaces and reacher, most of these activities can be initiated at the bedside in a chair without the use of a walker. See reference: Bernstein (ed): Bernstein Lewis, C and Daleiden, S: Clinical implications of neurologic changes in the aging process.

64. (B) Catching and bursting soap bubbles This activity involves visually tracking a slow-moving target and requires minimal fine motor precision to accomplish a successful "hit." Answers A, C, and D also require visual tracking and eye–hand coordination, but they involve more fast-moving targets and require immediate, more precise movements. These activities can therefore be used to promote more advanced skills. See reference: Case-Smith (ed): Dubois, SA: Preschool services.

65. (C) CARF. The Commission on Accreditation of Rehabilitation Facilities (CARF) is the regulatory agency for the provision of rehabilitation services. AOTA (answer A) was formed in March of 1917 as the National Society for the Promotion of Occupational Therapy. JCAHO (answer B) is the Joint Commission on Accreditation of Hospital Organizations. The JCAHO reviews the medical care provided by hospital organizations. The NBCOT (answer D) is the agency that develops and administers the examination for registration as an OT; therefore, answers A, B, and D are incorrect. See reference: Neistadt and Crepeau (eds): Bailey, DM: Legislative and reimbursement influences on occupational therapy: Changing opportunities.

66. (A) Prevent loss of joint and skin mobility During the acute stage, when burn wounds are partial or full thickness in nature, maintenance of joint range of motion and skin mobility is the primary goal of intervention. Providing adaptive equipment (answer B) is typically performed during the surgical or postoperative stage, and compression and vascular garments (answer C) and the prevention of scarring (answer D) are goals most commonly implemented during the rehabilitation phase. See reference: Pedretti (ed): Jordan, CL, and Allely, RR: Burns and burn rehabilitation.

67. (B) rinse the eye with an eye wash or water immediately. It is necessary to immediately wash the eye because the "backwash" fluid in the IV is uni-

dentifiable body fluid and universal precautions should be followed. It is recommended to flush an exposed area with warm water or normal saline immediately. Therefore, answers A, C, and D are incorrect. Following the cleansing of the eye, it is recommended to contact the immediate supervisor and report the exposure through the facility reporting system. See reference: Occupational Safety and Health Administration: Standard #1910. 1030, 1 FR 5507, February 13, 1996.

68. (B) show acceptance and understanding to the individual. Paraphrasing is used to clarify and relay acceptance of what an individual has communicated. The OT practitioner paraphrases by repeating in her or his own words what the client has said. Redirection (answer A) is used to promote healthier thoughts and behaviors. Forcing the individual to make a choice (answer C) may be accomplished by providing a question that includes two possible choices. A client is encouraged to provide additional information (answer D) when the OT practitioner asks open-ended questions. See reference: Denton: Treatment planning and implementation.

69. (D) Interdisciplinary care improvement teams Health care professionals who are part of an interdisciplinary care improvement team work together to "address such issues as patient flow, the discharge process, patient outreach, and promotion and cost-efficiencies" (p. 47). Quality improvement (answer A) is a systematic approach to monitoring patient care. Peer review (answer B) is a component of quality improvement. Cost accounting (answer C) is a method of tracking the costs of specific services or costs incurred by diagnosis-specific groups. See reference: Jacobs and Logigian (eds): Logigian, MK: Cost management.

70. (B) increase physical activity and fitness. Wellness programs focus on developing personal control of behaviors through educational approaches and active participation in activities that promote health, such as increasing level of physical activity to improve physical fitness. Answers A, C, and D reflect traditional occupational therapy therapeutic interventions to improve performance in specific deficit areas rather than promoting general good health. See reference: Cottrell (ed): Swarbrick, P: A wellness model for an acute psychiatric setting.

71. (C) " I'm just too tired." One of the main symptoms of severe depression is decreased energy; therefore, the response of "I'm too tired" indicates fatigue. Answer A reflects a level of feeling that is higher than the usual subdued feelings associated with depression. Answer B reflects the individual's perceptions of his or her ability or competence. Answer D is a response reflecting interests or values that conflict with the proposed activity. See reference: Bonder: Mental disorders.

72. (B) have at least 1 year of experience as a certified OT practitioner. An individual who passes the NBCOT examination becomes a certified OT practitioner. In order to be a primary supervisor for a level-II OT student, the individual must be a registered OT with at least 1 year of experience. To supervisor level-II OTA students, the individual must be a certified OT practitioner with at least 1 year of experience. There is no minimum experience requirement for supervising level-I students. Although it may help to develop supervisory skills to work with a level-I student before taking a level-II student (answer D), there is no such requirement. See reference: AOTA: Standards for an accredited educational program for the occupational therapist.

73. (A) repetition, high force, and awkward joint postures. Repetition, high force, and awkward joint postures are work-related risk factors that are frequently associated with cumulative trauma disorders. Answer B, progressive resistive exercises, joint mobilization, and weight bearing, are not considered to be primary factors that contribute to cumulative trauma disorders. Answers C and D, inflammation, swelling, pain, fatigue, cramps, and paresthesias, are all considered to be potential symptoms of cumulative trauma disorders, not factors that contribute to the condition. See reference: Pedretti (ed): Kasch, MC: Hand injuries.

74. (A) Use disposable cotton swabs and have clients bring their own cosmetics Universal precautions are related to the prevention of the spread of infection. Using disposable cotton swabs and having clients use their own cosmetics would be effective in reducing the risk of infection. Combing someone's hair (answer B) does not usually involve risks related to blood or bodily fluids. Washing equipment (answer C) that is used near eyes and mouths by several individuals is inadequate. Avoiding glass containers (answer D) is a safety precaution that is related to self-harm and not universal precautions. See reference: Early: Safety techniques.

75. (B) a tub bench and toilet rails. A tub bench and toilet rails make bathroom transfers easier and safer and allows the person with a unilateral LE amputation to transfer independently. Lightweight cooking utensils (answer A) are recommended for those with weakness or joint involvement of the upper extremities. Answers C and D are incorrect because long-handled dressing devices and reachers are more likely to be recommended when compensation for hip or trunk flexion is needed, and use of these devices might discourage the normal bending activity in the person with LE amputation. See reference: Pedretti (ed): Pasquinelli, S: Lower extremity amputations and prosthetics.

76. (D) determine the need for further evaluation. The purpose of screening is to determine whether further assessments are needed and, if so, which tests would be appropriate for that child. A screening test is not designed for planning programs (answer C) or consultation (answer A), and they do not test any skills (answer B) in a comprehensive way. See reference: Solomon (ed): Peralta, AM, and Kramer, P: General treatment considerations.

77. (D) An exposure has occurred; put on gloves, clean up the spill with paper towels, put the soiled paper towels in a plastic bag, seal the bag, disinfect the area, and finish the patient's session with whatever time is still left. The Occupational Safety and Health Administration (OSHA) has identified materials that require universal precautions to include blood, semen, vaginal secretions, cerebrospinal fluid, synovial fluid, pleural fluid, any body fluid with visible blood, any unidentifiable body fluid, and saliva from dental procedures. Items OSHA has identified as not needing universal precautions include feces, nasal secretions, sputum, sweat, tears, urine, and vomitus. Because the urine had blood in it, in this case it WOULD be considered an exposure (answer A). Hospitals have policies regarding response to exposures such as this. Answer A is incorrect because it indicates that an exposure has not occurred. Leaving the area unavailable for other therapists and their patients who might need to use it (answer B) would be inconsiderate. Contaminated linens and towels (answer B) need to be placed in a specially designated laundry area. See reference: Early: Safety techniques.

78. (C) A client with a C6 injury An individual with C6 quadriplegia has some use of the abductor pollicis longus, extensor pollicis longus, extensor digitorum communis, and extensor carpi ulnaris. The extensor tone of the muscles in conjunction with the splint will operate the power for prehension force. Individuals with CI or C3 injuries have higher level lesions and lack the wrist extension strength needed to operate the wrist-driven flexor hinge splint. An individual with a T1 injury is able to grasp and manipulate utensils without difficulty or need for assistance. See reference: Trombly (ed): Hollar, LD: Spinal cord injury.

79. (D) installation of a bidet with a spray wash and air-drying mechanism. Use of a bidet for hygiene after use of the toilet eliminates any upper extremity reach requirement. Answers A, B, and C describe adaptations appropriate for a child with poor postural control in need of external stability devices; these devices would not reduce reach requirements. See reference: Case-Smith (ed): Shepherd, J: Self-care and adaptations for independent living.

80. (A) total quality management. This model "encourages health care institutions to move away from a focus on compliance to standards and refocus on improvement goals in an effort to deliver high quality care" (p. 121). Answers B, C, and D, are all concepts that contribute to the model of total quality management and include finance, marketing, and operations. See reference: Jacobs and Logigian (eds): Logigan, MK: Quality management.

81. (A) Perform a job analysis. Job analysis identifies essential functions of a particular job. Based on the results, the OT practitioner can then work with the individual to maximize performance or request reasonable accommodation (answer B). Activities that promote self-efficacy (answer C) are beneficial for individuals with depression but should not be used at this stage of the individual's program. A weekly support group may be an effective way for the individual to obtain support and can be recommended by the OT practitioner, but it is not the FIRST action the OT practitioner would take. See reference: Early: Work, homemaking and childcare.

82. (B) The child's writing, dressing, and self-feeding skills Because the child was being treated for difficulties with fine motor skills, discharge criteria should focus on fine motor function. Answers A, C, and D describe information that is relevant in overall discharge planning but is not relevant in determining readiness for discharge. See reference: Case-Smith (ed): Case-Smith, J, Rogers, J, and Johnson, JH: School-based occupational therapy.

83. (A) attention-deficit hyperactivity disorder (ADHD). This behavior exemplifies the excessive fidgeting and restlessness, inattention, and impulsiveness characteristic of ADHD. Although some of the symptoms of overactivity and impulsiveness are part of a mood disorder of the manic type (answer B), there usually are also symptoms of grandiosity and inflated self-esteem. A child with a conduct disorder (answer C) would exhibit interference with the basic rights of other children or societal rules. A child with anxiety disorder (answer D) would show signs of uneasiness, apprehension, or dread associated with anticipation of danger. See reference: Neistadt and Crepeau (eds): Florey, L: Psychosocial dysfunction in childhood and adolescence.

84. (B) activity adaptation. Modifying how directions are provided is one way to adapt activities. Activity analysis (answer A) is the process of identifying the aspects, steps, and materials used in performing the activity. Grading activities (answer C) is a gradual progression of steps toward a goal. Clinical reasoning (answer D) is the problem-solving process that practitioners use in thinking about a client's treatment. See reference: Early: Analyzing, adapting, and grading activities.

85. (D) Ice application, immobilization, and splinting Ice, immobilization, and splinting are all interventions that are considered to be appropriate adjunct activities to be used during the acute stages of tennis elbow. Answers A, B, and C, are all contraindicated because of their potential to increase

edema, pain, and immobility. See reference: Cailliet: Elbow pain.

86. (B) Ask the individual to try some lacing with distant supervision and praise her for what she has been able to do All of the responses are increments of approaches used for decreasing dependency needs, but answer B is the best next step in this case because it allows the individual to attempt some lacing in the presence of the OT, who in turn offers reassurance that the individual is actually able to do the activity. The step in answer B would be followed by the step in answer D. Here the individual is required to attempt some lacing without benefit of the OT at her side; the OT is nearby, but working with another client. As the individual is able to do more of the activity independently, written instructions (answer A) replace the OT as instructor. Finally, when the individual is feeling comfortable with self-instruction, asking her to work on the project out of the presence of the OT (answer C) heightens the level of self-responsibility. See reference: Early: Analyzing, adapting, and grading activities.

87. (B) An activity exploring leisure opportunities and problems In the process of making choices about activities, the first step is developing awareness and knowledge. OT practitioners "... assist the clients in developing awareness of options and limits" (p. 387). This individual's leisure interests are already known, so answer A would be a duplication of information you already have. Magazine picture collages could be adapted to further examine interests and values, but this answer (answer C) does not describe such an adaptation. Answer D is premature at this point because the individual has not identified any goals around which to plan future leisure activities. See reference: Neistadt and Crepeau (eds): Knox, SH: Treatment through play and leisure.

88. (D) Use dust mitt to keep fingers fully extended Using dust mitts "keeps fingers straight and prevents the static contraction and potentially deforming forces of holding a dust cloth" (p. 644). Pushing the vacuum (answer A) forward by straightening the elbow completely, then pulling it back close to the body utilizes long strokes and promotes good elbow and shoulder range of motion. When ironing (answer B), trying to get the elbow into full extension helps to maintain elbow range of motion. Keeping lightweight objects (answer C) on high shelves encourages reaching, which helps maintain shoulder range of motion. See reference: Pedretti (ed): Hittle, JM, Pedretti, LW, and Kasch, MC: Rheumatoid arthritis.

89. (D) The effect of personal traits and the environment on role performance Evaluation according to the Model of Human Occupation would focus on the effect of personal traits and the environment on role performance. Evaluation according to the Behavioral frame of reference identifies problem behaviors that need to be extinguished (answer A). The Object Relations frame of reference seeks to clarify thoughts, feelings, and experiences that influence behavior (answer B). An OT using the Cognitive Disability frame of reference should evaluate cognitive function, including assets and limitations (answer C). See reference: Bruce and Borg: Model of human occupation.

90. (D) applesauce. Foods with even consistency, uniform texture, and increased density such as applesauce are the easiest to control and swallow. Foods with multiple textures like chicken noodle soup (answer A), sticky foods like peanut butter (answer B), and foods that are fibrous or break up in the mouth like carrot sticks (answer C) should be avoided. See reference: Case-Smith (ed): Case-Smith, J, and Humphry, R: Feeding intervention.

91. (B) flexed at all joints. When weight bearing, the fingers should be flexed at all joints (the fisted position). This preserves the tenodesis function by protecting the finger flexors from overstretching. Another reason for this position is to prevent claw-hand deformity by protecting the intrinsic hand muscles from overstretching. See reference: Pedretti (ed): Adler, C: Spinal cord injury.

92. (B) Dressing habits Certain dressing habits may indicate tactile defensiveness; for example, the child may show poor tolerance of certain textures or avoid wearing turtlenecks, socks, or shoes. Conversely, some children may never take off their shoes in order to avoid tactile overstimulation. Reading skills (answer A), friendships (answer C), and the choice of hobbies (answer D) could be affected secondarily, as a result of intolerance of certain textures or human touch or the inability to concentrate. However, because of the close connection between dressing and tactile tolerance, knowledge of the child's dressing habits (answer B) will give the OT practitioner the most reliable information. See reference: Case-Smith (ed): Parham, LD and Mailloux, Z: Sensory integration.

93. (D) Dynamometer This individual exhibits difficulty in the area of strength. A dynamometer measures grip strength through gross hand grasp. A volumeter (answer C) is a container used to measure edema in the hand by measuring the amount of water displaced when the hand is placed into the container. A goniometer (answer A) is a tool with two arms used to measure movement at a joint. One arm is held stationary while the other arm moves around an axis of 360 degrees. An aesthesiometer (answer B) measures two-point discrimination with a moveable point attached to a ruler that has a stationary point at one end. See reference: Trombly (ed): Trombly, CA: Evaluation of biomechanical and physiological aspects of motor performance.

94. (C) Provide project samples for clients to du-

plicate Individuals functioning at cognitive level 4 are able to copy demonstrated directions presented one step at a time. They find it easier to copy a sample than to follow directions or diagrams. Individuals functioning at cognitive level 3 are capable of using their hands for simple, repetitive tasks (answer A) but are unlikely to produce a consistent end product. Those functioning at cognitive level 5 can generally perform a task involving three familiar steps and one new one (answer B). Individuals functioning at cognitive level 6 can anticipate errors and plan ways to avoid them. These individual would be capable of following written directions (answer D). See reference: Early: Some practice models for occupational therapy in mental health.

95. (D) Alternate tasks that require standing with those that can be performed sitting The performance component at issue in this question is fatigue. When fatigue impedes occupational performance, energy conservation techniques should be considered. Alternating sitting and standing activities is one method that can be applied to conserve energy; others include avoiding bending and stooping, avoiding unnecessary trips, using an appropriate work height, and relaxing homemaking standards. Convincing the individual to do something she can't afford (answer A) may not be in her best interests and it is not an example consistent with the OT concept of collaborative decision making. Although increasing strength (answer B) may ultimately be useful, endurance is typically a more pressing issue for individuals with MS. Using the largest joint available for the task is a joint protection technique more appropriate for an individual with arthritis. See reference: Pedretti (ed): Hittle, JM, Pedretti, LW, and Kasch, MC, in Rheumatoid arthritis.

96. (D) distractibility. Distractibility involves losing one's focus because of other stimuli. Memory (answer A) is the ability to recall knowledge and past events. Problems with spatial operations (answer B) are generally observed when individuals attempt to fit objects into specific spaces. Generalization of learning (answer C) may be observed by asking the client to use existing knowledge in a new situation. See reference: Early: Responding to symptoms and behaviors.

97. (A) checking for irritation and pressure problems. Because a toddler cannot communicate discomfort effectively, skin irritation may go unnoticed for too long. A young child, therefore, is at higher risk for developing skin and pressure problems than an older, more verbal one. Although answers B, C, and D describe important factors in splint care, for the young child, primary emphasis should be placed on answer A. See reference: Case-Smith (ed): Exner, CE: Development of hand skills.

98. (C) visual agnosia. Visual agnosia is the inability to recognize common objects and demonstrate their use in an activity. Apraxia (answer A) is the inability to perform purposeful movement on command. A person with alexia (answer D) is unable to understand written language. Stereognosis (answer B) is the ability to identify an object by manipulating it with the fingers without seeing it. See reference: Trombly (ed): Quintana, L: Evaluation of perception and cognition.

99. (B) avoid use of power tools and sharp instruments. Individuals experiencing extrapyramidal syndrome, which may cause muscular rigidity, tremors, and/or sudden muscle spasms, should avoid using power tools or sharp instruments. Photosensitivity, an increased sensitivity to the sun, is another side effect often associated with neuroleptic medications that can be addressed by limiting sun exposure (answer A). Answer C is a strategy that can be used to avoid postural hypotension, a sudden drop in blood pressure resulting in feeling faint or loss of consciousness when moving from lying or sitting to standing. Dry mouth is a common side effect of many drugs and can be intensified by the dehydrating effects of caffeinated drinks and alcohol (answer D). All of the above are possible side effects of neuroleptic medications, but answer B is most important because it relates to the only side effect the client has experienced. See reference: Early: Psychotropic medications and somatic treatments.

100. (C) Program evaluation Program evaluation is the compilation of the intervention results for a population of individuals. Final evaluations of clients involved in the program and client satisfaction surveys (answers A and B) may both be components of the program evaluation. Utilization review (answer D) evaluates the care that is provided to ensure that services were appropriate and not overutilized or underutilized. Utilization review also analyzes the services to ensure that the interventions were provided in an economical manner. See reference: Neistadt and Crepeau (eds): Perinchief, JM: Management of occupational therapy services.

101. (A) incident report. Facilities use incident reports to document incidents such as this. Although the incident may be referred to in a daily progress note (answer B), an incident report must also be filed. An incident report form includes a level of detail that may not be achieved in a letter (answer C), and a verbal report (answer D) is not a form of documentation. See reference: Ryan (ed): Practice Issues in Occupational Therapy: Jones, RA: Service operations.

102. (C) Repeatedly squeeze with the hand against increasing amounts of resistance. The biomechanical approach is a treatment approach used when a person has a deficit in strength, endurance, or range of motion but has voluntary muscle control during performance of activities. The biomechanical approach focuses on decreasing the deficit

area to improve the person's performance of daily activities. Eliciting functional grasp using reflex inhibiting postures (answer A) is an example of a neurophysiologic approach, which emphasizes an understanding of the nervous system in a person with brain damage and how to elicit a desired response from that person. Muscles can be stimulated through a variety of neurodevelopmental techniques (answer B), using an understanding of the nervous system to elicit a response in a developmental sequence. Building up utensils (answer D) is an example of the rehabilitative approach, which teaches a person how to compensate for a deficit on either a temporary or permanent basis. See reference: Trombly (ed): Zemke: Remediating biomechanical and physiological impairments of motor performance.

103. (C) developmental dyspraxia. The motor problem described as it occurs during the evaluation is characteristic of developmental dyspraxia. Children with dyspraxia often learn tasks such as jumping rope with great difficulty, effort, and considerable practice. However, when the task is altered, such as in this case by asking the child to skip backwards, the child is unable to adapt the task for a long while. Answer A is incorrect because the child with delayed reflex integration would have difficulty with all aspects of the task. Answer B is incorrect because a problem of bilateral integration would affect both aspects of this task, jumping rope forward and backward. Answer D is also incorrect because general incoordination would probably affect performance of both forward and backward rope jumping. See reference: Case-Smith (ed): Parham, LD, and Maillous, Z: Sensory integration.

104. (A) collecting chart review information. After a certified OT has demonstrated service competency, it is appropriate for him or her to complete data collection through record reviews, interviews, general observations, and behavior checklists. Answers B, C, and D require interpretive and analytical skills in which OTs have received additional training. A certified OT assistant can collaborate with an OT, but it is inappropriate to have a COTA complete these portions independently. See reference: AOTA: Occupational therapy roles.

105. (A) Plaster cylindrical splint A plaster cylindrical splint would encourage a static stretch of the PIP joint contracture. Answer B is a form of PIP extension and is considered to be a dynamic splint. Answer C is used to isolate tendon and joint range of motion, and answer D is also a form of dynamic splinting. See reference: Pedretti (ed): Belkin, J, and English, CB: Orthotics.

106. (A) Thumb against the tip of the index finger The correct position for tip pinch is the thumb against the tip of the index finger. The thumb against the side of the index finger describes the position for lateral pinch. The thumb against the tips of the index and middle fingers describes the test position for three-jaw chuck, or palmar pinch. The thumb against the tips of all the fingers is not a standard test position. See reference: Trombly (ed): Trombly, CA: Evaluation of biomechanical and physiological aspects of motor performance.

107. (C) Interpret the results based on data collected by the COTA Once the OTR has assigned performance of an evaluation to a COTA, the OTR is responsible for analyzing and interpreting the results. Service competency (answer A) would need to be established prior to the COTA administering the evaluation. Collecting data (answer B) is the responsibility of the COTA in this scenario. Developing the treatment plan (answer D) would follow analysis of the data. See reference: Early: Data collection and evaluation.

108. (B) measure the distance from the fingertip to the distal palmar crease with the hand in a fist. The distance from the fingertip to the distal palmar crease with the hand fisted may be measured in either inches or centimeters. This measures how close the fingertip comes to the palm. A person who has full flexion would have a measurement of 0. Answers A and C are incorrect as actively or passively measuring the flexion at each joint and totaling them are measurements taken with a goniometer and recorded in degrees. Answer D, measuring the distance between the tip of the thumb and the fourth phalanx, is incorrect because it is a measurement of opposition. See reference: Hunter, Schneider, Mackin, and Bell (eds): Cambridge, C: Range of motion measurements of the hand.

109. (C) Use the handout only as a resource while developing the presentation. The OT Code of Ethics states that "Occupational therapy personnel shall accurately represent the qualifications, views, contributions, and findings of colleagues" (p. 1038). The options presented in answers A and B do not give the necessary credit to the author for his or her contribution. It is not necessary to discard the article altogether (answer D). See reference: AOTA: Occupational therapy code of ethics.

110. (A) Postural hypotension A frequent side effect of neuroleptic drugs is a decrease in blood pressure in response to sudden movements, specifically up and down movements, resulting in faintness or loss of consciousness. The parachute activity involves significant up-and-down body movements and therefore warrants the therapist's attention with this patient population. Answers B, C, and D are also potential side effects of antipsychotic medications but would usually not be problematic with parachute activities. See reference: Early: Psychotropic medications and other biological treatments.

111. (B) the OTR must assume responsibility for all OT services delivered. An OTR is always responsible for services provided by the COTA under his or her supervision. The AOTA does not require that the patient have a referral for provision of services. However, it is important to note that state licensure laws and accrediting agencies may require a formal referral. Answer A is incorrect because the OTR is operating within AOTA standards. A written letter of consent (answer C) is not required by either state or accrediting agencies. A COTA would not initiate contact with the physician (answer D) without discussing the case with the supervising OTR. See reference: Ryan (ed): Practice Issues in Occupational Therapy: Ryan, SE: Therapeutic intervention process.

112. (A) improving accessibility in building access, building interiors, and rest rooms. Title III of the ADA addresses accessibility of facilities used by the public and focuses on removal of structural barriers to allow access to the premises and use of the facilities, including, parking areas, walks, ramps, entrances, etc. Answers B, C, and D may be relevant areas for OT consultation; however, these relate to Title I of the ADA which addresses employment of persons with disabilities. See reference: Pedretti (ed): Smith, P: Americans with Disabilities Act: Accommodating persons with disabilities.

113. (C) recommend activities to develop fine coordination that teachers can incorporate into classroom programming. Recommending classroom activities that will develop the performance component of fine coordination would be the best population-based intervention since it involves addressing the occupational performance needs of many students. Answers A, B, and D focus OT efforts toward individual intervention approaches. See reference: AOTA: Guide To Occupational Therapy Practice: .

114. (C) swimming in a cool water pool. Swimming is an excellent activity for promoting physical fitness, and the cool water pool (temperature under 84 degrees) will prevent the overheating that is contraindicated for individuals with MS. Jogging and volleyball (answers A and D) are both likely to result in overheating, and volleyball would probably fatigue weak hand muscles. Painting (answer B) is a lightweight activity that would probably appeal to an artist, but would do very little to promote physical fitness. See reference: Pedretti (ed): Hietpas, J, Hooks, ML, Atchison, P, et al, in Degenerative diseases of the central nervous system.

115. (C) Both OTRs and COTAs should have liability insurance. Liability insurance protects OT practitioners from financial damage should they be sued for negligence or misconduct. Most facilities maintain coverage for licensed professionals, but the level of coverage may not be sufficient to cover the amount sought for by the claimant. Therefore, OT practitioners may chose to insure themselves at a higher level. See reference: Ryan (ed): Practice Issues in Occupational Therapy: Jones, RA: Service operations.

116. (A) Complete independence with self-care and transfers An individual with T4 paraplegia will have sufficient trunk balance and upper extremity strength and coordination to complete self-care and transfers independently. See reference: Pedretti (ed): Adler, C. Spinal cord injury.

117. (B) holding a class about job-seeking strategies. The purpose of applying remedial strategies is to enhance underlying abilities. Teaching and training methods are commonly used techniques. Answer A, an interest checklist, is a tool used to identify the degree of an individual's interest in a variety of leisure areas. Answer C is an example of a compensatory strategy. Answer D provides opportunities for exploration and expression. See reference: Early: Data collection and evaluation.

118. (D) apply the stimuli to the uninvolved area proximally to distally in a random pattern. The general guidelines for sensation testing are that the person's vision should be occluded, the stimuli should be randomly applied with false stimuli intermingled, a practice trial should be performed before the test, and the unaffected side or area should be tested before the affected side or area. Also, the amount of time a person has to respond should be established. See reference: Trombly (ed): Bentzel, K: Evaluation of sensation.

119. (C) Avoid resistive materials. For a child with acute juvenile rheumatoid arthritis, the OT practitioner should always use techniques for joint protection and energy conservation. Activities requiring the manipulation of highly resistive materials such as clay, leather, and copper sheets should be avoided; the pressure applied to the joints could exacerbate the condition. Avoiding light touch (answer A) is a precaution more relevant in the treatment of a child with tactile defensiveness. Rapid vestibular stimulation (answer B) is contraindicated for a child who is prone to seizures. The need to avoid above-normal body temperature (answer D) is more relevant to a client with MS because high temperature exacerbates the symptoms. See reference: Case-Smith (ed): Rogers, SL, Gordon, CY, Schanzenbacher, KE, and Case-Smith, J: Common diagnosis in pediatric occupational therapy.

120. (D) strength. Exerting enough pressure to twist off the lid requires strength. He demonstrates adequate range of motion (answer A) when he grasps the knife. He demonstrates adequate coordination (answer B) by spreading peanut butter on the bread and accurately positioning the lid onto the jar opening. He demonstrates adequate endurance (answer C) by standing during the entire activity of making a peanut butter sandwich. See reference: AOTA:

Uniform Terminology for Occupational Therapy, third edition.

121. (D) A sheltered workshop Sheltered workshops are designed to help individuals master basic work skills. Answers B and C are similar in that they incorporate actual job sites for developing work skills. Answer A focuses on work-related and leisure activities. See reference: Neistadt and Crepeau (eds): Baloueff, O: Developmental delay and mental retardation.

122. (A) fail the student. Students should be evaluated at the midpoint of each level-II fieldwork experience as well as at the conclusion. The purpose of the final evaluation is to provide the student with feedback regarding performance during fieldwork as well as to document that entry-level competence has been achieved. A student who does not demonstrate entry-level competence should not be passed. Therefore, answers B, C, and D are incorrect. See reference: Neistadt and Crepeau (eds): Interdisciplinary communication and supervision of personnel.

123. (D) plan new motor tasks. Dyspraxia refers to difficulty planning new motor tasks (answer D). Inability to print or write (answer A) is termed "dysgraphia." The term "dyslexia" (answer B) literally means dysfunction in reading. Inability to perform mathematics (answer C) is known as dyscalcula. See reference: Case-Smith (ed): Rogers, SL, Gordon, CY, Schanzenbacher, KE, and Case-Smith, J: Common diagnosis in pediatric occupational therapy practice.

124. (A) apply the stimuli beginning at an area distal to the lesion progressing proximally. The general guidelines for sensation testing are that the person's vision should be occluded, the stimuli should be randomly applied with false stimuli intermingled (opposite of answer C), a practice trial should be performed before the test, and the unaffected side or area should be tested before the affected side or area (opposite of answer B). Also, the tested individual should be given a specified amount of time in which to respond; therefore, answer D is incorrect. See reference: Trombly (ed): Bentzel, K: Evaluation of sensation.

125. (C) needs assessment. Needs assessment is the necessary first step of gathering data about the population, treatment needs, and resources available. Program planning (answer A) involves establishing goals and objectives based on the results of the needs assessment. Program implementation (answer B) occurs following program planning and involves coordination, assessment, and intervention selection. Program evaluation (answer D) occurs after implementation and involves systematic review and analysis of the program based on achievement of program goals. See reference: Cottrell (ed):

Grossman, J, and Bortone, J: Program development.

126. (D) adapted teaching techniques. Answer D is correct because a child with this type of disability characteristically has learning problems that require such teaching methods as "chaining" or behavior modification. Answers A, B, and C are of secondary importance because physical coordination may be impaired or other physical limitations such as abnormal muscle tone or significant problems with balance could also be present. These additional problems may require adaptive equipment, clothing, or techniques. However, all aspects of dressing depend on the child's ability to learn procedures of dressing; therefore, it is necessary to consider task analysis and teaching approach first. See reference: Case-Smith (ed): Shepherd, J: Self-care and adaptations for independent living.

127. (A) a cotton ball. When retesting it is important to use the method used initially in order to make an accurate comparison of status before and after treatment. In addition, evaluation results are more consistent when the individual who performed the initial evaluation performs subsequent reevaluations. An aesthesiometer (answer B) is used to measure two-point discrimination, not light touch. Semmes-Weinstein monofilaments (answer C) are a good tool for assessing light touch thresholds but the results may not be as useful for comparison purposes. A pin or straightened paper clip (answer D) is used for testing superficial pain. See reference: Pedretti (ed): Pedretti, LW: Evaluation of sensation and treatment of sensory dysfunction.

128. (D) Treat the patient as scheduled and charge for the 1 hour of direct time spent with the patient. This answer is correct in that this meeting was not part of the planned intervention and had occurred spontaneously and without measurable goals. Based on the Standards of Practice, if collaboration with the individual or family was included as a part of the intervention plan, the patient could be billed for the time. See reference: Kornblau and Starling: Legal issues in ethical decision making.

129. (D) (1) gather shirt up at the back of the neck; (2) pull gathered back fabric off over head; (3) remove shirt from unaffected arm; (4) remove shirt from affected arm. Answers A, B, and C are examples of incorrect sequences that would result in failure to remove the shirt successfully. See reference: Pedretti (ed): Foti, D, Pedretti, LW, and Lillie, S: Activities of daily living.

130. (C) Notify NBCOT of the situation and reassign the patient to a different therapist According to the Code of Ethics, therapists are responsible for maintaining relationships that "do not exploit the recipient of services sexually, physically, emotionally, financially, socially or in any other manner." The pa-

tient–therapist relationship is compromised when the therapist enters into a social or intimate relationship with a patient. Every therapist is responsible to report "any breaches of the Code of Ethics to the appropriate authority," whether they are a supervisor or not. Because the issue is practice related, the NBCOT is the appropriate authority. It is then the responsibility of the NBCOT to determine if and what type of disciplinary action should be taken. Maintaining a relationship with a patient (answer A) is unacceptable. The Code of Ethics does not require the supervisor to take a disciplinary action, such as terminating or reassigning the employee (answers B and D), but the facility might. See reference: AOTA: Occupational therapy code of ethics.

131. (B) Pass around a scent box and ask each patient to smell the contents. Sensory integration theory holds that individuals can learn by receiving, processing, and responding to sensory stimulation. Starting a group for regressed individuals with sensory stimuli such as touch and smell helps to get the individuals' attention and arouse their interest. Asking individuals in this type of a group to introduce themselves (answer A) can be confusing and time consuming, especially when dealing with regressed individuals with limited attention spans. Reading favorite poems (answer C) and discussing lunch menus (answer D) are activities more suited to patients functioning on higher levels than the group described here. See reference: Early: Group concepts and techniques.

132. (C) Avoid having these individuals in close proximity to others to reduce opportunities for physical contact Avoiding close proximity situations is the recommended environmental modification for sexual acting-out behaviors. Advising the client of your expectations (answer D) is an appropriate use of self in such situations. Standing to the side (answer B) is a recommended environmental modification for highly aggressive and hostile behavior risks. Providing real-life activities in a stimulating environment (answer A) has been found to be helpful with reducing some delusions. See reference: Early: Safety techniques.

133. (B) The patients' written consents to take the photographs and use them for publicity A photograph of a person who is being treated at a health care facility would release privileged information and would violate confidentiality just as much as releasing the individual's name or diagnosis (answers A and D). No information about a person may be released without a written consent. It is not necessary to obtain permission of the department head to use a photograph to promote a positive image for the facility (answer C). See reference: Bailey: Final preparation before implementing the research plan.

134. (C) Assertiveness training Broken record is a specific assertiveness skill concerned with repeating your position without losing control. Music therapy (answer A) is a creative arts discipline. Psychodrama (answer D) is a group technique for expressing catharsis. Self-awareness groups (answer B) tend to focus on feeling identification and expression versus skill building. See reference: Posthuma: Process and leadership.

135. (C) A COTA contributes to the process but does not complete the task independently. The COTA participates in this process by providing factual information to the OTR and collaboratively identifying discharge needs (answer C). However, because of the analytical nature of provision of discharge recommendations, the COTA does not complete this activity independently. Answers A and B are incorrect because they do not take into account the analytical nature of the task. Answer D is incorrect because it does not allow for the input of data from the COTA. See reference: AOTA: Occupational therapy roles.

136. (D) rationalization. Making excuses for or justifying others' behaviors that are generally considered to be unacceptable is called rationalization. Identification (answer A) occurs when one takes on the characteristics of another person. Projection (answer B) is the blaming of other people for performing the behaviors. Denial (answer C) is refusing to acknowledge that the behavior occurred. See reference: Christiansen and Baum (eds): Bonder, B: Coping with psychological and emotional challenges.

137. (C) interpreting results of assessments for the purposes of treatment planning. Interpretation of assessment results for purposes of treatment planning must be performed by the OTR. The functions noted in answers A, B, and D may all be performed by the COTA in a long-term care facility. See reference: AOTA: Occupational therapy roles.

138. (A) Modifying the environment to protect the infant from overstimulation and inappropriate stimuli Answers B and D represent traditional OT rehabilitation with an emphasis on specific diagnoses, developmental delay, immature sleep-wake state acquisition, limited range of motion, and splint fabrication. This approach will continue to be of importance within the NICU. The developmental support care approach, however, has expanded the traditional rehabilitation model to include and focus upon a protective and preventative component, which best defines occupational therapy in the NICU at the present time. Therefore, answer A best describes a protective and preventative approach to intervention in the NICU. Answer C, educating parents and staff, is a crucial aspect of both the traditional rehabilitation model and the developmental support care approach to implementing services in the NICU. However, it is not the best descriptor of an OT's scope of practice. See reference: Case-Smith (ed): Hunter, JG: Neonatal Intensive Care Unit.

139. (A) A vacuum feeding cup Individuals with impulsive behavior or poor judgment often attempt to drink too quickly. The rate of intake can be limited by using a drinking spout with a small opening, pinching a straw, or using a vacuum feeding cup with a control button. A cup with a large drinking spout (answer D) would increase the rate of intake, which could result in choking or spills. A "nosey cup" (answer B) allows individuals with dysphagia to maintain a tucked-chin position while drinking, which is necessary for a good swallow. A mug with two handles (answer C) would benefit an individual with limited grasp or coordination. See reference: Trombly (ed): Konosky, KA: Dysphagia.

140. (C) complete a review of the literature. Review of the written material is necessary in preparing the design of the research project. The literature review helps the researcher to state the purpose clearly and establish boundaries. Stating the purpose and the hypothesis follows the identification of the research question; therefore, answer A is incorrect. The design of the research and the establishment of the boundaries are affected by information from the literature review; therefore, answers B and D are incorrect. See reference: DePoy and Gitlin: Developing a knowledge base through review of the literature.

141. (C) radial nerve. Injury to the radial nerve in the wrist area causes sensory damage only. This damage occurs to the radial two thirds of the dorsum of the hand. Damage to the median nerve at the wrist causes decreased thumb and prehensile strength and complete or partial loss of sensation in the distal portion of the second digit (index finger) and third digits (long finger) with some loss in the fourth digit (ring finger). Damage to the ulnar nerve at the wrist causes decreased grip strength and complete or partial loss of sensation to half of the fourth digit (ring finger) and all of the fifth digit (little finger) as well as the proximal hypothenar region. The ulnar and median nerves are frequently entrapped together. A brachial plexus injury causes peripheral nerve damage to any or all of the fibers from C5 to T1. See reference: Pedretti (ed): Kasch, MC: Hand injuries.

142. (D) suggesting furniture and accessories that promote better positioning at work. The best recommendation is for ergonomically correct furniture and accessories. Additional adaptations may include tool modification and the training of workers in appropriate positioning. Answers A and C, setting up stress management and smoking cessation programs, are not considered to be ergonomic adaptations. Answer B is not an example of an ergonomic adaptation but is a treatment intervention. See reference: Pedretti (ed): Kasch, MC: Hand injuries.

143. (D) Explain to the administrator this is not

an appropriate solution and then develop an alternate solution. OT departments frequently are understaffed and need to operate as efficiently as possible. The collaborative teamwork between an OTR and a COTA is vital in treatment planning and implementation. When a collaborative relationship is operational, the COTA may participate in evaluation and treatment planning, provide treatment, and carry out documentation. Complying with the administrator's instructions (answers A, B and C) would result in inadequate supervision and would violate both the Standards of Practice and Code of Ethics. It is not within the OTA's scope of practice to carry out treatment planning and implementation without supervision. See reference: Neistadt and Crepeau (eds): Sands, M: Practitioners' perspectives on the occupational therapist and occupational therapy assistant partnership.

144. (D) provide wrist extension, MCP extension, and thumb extension. The purpose of this splint is to prevent the extensor tendons from overstretching as well as provide proper positioning of the hand for functional use. Answers A, B, and C are inappropriate functions for a dynamic radial nerve splint. See reference: Pedretti (ed): Kasch, MC: Hand injuries.

145. (D) weight-bearing over a small bolster in prone. Weight-bearing on the arms can help with overall inhibition of tone before participating in hand skill activities. Inhibition of flexor spasticity occurs through slow joint compression from weight bearing, as well as facilitation of ulnar to radial function in the hand. Answers A and B are incorrect because they require voluntary control of release of objects without inhibition. Answer C is incorrect because traction on the finger flexors would increase spasticity in the flexor muscles and make opening of the hand more difficult. See reference: Case-Smith (ed): Exner, CE: Development of hand skills.

146. (C) The client should enroll in a work-hardening program. Work-hardening programs are designed to "incorporate job-specific work tasks that progress the client to the physical demand levels of the actual job" (p. 380). Continuing to perform her home program (answers A and D) or discontinuing OT services would probably not enable the client to return to the work force after a 3-month absence. Home health OT (answer B) is appropriate for individuals who are unable to leave their homes to attend outpatient therapy. See reference: Ryan (ed): Practice Issues in Occupational Therapy: Engh, J, and Taylor, S: Work hardening.

147. (C) Describe how using a shower chair improves safety Informing the patient of various options is the first response. By describing the shower chair and how it make showering safer, the OT practitioner is conveying the concept that occupational performance is based on the interaction of perfor-

mance contexts (physical environment) and performance components (balance) and that there are methods to ensure safety. The OT practitioner would then inquire as to the patient's interest in purchasing a shower chair (answer B). Getting into the bathtub is even more risky than getting into the shower (answer A); therefore, that is not an option for the patient. With a patient who is very focused on deficits and expects therapy to completely remediate these deficits (answer D), answer C refocuses the emphasis on performance of the activity. See reference: Piersol and Ehrlich (eds): Seibert, C: The clinic called home.

148. (C) has a standard format. Standardization of a test means that the test is administered in a prescribed manner and that scoring and interpretation of scores are also completed in a prescribed way. The presence of data concerning the test's "norms" and the establishment of reliability and validity (answers A, B, and D) may be, and often are, provided with standardized tests but are not assumed to be part of the test unless this information is included. The aspects of standardized tests that are always assumed is the specific and standardized method of administration, scoring, and interpretation. See reference: Case-Smith (ed): Richardson, PK: Use of standardized tests in pediatric practice.

149. (C) steps, width of doorways, and threshold heights. The first area of evaluation would be the steps, width of doorways, and presence and height of door thresholds to determine whether the wheelchair user will be able to enter or exit interior spaces in the wheelchair or whether structural modifications are required. Answers A, B, and D reflect areas that will also need to be evaluated; however, they are not as critical to initial interior access. See reference: Pedretti (ed): Foti, D, Pedretti, LW: Activities of daily living.

150. (D) Program evaluation Program evaluation is a systematic collection and reporting of outcomes data to document program effectiveness and cost efficiency. Quality assurance (answer A) identifies problems and implements corrective actions. Peer review (answer B) is the system of other service providers' assessing the provision of care to ensure appropriate interventions and documentation practices. Answer C, utilization review, is the process of analyzing the provision of services to promote the MOST economical delivery of service. See reference: Neistadt and Crepeau (eds): Perinchief, JM: Management of occupational therapy services.

151. (B) wear noisy bracelets on the wrist as a reminder to visually scan toward the affected side. Although hazards may be removed from the environment, or padded to prevent injury to an individual, use of these interventions is only feasible in a person's home. It is best to teach the individual visual scanning of the affected area and the environment, a technique that the person may use anywhere. An individual may avoid using sharp tools or extreme water temperature, but this avoidance does not teach him or her how to monitor the affected side visually, because it is a precaution that addresses only the problem with sensation. Noisy bracelets are one technique that may be used to accomplish compensation for both unilateral neglect and absence of sensation. Visual impairments that are not accompanied by sensory or perceptual deficits are more readily overcome with retraining. See reference: Trombly (ed): Quintana, LA: Remediating perceptual impairments.

152. (C) Stabilizing the pelvis, hips, and legs Answer C is correct because when the pelvis, hips, and legs do not provide a good central base of support, the child resorts to compensatory movements. Stabilizing the trunk (answer A) is not correct because unless the pelvis is stabilized, arm movements may still be compromised. Answer B is not correct because use of a lap board or chair arms for weight bearing of the upper extremities will compromise the use of the arms and hands to stabilize the body. Stabilizing the head and neck (answer D) is not correct because the pelvis continues to be unstable and therefore is not a good base for arm movements. See reference: Case-Smith (ed): Nichols, DS: Development of postural control.

153. (D) provide a stockinet for the individual to wear inside the splint. A stockinet liner worn inside the splint keeps the perspiration from irritating the skin by absorbing the perspiration and keeping the skin away from the damp plastic. A stockinet liner is inexpensive enough to have several, so the individual can always have a clean one available. Answer A, putting talcum powder in a splint, works well with a small splint, but in a large splint would require a larger amount, and feel muddy when an individual perspires. Answer B, moleskin as a liner, does not clean well after wearing for a short time, and although it may be comfortable, it usually is discarded because of the soiled appearance and smell. Answer C, an individual using a splint made with perforated material, will continue to have perspiration and will need to use another method to keep the damp plastic from irritating the skin. See reference: Ryan (ed): The Certified Occupational Therapy Assistant: Schober-Branigan, P: Thermoplastic splinting of the hand.

154. (C) follow administration instructions and note changes in behavior. Although the tester may not deviate from the protocol, changes in behavior represent important test data and should be recorded. The responses described in (answers A, B, and D) may make the test results invalid by altering the sequence of test items, the grouping of items, or the actual test item itself. These may not be changed unless it is specified in the test manual. See reference: Case-Smith (ed): Richardson, PK: Use of standardized tests in pediatric practice.

155. (A) soft to hard to rough. Hypersensitivity stimuli is graded by texture and force. Texture begins with soft, progresses to hard, and moves to rough. The force begins with touch, progresses to rub, and moves to tapping. The texture and force of the stimuli are graded together. Light, medium, and heavy do not specify what the texture and force of the stimuli would be during training. A person with hypersensitivity would be unable to tolerate training beginning with a rough texture. See reference: Trombly (ed): Bentzel, K: Remediating sensory impairment.

156. (D) Home observation and parent interview "Observation of children in familiar settings and routines allows more characteristic views of their abilities and may be actually more reflective of how children can be expected to perform. . ." (p. 207). Parent interviews provide information about the child's abilities from the parent's point of view and can identify the priorities of the child's caregiver. Answers A, B, and C provide necessary information about performance components, development, and other parameters but are not as effective in helping the evaluator learn about the child's self-care functioning. See reference: Case-Smith (ed): Stewart, KB: Purposes, processes, and methods of evaluation.

157. (C) to both sides of the client's body. Answer C is correct because the client must be able to transfer to both sides of the body. It is usually difficult or impossible to arrange the home environment so that the all transfers can be done from one side only. For instance, if the toilet at home is close to the wall, getting on and off the toilet will require transfer first to one side of the body and then to the opposite side. The family also needs to know the different kinds and amounts of support they must use on each side of the client's body. Thus, answers A, B, and D are incorrect because they all involve transfer to only one side. See reference: Trombly (ed): Retraining basic and instrumental activities of daily living.

158. (A) A mutual process The supervisory process is one that requires the attention of both parties involved. The COTA needs to develop his or her own role and identity within the institution and profession. In addition, the OTR supervisor needs to provide the COTA with opportunities for growth and development. As part of this relationship, ongoing evaluation and counseling may take place to enhance learning and role development. Although answers B, C, and D are necessary to the supervisory process, the best answer is A. See reference: Early: Supervision.

159. (C) AC MRDD The AC MRDD stands for Accreditation Council for services for the Mentally Retarded and other Developmentally Disabled persons. JCAHO (answer A) stands for the Joint Commission of Accreditation of Hospital Organizations. The JCA-

HO is an agency that reviews medical care of hospitals, psychiatric facilities, hospices, long-term care agencies, and MR/DD programs seeking accreditation. CARF (answer B) stands for the Commission on Accreditation of Rehabilitation Facilities; CARF reviews programs in free-standing facilities as well as those that are part of a hospital system. The NLN/APHA stands for the National League for Nursing, American Public Health Association; the NLN/APHA surveys nursing homes. See reference: AOTA: The Occupational Therapy Manager: MacRae, N: Accreditation council on services for people with disabilities.

160. (A) pull-to-sit, leaning back against therapy ball. While all answers involve antigravity control, answer A addresses beginning control in neck and shoulders. Since control develops cephalocaudally, neck and shoulder control should be addressed first. By using an incline, the pull of gravity can be reduced, thus facilitating maximum control. See reference: Case-Smith (ed): Nichols, DS: The development of postural control.

161. (A) learn to type. Typing would allow the individual to communicate legibly in writing, while circumventing the individual's poor handwriting skills. Answer B, fine motor coordination exercises, and answer C, practicing letter or shape formations, are both ways to improve control of the writing utensils by improving coordination through exercises that will provide a greater smoothness to the writing. Answer D, exercises or activities for strengthening flexors and extensors in the finger, also allows improved use of the writing utensil by providing enough strength to properly position the writing tool. However, answers B, C, and D do not bypass the individual having to perform handwriting with a pen or pencil. See reference: Fisher, Murray, and Bundy (eds): Cermak, S: Somatodyspraxia.

162. (B) Developing vocational interests, social skills, and community mobility skills Answer B is correct because these skills are essential in functioning in the environment after school. Answer A, leisure interests, is not correct because, although they are important to the student's life, leisure skills and interest knowledge are not as essential. Answer C is not correct because, although it describes the student's motor control function, which may influence the type of job the adolescent performs, adaptation can be made in this area of need. Although developing fine motor skills (answer D) is a traditional OT role in school settings, it would not be an appropriate focus for transition planning intervention, of which the case described is an example. See reference: Case-Smith (ed): Rogers, SL, Gordon, CY, Schanzenbacher, KE, and Case-Smith, J: Common diagnosis in pediatric occupational therapy practice.

163. (A) further observation and evaluation of right-sided dysfunction is indicated. Answer A is correct because infants usually use a bilateral approach at this age. Although unilaterality occurs several months later, most children alternate hands in many activities until age 6 years. This means that this infant should be observed for possible right-sided dysfunction. Answer B is incorrect because unilaterality at age 4 months is not typical development. Answer C is incorrect because hand dominance begins to develop at age 3 to 6, and answer D is incorrect because bilaterality precedes unilaterality in the course of infant development. See reference: Neistadt and Crepeau (eds): Kohlmeyer, K: Evaluation of sensory and neuromuscular performance components.

164. (A) refine the question and develop the background. Once the question has been identified, a review of the literature should occur. The next step in research is to refine the question and develop the background. Answer B is the next step of the process, which is deciding on the methodology. Answers C and D come later in the research, as the researcher establishes the boundaries and then collects and analyzes data. See reference: Royeen: Quality in research.

165. (C) by tilting backwards up to 60 degrees while rocking. By lowering the child backwards from the sitting position, the child is required to activate increasing degrees of antigravity control in the neck musculature. As the child's strength increases, the degree of incline can be increased. Answers A, B and D do not address antigravity control using neck flexor musculature. See reference: Case-Smith (ed): Nichols, DS: Development of postural control.

166. (B) wearing permanent-press clothing. Using a wrinkle-resistant fabric eliminates or decreases the amount of ironing needed. The side-loading washer (answer A) is an example of household equipment adapted to eliminate excessive reaching from a wheelchair. An extended-handle dustpan (answer C) eliminates bending or stooping from a standing or sitting position. Neither the dustpan nor the washer, however, eliminates or reduces the amount of work needed for the tasks. Good body mechanics (answer D) are necessary to protect or maintain physical health, but they do not eliminate or reduce the amount of work. See reference: Trombly (ed): Trombly, CA: Retraining basic and instrumental activities of daily living.

167. (A) Arrhythmic and unexpected Sensory integration treatment is complex and highly individualized and must be monitored carefully to observe the effects of sensory input of varying types on the individual. The characteristics of facilitatory sensory input are unexpected, arrhythmic, uneven, or rapid input. Answer B is not correct because, although arrhythmic input is excitatory, slow sensory input is inhibitory. Sustained and slow sensory input (answer C) is inhibitory, not facilitatory. Answer D is incorrect because, although facilitatory input is unexpected, rhythmic input is inhibitory. See reference: Bruce and Borg: Movement-centered frame of reference.

168. (B) Back up the body to the passenger seat, hold onto a stable section of the car, extend the involved leg, and slowly sit in the car This is the safest way to perform a car transfer after surgery for a total hip replacement. Answers A, C, and D would all be contraindicated and are not representative of total hip precautions. See reference: Pedretti (ed): Adler, C, and Tipton-Burton, M: Wheelchair assessment and transfers.

169. (B) club foot. Pes varus or equinovarus is also called club foot. This deformity involves forefoot inversion and supination, heel varus, equinus through the ankle, and medial deviation of the foot in relationship to the knee. See reference: Smith, Weiss, and Lehmkuhl: Ankle and foot.

170. (B) Use a walker Ambulatory aids may be used to substitute for lost motion, reduce weight bearing on the lower extremities, or widen the base of support to increase stability. An individual with a balance deficit requires a wider base of support, which is provided by walkers and quad canes. A standard cane (answer A) is effective for reducing weight bearing, and does not provide as much stability as a walker or quad cane. This individual is ambulatory; therefore, working on meal preparation from a wheelchair (answer C) in a home without kitchen modifications would create an unnecessary hardship. See reference: Dutton: Rehabilitation postulates regarding intervention.

171. (C) National Alliance for the Mentally Ill This is a support group that is open to clients and families and focuses on education and support related to all mental illnesses. Al-Anon (answer A) is a support group for alcohol use among family members. Family therapy (answer B) is not a support group. Recovery, Inc. (answer D) is a self-help support group for clients with mental disorders. See reference: Early: Who is the consumer?.

172. (B) reflex sympathetic dystrophy. This diagnosis is typically "a disabling reaction to pain that is generated by an abnormal sympathetic reflex" (p. 680). Signs include pain, edema, coolness of the hand, and blotchy skin. The level of trauma does not typically correlate to the amount of pain that the client is experiencing. Answer A is more commonly associated with a nerve repair or amputation and presents with symptoms of shooting or sharp pains. Answers C and D do not typically correlate with the symptoms described by patients with reflex sympathetic dystrophy. See reference: Pedretti (ed): Kasch, MC: Hand injuries.

173. (C) I think baking would be a helpful activity to try. Baking something you like offers you sev- eral choices and decisions. These choices and decisions can help you feel more positive about making other decisions. You can choose a cake mix or a cookie mix. Which would you like? Answer C limits options as well as provides the rationale for the choices. Answer A is a leading question that really offers only one choice. Answer B does not provide any options. Answer D is a closed question, offering no real choice for the individual. See reference: Denton: Effective communication.

174. (B) observe him in his home during feeding time. "Considering the context of the child's environments is a critical process in occupational therapy assessments" (p. 167). The reason he does not feed himself may be environmental—for instance, his parents may have taught him not to touch food with his fingers or he may not have learned to feed himself because his grandmother always feeds him. Or the child may not be able to transfer skills learned at home to the clinic—that is, he may believe that "the place to eat is home, not the clinic." Although answers A and C provide useful information for treatment planning, they do not address feeding skills. Answer D does not put the skill to be assessed into an environmental context. See reference: Case-Smith (ed): Stewart, KB: Occupational therapy assessment in pediatrics.

175. (B) assisted stand pivot transfer. An assisted stand pivot transfer is implemented when the client assists with the transfer. Answer A, an independent transfer from a wheelchair to an elevated mat or plinth, is done independently without the assistance of the practitioner. Answer C, a pneumatic lift, is a device that may be used when the client is larger than the therapist. Answer D, a dependent stand pivot transfer, is one in which the therapist assists with more than 50% of the transfer. See reference: Pedretti (ed): Adler, C, and Tipton-Burton, M: Wheelchair assessment and transfers.

176. (D) Scoop dish This is the most correct answer because the sides of the scoop dish provide a shape that aids the scooping movement. A high back to the plate provides a surface to push the food against to aid in getting the food onto the spoon. The swivel spoon (answer A) helps primarily when supination is limited. The nonslip mat (answer B) helps stabilize the plate itself, and the mobile arm support (answer C) positions the arm and helps the weak shoulder and elbow muscles to position the hand. See reference: Case-Smith (ed): Case-Smith, J, and Humphrey, R: Feeding intervention.

177. (C) Activities which provide tapping, application of textures, and weight bearing to the residual limb Massage, tapping, use of textures and weight bearing on the distal end of the residual limb are techniques used to develop tolerance to touch and pressure in the hypersensitive limb. Answers A and B will not affect hypersensitivity and answer D is incorrect because the patient is in the preprosthetic phase and does not have access to the prosthesis. See reference: Trombly (ed): Celikol, F: Amputation and prosthetics.

178. (D) disorganized psychosis. Directive group treatment is a highly structured approach that is used in acute care psychiatry for minimally functioning individuals. This approach is useful for disorganized and disturbed functioning with patients with psychoses and other neurological disorders. Task groups are more appropriate for substance abuse disorders (answer A), and psychoeducation groups are most appropriate for eating and adjustment disorders (answers B and C). See reference: Early: Group concepts and techniques.

179. (B) Implement a pureed diet and allow adequate time for eating As ALS progresses, speaking and swallowing become more difficult and a pureed diet becomes necessary. The individual runs the risk of aspiration or choking if meals are rushed. Adaptive equipment (answer A) is provided much earlier in the disease process. The independence achieved with adaptive equipment has a positive psychological effect on the individual who sees his or her independence slipping away. See reference: Pedretti (ed): Pedretti, LW, and McCormack, GL: Amyotrophic lateral sclerosis.

180. (C) Hallucinations The symptoms of schizophrenia are generally classified as either negative or positive. Negative symptoms tend to persist after the positive, or acute, symptoms are treated with medications. Negative symptoms greatly impact an individual's level of functioning. Answers A, B, and D are all negative symptoms. See reference: Early: Understanding psychiatric diagnosis: The DSM-IV.

181. (B) Bend both knees, keep the back straight and bring object close to the body when lifting Bending with both knees while keeping the back straight and the object close to the body will prevent low back bending and strain. Answers A, C, and D are all incorrect methods for lifting and carrying objects. Answers A and C will actually increase an individual's chance of increasing low back strain. See reference: Pedretti (ed): Smithline, J: Low back pain.

182. (A) "It sounds as if you're not sure whether you are ready to be discharged." Paraphrasing is repeating what someone has said in your own words. Chitchat (answer B) is a conversational response unrelated to what the individual said. Confrontation (answer D) is a response that requires the individual to acknowledge difficult or painful issues. Proposing a solution (answer C) does not help the individual improve his or her decision-making skills or sense of competence. See reference: Denton: Effective communication.

183. (B) use moderately heated water. Hot water may contribute to fatigue in individuals with MS and should therefore be avoided. Moderate water temperature is recommended. Bathing in cool water (answer A) is unnecessary and may cause chilling and increase spasticity. Bathing rather than showering (answer C) may be recommended for individuals with poor balance or standing tolerance, such as those with MS or COPD. Bathing at the sink (answer D) may be recommended for individuals who experience difficulty bending, such as those with hip or knee replacements or back pain, but durable medical equipment is typically available for all of these diagnoses so that bathing in the tub would be possible through the use of a tub bench and handheld shower. See reference: Ryan (ed): Practice Issues in Occupational Therapy: Jensen, D, and Linroth, R: The adult with multiple sclerosis.

184. (A) restore and maintain functional performance of self-chosen occupations that enhance competent performance of valued occupational roles. The depression is likely to be in reaction to the individual's AIDS disease and major loss of functioning at stage 4. Stage 4 of AIDS generally means severe physical and neurological changes. Because the change of function can be broad, answer A is the most comprehensive approach. Answers B, C, and D are too restrictive to be a "major focus." Also, restoration of work is typically unrealistic at stage 4 of AIDS. See reference: Neistadt and Crepeau (eds): Pizzi, M and Burkhardt, A: Occupational therapy for adults with immunological diseases.

185. (C) increase swimming time to 25 minutes or to tolerance. This individual's goal is to maximize strength and endurance. Although ALS is a progressive degenerative disease, improvements in strength and endurance are possible if the individual was not previously functioning at maximum capacity. This individual's performance indicates potential for further improvement. The program should therefore be upgraded, not downgraded (answer B). Methods for improving endurance include increasing the frequency, intensity, or duration of the activity. The correct answer (C) increases the duration of the activity while recognizing the importance of avoiding fatigue. Answer A continues the program at a maintenance level. Using adaptive equipment (answer D), such as a flotation belt, is an energy-saving strategy that would be appropriate if the individual were experiencing fatigue during swimming. See reference: Dutton: Biomechanical postulates regarding intervention.

186. (C) lower back. Touching the lower back requires shoulder abduction and internal rotation. Answer A, back of the neck, and answer B, top of the head, are incorrect because they would require external shoulder rotation. Answer D, opposite shoulder, is also incorrect because horizontal adduction is required for this motion. See reference: Trombly (ed): Trombly, CA: Evaluation of biomechanical and physiological aspects of motor performance.

187. (C) have the patient get dressed in a certain way, then change the task at the next session. Giving the patient a functional task, then changing and observing how he responds will tell the therapist how well the patient can transfer learning to new situations. If the patient can't perform the activity when it is changed slightly, it suggests there may be difficulty with new learning. If the patient can perform the activity with many changes and in a different setting, it suggests that he has more capacity for transfer of learning to new situations. Answers A, B, and D could be ways of assessing different aspects of cognition (judgment, perceptual problem solving and ability to calculate figures), but as described, would not provide evidence of transfer of learning. See reference: Neistadt and Crepeau (eds): Neistadt, ME: Theories derived from learning perspectives.

188. (C) righting reactions. Righting reactions develop after the integration of primitive reflex patterns, which are thought to be necessary for survival in the normal newborn. Righting reactions allow children to right their heads against gravity and to realign their bodies around the movement of the head in that process. Prehensile reactions refer to grasping patterns and reach, which differentiate humans from other primates. Equilibrium reactions develop after righting reactions and allow the child to maintain a standing and walking posture. See reference: Neistadt and Crepeau (eds): Kohlmeyer, K.: Evaluation of sensory and neuromuscular performance components.

189. (D) hold him firmly when picking him up. Holding the child firmly inhibits responses to light touch, which are usually uncomfortable for children with tactile defensiveness. Tickling (answer A) and light stroking (answer C) are also uncomfortable or intolerable for a child with tactile defensiveness. A strong stimulus such as loud music causes further startling and discomfort during a time when the child is MOST vulnerable to the sensation of light touch (i.e., when clothing is being removed). See reference: Case-Smith (ed): Parham, LD, and Mailloux, Z: Sensory integration.

190. (C) Tip Tip prehension is accomplished by flexing the IP joint of the thumb and the PIP and DIP joints of the finger and bringing the tips of the thumb and finger together. This type of prehension is used to pick up objects such as a pin, nail, or coin. Lateral prehension (answer A) is formed by positioning the pad of the thumb against the radial side of the finger. This prehension pattern is used for holding a pen, utensil, or key. Palmar prehension (answer B), also known as three-jaw chuck (answer D), is formed by positioning the thumb in opposition to the tips of the index and middle fingers, forming a pad-to-pad oppo-

sition. This form of prehension is commonly used to lift objects from a flat surface and tie a shoelace. See reference: Pedretti (ed): Belkin, J, English, CB, Adler, C, and Pedretti, LW: Orthotics.

191. (C) texture of the cords she will be using. Coarse materials like jute may shred and give splinters or injure the skin on hands and fingers. This is particularly important for individuals with diabetes who frequently have poor sensation and circulation in their extremities. Skin damage must be avoided since healing is compromised. The length of the cord (answer A) would be significant for an individual with limited range of motion. The thickness of the cord (answer B) would be significant for an individual with limited hand function. The type of surface the individual stands on (answer D) would be important to an individual with back pain. See reference: Reed and Sanderson (eds): Diabetes mellitus—type II.

192. (C) precipitating conditions and events that elicit stress reactions. The conditions and events that elicit stress reactions are known as stressors (answer C). Stressors can be either short term or long term. Answer A describes coping, answer B describes stress, and answer D describes adaptation. See reference: Christiansen and Baum (eds): Christiansen, C: Performance deficits as sources of stress.

193. (C) altered task method. "When the task method is altered, the same task objects are used in the same environment, but the method of performing the task is altered to make the task feasible given the performance deficits" (p. 338). An example would be substituting one-handed techniques for someone who previously used both hands (i.e., one-handed shoe tying for an individual who recently had an above-elbow amputation). Problem solving is the ability to organize information from several levels to generate a solution to a problem. Retraining teaches the same skills of an activity to the person who previously had mastery of those skills. (e.g., having a person with hand weakness practice tying knots). Compensation would be avoiding performance of the activity entirely by using an alternative piece of equipment or method. See reference: Neistadt and Crepeau (eds): Holm, MB, Rogers, JC, and James, AB: Treatment of activities of daily living.

194. (C) Change to a power wheelchair to reduce effort Considering the progressive nature of the child's disease, as well as strength and endurance, the best recommendation would be to change to a power wheelchair. The child would be better able to participate in the cognitive tasks of school if less effort was required for mobility. Answer A, retaining the manual chair, would be counterproductive to functioning well at school, and strength will not be improved with this child's condition. Answer B might make mobility a little easier but will not solve the long-term problem of decreasing strength and endurance. Answer D would still make demands on strength and energy that would appear unwise considering the nature of Duchenne muscular dystrophy. The team's recommendation should also be integrated with the family's needs and resources. See reference: Case-Smith (ed): Case-Smith, J, Rogers, J, and Johnson, JH: School-based occupational therapy.

195. (D) 5 feet by 5 feet An outward opening door needs a space of 5 feet by 5 feet to allow for the wheelchair to be maneuvered around the door. A standard wheelchair requires 5 feet of turning space for a 180- or 360-degree turn. An area that is 3 feet by 5 feet (answer A), 4 feet by 4 feet (answer B), or 4.5 feet by 3 feet (answer C) would not provide enough space to allow the wheelchair to be turned. See reference: Pedretti (ed): Smith, P: Americans with disabilities act: accommodating persons with disabilities.

196. (D) instruction in how to perform the activities safely. Instructing caregivers in methods that will promote safe performance of functional activities, such as locking wheelchair brakes before standing up, is the first focus for caregiver training. Answers A, B, and C are also useful areas of caregiver instruction, however, safety is the first priority. See reference: Neistadt and Crepeau (eds): Hom, MB, Rogers, JC, and James, AB: Treatment of activities of daily living.

197. (C) Provide a screen to reduce peripheral visual stimuli Although all the answers describe techniques that could assist the student, the use of a carrel is most appropriate in a mainstreamed classroom, because the other methods or adaptations (answers A, B, and D) could have a negative impact on the other children's ability to learn. See reference: Case-Smith (ed): Schneck, CM: Visual perception.

198. (C) get the shirt all the way on, then line up the buttons and holes and begin buttoning from the bottom. It is easier to see the buttons and buttonholes at the bottom of the shirt than at the top (answer B); therefore, beginning to button from the bottom is more likely to result in success for the individual with motor or visual-perceptual deficits. Buttoning first (answer A) may result in ripping off the buttons as the shirt is pulled over the head. A buttonhook with a built-up handle (answer D) would be helpful for an individual with finger weakness or incoordination (e.g., quadriplegia), not hemiparesis. See reference: Pedretti (ed): Foti, D, Pedretti, LW, and Lillie, S: Activities of daily living.

199. (C) IEP The individual education plan is a form that must be completed for children receiving services in the school system. This documentation standard was defined in the Education of the Handicapped Act (1975 and 1986). The UB-82 form (answer A) is used to process insurance claims. FIM (answer B), which stands for "functional independence measure" is a method used on rehabilitation units to measure an individual's level of independence. The HCFA-1500 form (answer D) is used to bill Medicare and other insurance carriers for health care services. See reference: Neistadt and Crepeau (eds): Perinchief, JM: Management of occupational therapy services.

200. (B) identify and analyze the tasks and occupations that the client will be performing in the home. The first step in the process is to analyze the tasks and occupations that the client will be performing at home because this forms the basis of the entire assessment and recommendations that will be offered. This will also provide a framework for determining how well the client can perform the tasks within the particular environment being surveyed. Answers A, C, and D are also important aspects of the process but occur after the initial step. See reference: Pedretti (ed): Smith, P: Americans with Disabilities Act: Accommodating persons with disabilities.

BIBLIOGRAPHY

Allen, CK, Earhardt, CA, and Blue, T: Occupational Therapy Treatment Goals for the Physically and Cognitively Disabled. The American Occupational Therapy Association, Rockville, MD, 1992.

American Occupational Therapy Association Inc: Commission on Practice: Guide for supervision of occupational therapy personnel in the delivery of occupational therapy services. Am J Occup Ther 53:592-594, 1999.

American Occupational Therapy Association Inc: Commission on Standards and Ethics: Occupational Therapy Code of Ethics. Am J Occup Ther 48:1037-1038, 1994.

American Occupational Therapy Association Inc: Effective Documentation For Occupational Therapy. American Occupational Therapy Association, Rockville, MD, 1991.

American Occupational Therapy Association Inc: Guidelines for the use of aides in occupational therapy practice. Am J Occup Ther 53:595-597, 1999.

American Occupational Therapy Association Inc: Intercommission Council: Occupational Therapy Roles. Am J Occup Ther 47:1087-1099, 1993.

American Occupational Therapy Association Inc: Intercommission Council: Occupational Therapy Roles. Am J Occup Ther 47:1087-1099, 1993.

American Occupational Therapy Association Inc: Policy: Registered Occupational therapists and certified occupational therapy assistants and modalities. Am J Occup Ther 45:1112-1113, 1991.

American Occupational Therapy Association Inc: Standards for an accredited educational program for the occupational therapist. Am J Occup Ther 53:575-582, 1999.

American Occupational Therapy Association Inc: Statement: Purpose and value of occupational therapy fieldwork education. Am J Occup Ther 50:845, 1996.

American Occupational Therapy Association Inc: Statement: The role of occupational therapy in the independent living movement. Am J Occup Ther 47:1079-1080, 1993.

American Occupational Therapy Association Inc: The Guide to Occupational Therapy Practice. Am J Occup Ther 53:247-322, 1999.

American Occupational Therapy Association Inc: The Occupational Therapy Manager, revised edition. American Occupational Therapy Association, Rockville, MD, 1996.

American Occupational Therapy Association, Inc: Essentials and guidelines for an accredited educational program for the occupational therapy assistant. Am J Occup Ther 45:1085-1092, 1991.

Americans with Disabilities Act. Appendix to Part 1191 ADA - Accessibility Guidelines for Buildings and Facilities. Federal Register/ Vol 56. No 134, 1991. US Architectural & Transportation Bariers Complinace Board.

Angelo, J (eds): Assistive Technology for Rehabilitation Therapists. FA Davis, Philadelphia, 1997.

Bailey, DM: Research and the Health Professional: A Practical Guide, ed 2. FA Davis, Philadelphia, 1997.

Bernstein Lewis, C (ed): Aging: The Health Care Challenge, ed 2. FA Davis, Philadelphia, 1990.

Bonder, BR and Wagner, MB (eds): Functional Performance in Older Adults. FA Davis, Philadelphia, 1994.

Bonder, BR: Psychopathology and Function, ed 2. Slack, Thorofare, NJ, 1995

Borcherding, S: Documentation Manual for Writing SOAP Notes in Occupational Therapy. Slack, Thorofare, NJ, 2000.

Breines, EB: Occupational Therapy Activities from Clay to Computers: Theory and Practice. FA Davis, Philadelphia, 1995.

Bruce, MA and Borg, B: Psychosocial Occupational Therapy: Frames of Reference for Intervention, ed 2. Slack, Thorofare, NJ, 1993.

Cailliet, R: Soft Tissue Pain and Disability, ed 3. FA Davis, Philadelphia, 1996.

Case-Smith, J (ed): Occupational Therapy for Children, ed 4. CV Mosby, St. Louis, 2001.

Christiansen, C (ed): Ways of Living: Self-Care Strategies for Special Needs. American Occupational Therapy Association, Bethesda, MD, 1994.

Christiansen, C and Baum, C (eds): Occupational Therapy: Enabling Function and Well-Being (2nd ed). Slack: Thorofare, NJ, 1997.

Cole, MB: Group dynamics in occupational therapy, ed. 2. Slack, Thorofare, NJ, 1998.

Cottrell, RP (ed): Proactive Approaches in Psychosocial Occupational Therapy. Slack, Thorofore, NJ, 2000.

Denton, PL: Psychiatric Occupational Therapy: A Workbook of Practical Skills. Little, Brown, Boston, 1987.

DePoy, E and Gitlin, LN: Introduction to Research: Multiple Strategies for Health and Human Services, 1994, Mosby, St. Louis.

Dutton, R: Clinical Reasoning in Physical Disabilities. Williams & Wilkins, Baltimore, 1995.

Early, MB: Mental Health Concepts and Techniques for the Occupational Therapy Assistant. Lippincott Williams & Wilkins, Philadelphia, 2000.

Emlet, CA, Crabtree, JL, Condon, VA and Treml, LA (eds): In-Home Assessment of Older Adults: An Interdisciplinary Approach. Aspen, Gaithersburg, MD, 1996.

Fisher, AG, Murray, EA, and Bundy, AC (eds): Sensory Integration: Theory and Practice. FA Davis, Philadelphia, 1991.

Gillen, G and Burkardt, A (eds): Stroke Rehabilitation: A Function-Based Approach. Mosby, St. Louis, 1998.

Griffin ER and Lember S: Sexuality and the Person with Traumatic Brain Injury: A Guide for Families. FA Davis, Philadelphia, 1993.

Hellen, CR: Alzheimer's Disease: Activity-Focused Care, ed 2. Butterworth-Heinemann: Boston, 1998.

Hemphill, BJ (ed): Mental Health Assessment in Occupational Therapy. Slack, Thorofare, NJ, 1988.

Hunter, J, Schneider, M, Mackin, E, and Bell, J (eds): Rehabilitation of the Hand: Surgery and Treatment, ed 3. CV Mosby, Philadelphia, 1990.

Jacobs, K and Logigian, M (eds): Functions of a Manager in Occupational Therapy, ed 3. Slack, Thorfare, NJ, 1999.

Kettenbach, G: Writing SOAP Notes, ed 2. FA Davis, Philadelphia, 1995.

Kornblau and Starling: Ethics in Rehabilitation: A Clinical Perspective. Slack, Thorofare, NJ, 2000.

Kramer, P, and Hinojosa, J (eds): Frames of Reference for Pediatraic Occupational Therapy, ed 2. Lippincott Williams & Wilkins, Philadelphia, 1999.

Larson, O, Stevens-Ratchford, RG, Pedretti, LW, and Crabtree, J (eds): ROTE: The Role of Occupational Therapy with the Elderly. American Occupational Therapy Association Inc., Bethesda, MD, 1996.

Logigian, MK and Ward, JD, (eds): A Team Approach for Therapists: Pediatric Rehabilitation. Little Brown, Boston, 1989.

Mattingly, C and Fleming, MH: Clinical Reasoning: Forms of Inquiry in a Therapeutic Practice. FA Davis, Philadelphia, 1994.

Mosey, AC: Activities Therapy. Raven Press, NY, 1973.

Neistadt, ME and Crepeau, EB (eds): Williard & Spackman's Occupational Therapy, ed 9. Lippincott Williams & Wilkins, Philadelphia, 1998.

Norkin, CC and Levangie, PK: Joint Structure and Function: A Comprehensive Analysis, ed 2. FA Davis, Philadelphia, 1992.

Norkin, CC, and White, DJ: Measurement of Motion: A Guide to Gonionmetry, ed 2. FA Davis, Philadelphia, 1995.

Occupational Safety and Health Administration: Standard #1910.1030,1 FR 5507, February, 1996

Palmer, ML and Toms, JE: Manual for Functional Training, ed 3. FA Davis, Philadelphia, 1992.

Pedretti, L (ed): Occupational Therapy: Practice Skills for Physical Dysfunction, ed 4. Mosby-Yearbook, St. Louis, 1996.

Piersol, CV and Ehrlich, PL (eds): Home Health Practice: A Guide for the Occupational Therapist. Imaginart, Bisbee, AZ, 2000.

Posthuma, BW: Small Groups in Counseling and Therapy: Process and Leadership, ed 3. Allyn and Bacon, Boston, 1999.

Reed, KL and Sanderson, SN (eds): Concepts of Occupational Therapy, ed 3. Williams and Wilkins, Baltimore, 1992.

Reed, KL: Quick Reference to Occupational Therapy, ed 2. Aspen, Gaithersburg, MD, 2001.

Richard, RL. Staley, MJ (eds): Burn Care and Rehabilitation: Principles and Practice. FA Davis, Philadelphia, 1994.

Ross, M and Bachner, S (eds): Adults with Developmental Disabilities: Current Approaches in Occupational Therapy. American Occupational Therapy Association, Bethesda, MD, 1998.

Rothstein, JM, Roy, SH, and Wolf, SL: The Rehabilitation Specialist's Handbook. FA Davis, Philadelphia, 1991.

Royeen, CR: A Research Primer in Occupational and Physical Therapy. American Occupational Therapy Association, Bethesda, MD, 1997.

Ryan, SE (ed): Practice Issues in Occupational Therapy: Intraprofessional Team Building. Slack, Thorofare, NJ, 1993.

Ryan, SE (ed): The Certified Occupational Therapy Assistant: Principles, Concepts and Techniques, ed 2. Slack, Thorofare, NJ, 1993.

Sabonis-Chafee, B and Hussey, SM: Introduction to Occupational Therapy, ed 2. Mosby, St. Louis, 1998.

Smith, LK, Weiss, EL, and Lehmkuhl, LD: Brunnstrom's Clinical Kinesiology, ed 5. FA Davis, Philadelphia, 1996.

Solomon, JW (ed): Pediatric Skills for Occupational Therapy Assistants. Mosby, St.Louis, 2000.

Trombly, CA (ed): Occupational Therapy for Physical Dysfunction, ed 4. Williams and Wilkins, Baltimore, 1995.

Unsworth, C (ed): Cognitive and Perceptual Dysfunction: A Clinical Reasoning Approach to Evaluation and Intervention. FA Davis, Philadelphia, 1999.

Zoltan, B: Vision, Perception and Cognition: A Manual for the Evaluation and Treatment of the Neurologically Impaired Adult, ed 3. Slack, Thorofare, NJ, 1996.